PREVENTION'S
ULTIMATE GUIDE TO
WOMEN'S
HEALTH
AND
WELLNESS

ACTION PLANS FOR MORE THAN 100 WOMEN'S HEALTH PROBLEMS

By the Editors of
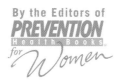

RODALE

Prevention and *Prevention* Health Books are registered trademarks of Rodale Inc.

Printed in the United States of America
Rodale Inc. makes every effort to use acid-free ∞, recycled paper ♻.

Book design by Carol Angstadt

Library of Congress Cataloging-in-Publication Data

Prevention's ultimate guide to women's health and wellness : action
   plans for more than 100 women's health problems / by the editors of
   Prevention Health Books for Women.
     p.   cm.
   Includes index.
   ISBN 1–57954–491–6 hardcover
   1. Women—Health and hygiene.   2. Women—Diseases—Prevention.
I. Title: Guide to women's health and wellness.   II. Prevention Health Books
for Women.
RA778 .P8857   2002
613'.04244—dc21   2002006637

Distributed to the book trade by St. Martin's Press

2 4 6 8 10 9 7 5 3 1 hardcover

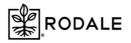

RODALE

WE **INSPIRE** AND **ENABLE** PEOPLE TO IMPROVE
THEIR LIVES AND THE WORLD AROUND THEM

FOR PRODUCTS & INFORMATION
WWW.RODALESTORE.COM
WWW.PREVENTION.COM
(800) 848-4735

Photo Credits

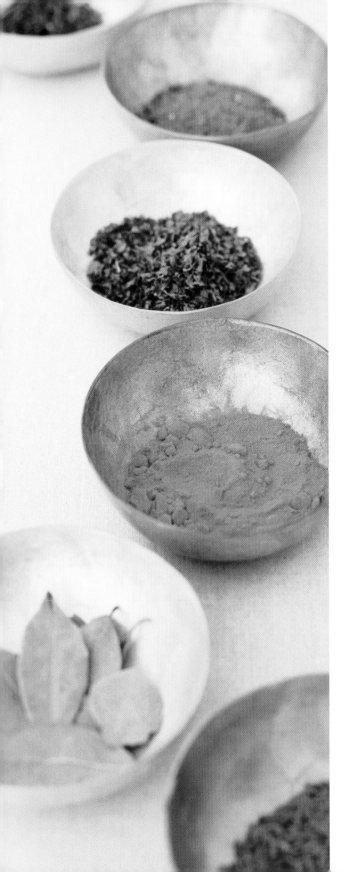

About *Prevention* Health Books

The editors of *Prevention* Health Books are dedicated to providing you with authoritative, trustworthy, and innovative advice for a healthy, active lifestyle. In all of our books, our goal is to keep you thoroughly informed about the latest breakthroughs in natural healing, medical research, alternative health, herbs, nutrition, fitness, weight loss, and well-being. We cut through the confusion of today's conflicting health reports to deliver clear, concise, and definitive health information that you can trust. And we explain in practical terms what each new breakthrough means to you, so you can take immediate, practical steps to improve your health and well-being.

Every recommendation in *Prevention* Health Books is based upon reliable sources, including interviews with qualified health authorities. In addition, we retain top-level health practitioners who serve on our board of advisors. *Prevention* Health Books are thoroughly fact-checked for accuracy, and we make every effort to verify recommendations, dosages, and cautions.

The advice in this book will help keep you well-informed about your personal choices in health care—to help you lead a happier, healthier, and longer life.

Notice

This book is intended as a reference volume only, not as a medical manual. The information given here is designed to help you make informed decisions about your health. It is not intended as a substitute for any treatment that may have been prescribed by your doctor. If you suspect that you have a medical problem, we urge you to seek competent medical help.

Mention of specific companies, organizations, or authorities in this book does not imply endorsement by the publisher, nor does mention of specific companies, organizations, or authorities in the book imply that they endorse it.

Internet addresses and telephone numbers given in this book were accurate at the time it went to press.

Board of Advisors

Contents

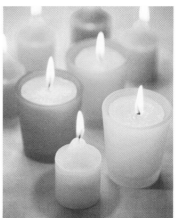

PART ONE: What's Going On?
The Savvy Woman's Health Planner

PART TWO: Your Stay Well, Stay Young "To Do" List

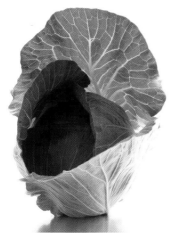

PART THREE: Primary Care:
Essential Protection against Major Health Threats

PART FOUR: Hormonal Wellness: The Best-Ever Life-Stage Strategies

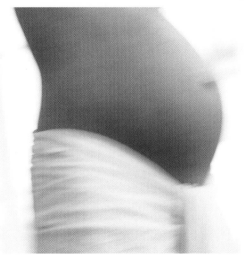

PART FIVE: Doctors' Best Symptom Solvers

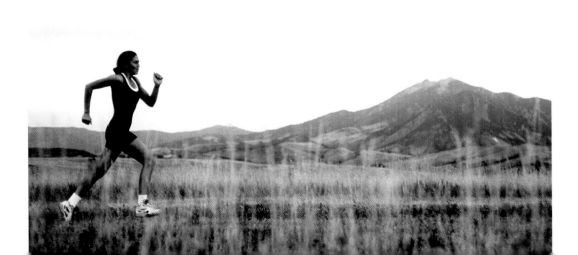

Foreword

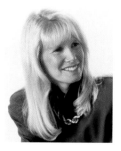

Over the past century, remarkable advances in women's health care have almost doubled the average woman's life span, dramatically reduced maternal and infant mortality, and resulted in the development and delivery of medical services and treatments that previous generations could not have imagined. Women are not only living longer, they are also healthier than at any time in history. A new national focus on women's health in our country has provided women with greater knowledge and access to information about their health. Women's health issues have been integrated into medical research, health care professional training, and clinical practice. Additionally, one of the most important accomplishments over the past decade has been the recognition that women and men have different health needs, and that gender matters in understanding health and disease.

Consider this: In the year 1900, a woman had beaten the odds if she saw her 49th birthday; the average life expectancy for Americans was 48 years. The leading killers then were infectious diseases such as tuberculosis, smallpox, diphtheria, and influenza, and complications of childbirth. But thanks to the triumph of public health interventions including sanitation, vaccinations, health education, preventive health practices, safety and environmental regulations, increased access to health care, new medical diagnostic and treatment interventions, and the implementation of national public health policies, at the dawn of the 21st century American women are living 30 years longer on average than they did a century ago. In fact, last year's census forms offered a three-digit space for entering one's age to accommodate the more than 50,000 Americans who are more than 100 years old. It is estimated that a baby born today has a one in three chance of living to be 100. Consequently, the challenge is to keep women healthy over the course of their longer life spans.

You see, the very success of public health interventions over the past century has resulted in a shift in the threats to American women's health. Today, the major killers of women are chronic illnesses, including cancer, diabetes, heart and lung disease, and stroke, as well as injuries and violence. As much as 50 percent of the causes of these conditions are linked to preventable behavioral, lifestyle, and environmental factors, including smoking (400,000 Americans die annually from tobacco-related illnesses), overweight and lack of physical exercise (300,000 people in the United States die each year from illnesses caused by or linked to obesity), injuries, unsafe sexual practices, and alcohol and substance abuse (more than 129,000 deaths). The simple fact is that more than any miracle drug that could be discovered, reducing health-damaging behaviors by every American woman could reduce premature deaths by as much as one half, significantly decrease disability, increase quality of life, and dramatically cut health care costs.

That's why improving the nation's health today means focusing like a laser on prevention, putting it at the forefront of our country's health care agenda. It also means intensifying the national focus on women's health—a cause that for too long was neglected in the halls of public policy, in research, and in the delivery of clinical and preventive services.

Despite the tremendous progress that has been made in advancing women's health, many challenges still remain. They include rectifying health disparities for women of color, providing access to health care services for all Americans, and decreasing the toll that chronic diseases and conditions take, particularly on the health of senior women.

In the 21st century, improving women's health means addressing the social, biomedical, and environmental issues that will shape the health landscape of the future. Worldwide, a woman's income and level of education are the most powerful predictors of her health. So, prevention means ensuring economic and educational equity for all of our nation's women. Prevention also means addressing mental illness, diseases that affect one out of five Americans each year, and developing strategies to eliminate environmental hazards from women's lives. It means safeguarding our nation's future by ensuring that every girl has a healthy start and healthy self-esteem and is protected from violence, tobacco, and drugs.

So at the dawn of the 21st century, let's remember the public health lessons of the past and apply them with advances from science to new health challenges facing us today and in the future. Let's do it by emphasizing the power of disease prevention and health promotion for communities and for individuals, by fostering and disseminating advances from research, and by increasing access to health care services for all Americans.

Knowledge is power when it comes to your health. Put prevention into practice and take an important step toward a healthier future for you and your family.

Susan J. Blumenthal, M.D., M.P.A.

U.S. Assistant Surgeon General

U.S. Department of Health and
Human Services

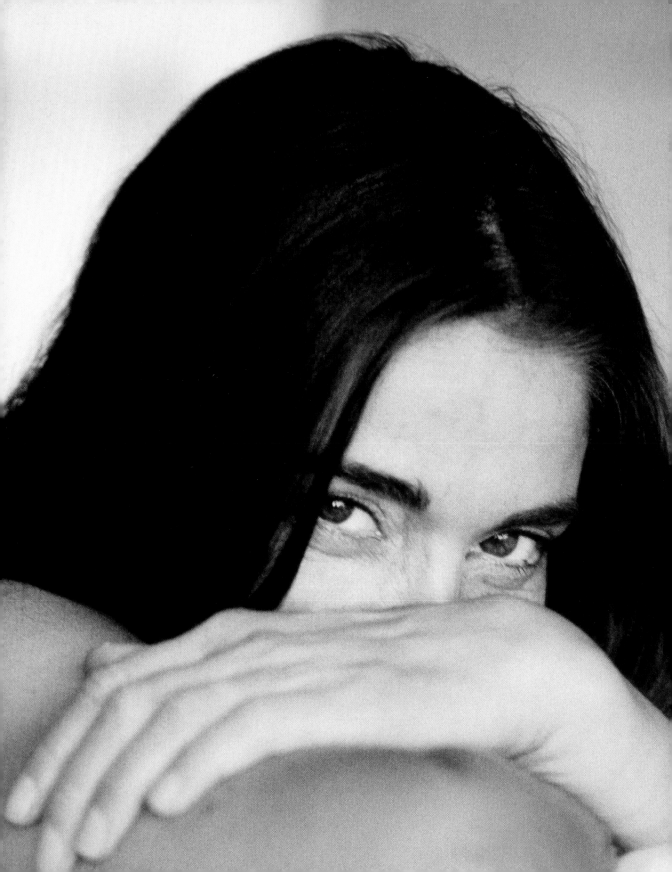

WHAT'S

GOING ON?

THE SAVVY

WOMAN'S

HEALTH

PLANNER

The Female Body, Decade by Decade

Centuries from now, anthropologists might look at today's "over the hill" birthday cards as cultural indicators of women's attitudes toward getting older. Snide remarks about sagging breasts, expanding waistlines, and disappearing sex lives may serve to help women shrug off changes as shared—and inevitable—declines.

Imagine, for a moment, an alternative Birthday Card Universe—an equally fertile market where the prevailing message is positive and congratulatory, applauding well-toned muscles, glowing skin, sparkling teeth, sharp eyesight, and a reliable memory.

A fantasy, you say? Maybe; maybe not. Take the right steps and, with every birthday you celebrate, you can maintain the vibrancy and healthy glow you had at 20. And it's easier than you might think. Start with *Prevention*'s "Wellness Checklists" for every stage of a woman's life, from high school graduation through career, marriage, kids, menopause, retirement, and beyond.

At each life stage, you'll start with the building blocks of wellness: Self-Care Checklists, which cover a healthy diet and nutritional solutions to problems that may pop up along the way—such as weight gain, high blood pressure, or hot flashes—plus Doctor's Office Checklists, with special attention to conditions to watch for and medical screens and tests that can help you detect and manage small problems before they become unmanageable.

Once you get oriented, depending on your current age, turn to part 2, Your Stay Well, Stay Young "To Do" List, to learn more about getting the right exercise and the right vitamin and mineral supplements, and other preventive steps on your course to good health and well-being. You'll find step-by-step action plans for customizing medical advice for your personal needs.

Skeptical? If you don't think any of these strategies can really make a difference in 20 or 30 years, ask gerontologist Michael Lichtenstein, M.D., at the University of Texas Health Science Center in San Antonio. "People who have lifelong health maintenance habits like exercising and eating healthy will live long and healthy lives," he says.

Whatever stage of life you're in, you can take the road to lifelong health and end up being a 70-year-old who may never lay eyes on another "over the hill" birthday card.

AGES 18 *to* 35

Imagine a group of runners at the start of a race. Their bodies are in superior shape, they're focused, and they're primed to do their best.

As a young woman, you're at a similar starting line. You have every reason to expect a long and healthy life. Women's life expectancy has increased by nearly 61 percent in the past century, from 48.3 years in 1900 to 79.5 years in 1998. Women aren't letting disease slow them down, either. In the past, a cancer diagnosis meant a slim chance of survival. But now, thanks to improved methods of prevention, detection, and treatment, more than half of the 8 million Americans who have cancer are outliving the disease.

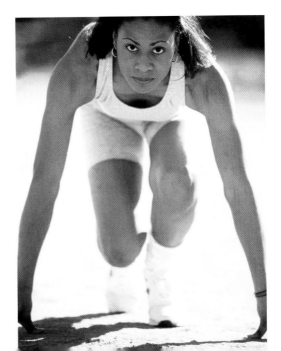

What's the best way to get to the finish line? Start with a base of healthy habits that continue throughout your journey.

The medical screens and tests you'll find here help detect cancer and other diseases early, when they're easier to treat, or even cure. Even better, take steps to prevent illness. For instance, fruit and vegetables contain phytochemicals, substances that actually fight cancer. Whole grains provide fiber, which lowers risk for diabetes, heart disease, and cancer. And omega-3 fatty acids, which are good for the heart, also help lift your mood.

And the sooner you take steps to keep your weight in check, the better. Putting this step off will make weight control harder, as your metabolism tends to slow once you approach the age of 40. Being obese—more than 30 percent over your ideal body weight—puts you at greater risk for many conditions, including diabetes, high blood pressure, heart and artery disease, sleep disruptions, varicose veins, osteoarthritis, some cancers, respiratory problems, and complications during pregnancy and surgery. If you're overweight, the nutritional guide-

lines here will help you get started on eating a healthy diet. And for a more thorough program on losing weight, see chapter 6.

Even if you don't have a weight problem, eating healthfully throughout your lifetime is still important. Proper nutrition can increase your energy levels, improve your mood; eating healthfully when pregnant could help you avoid birth defects in your baby.

The sooner you practice good health habits, the better off you'll be in the future.

"Most of us have eating patterns that were formed when we were very young," says Terri Brownlee, R.D., nutrition director of the Duke University Diet and Fitness Center in Durham, North Carolina. "Even at 20 years old, it's difficult to make changes. But it's certainly harder the longer you wait. If you wait until you're 50 or 60 years old, bad habits are much harder to break."

Studies on people who have adopted a healthy diet and continued with it for years have shown that true lifestyle changes are the only way to do it.

Your Self-Care Checklist

◯ **Multivitamins and mineral supplements**
To be extra sure you're getting the vitamins and minerals you need, get in the habit of taking a multivitamin and mineral supplement that provides 100 percent of the Daily Value for most nutrients, including vitamin A or beta-carotene, vitamin D, vitamin B_6, copper, and zinc.

Consider taking separate supplements of 100 to 500 milligrams of vitamin C and 100 to 400 IU of vitamin E. They act as antioxidants, counteracting the natural effects of aging and environmental damage at the cellular level.

Also, make sure your multivitamin has a USP (United States Pharmacopeia) label on it. It means the manufacturer guarantees the supplement contains the amount of vitamins listed on the label.

For all women under 50, *Prevention* magazine recommends 500 milligrams of a calcium supplement. One type, calcium carbonate, should be taken with meals, while you may take calcium citrate on an empty stomach.

◯ **Folate/folic acid** The B vitamin folic acid (the supplement form of folate) prevents a serious type of birth defect called neural tube defects. Women are advice to get 400 micrograms of folic acid from a supplement. While pregnant, your doctor may advise you to increase your intake to 600 micrograms.

Along with your supplements, eat two folate-rich foods a day, like spinach, kidney beans, or orange juice.

◯ **Iron** One out of five premenopausal women doesn't get the Daily Value of 18 milligrams of iron. Without enough iron, you'll feel tired and have trouble concentrating.

To battle that fatigue, eat iron-rich foods, such as legumes, dark green leafy vegetables, and extra-lean meat. Consuming vitamin C, like orange juice, with iron-rich foods boosts absorption.

◯ **Good-mood foods** Women in their thirties who battle mood problems may be reacting to the food they eat, nutrients they're missing, or drugs they take.

■ Premenstrual symptoms may be worse if you're not getting enough calcium, so make sure you're eating three servings of dairy that add up to 1,000 milligrams of calcium a day, from milk, yogurt, or calcium-fortified orange juice. This will help minimize mood swings from PMS.

■ Women who take birth control pills are usually low on vitamin B_6, which helps manufacture the mood-boosting chemical serotonin. Make sure you're getting enough by eating bananas and extra-lean meat.

Your Doctor's Office Checklist

◯ **Dental checkups** Go to the dentist every 6 months to help prevent cavities, gum disease, and other oral problems.

◯ **Eye exams** If you haven't already done so, get an initial comprehensive eye exam that tests for glaucoma, cataracts, and macular degeneration. Follow up with your eye doctor if your vision changes. You'll need more frequent checkups when you're in your forties.

◯ **Serum ferritin test and transferrin saturation test** If waning energy makes you suspect you're getting too little iron, talk to your doctor about getting a serum ferritin test, a blood test that

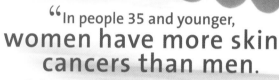

measures the amount of iron in the body. Iron deficiency is the most common known form of nutritional deficiency, and it's highest among women of childbearing age. Eleven percent of nonpregnant women ages 16 to 49 are deficient in iron, and 3 to 5 percent have iron deficiency anemia.

Iron overload, or hemochromatosis, is also a common genetic disease. Get screened for it at age 18 with a serum ferritin test and a transferrin saturation test, especially if you're frequently fatigued or have liver disease, diabetes, arthritis, or a family history of hemochromatosis.

○ **Skin exam** Just one or two blistering sunburns in youth can set the stage for skin cancer later in life, though it might take decades for the signs to surface. Today more than 1 million cases of skin cancer are diagnosed each year in North America, but most are curable if detected early enough.

Starting at age 18, examine your skin at least once a year for signs of skin cancer. "Check your birthday suit every year on your birthday," says Ira Davis, M.D., assistant professor of dermatology at New York Medical College in Valhalla.

Use a mirror if you have to and look for:

- Pearly white bumps or spots that may bleed, may break down, or don't heal, usually on the face or the arms (but they can appear anywhere on the body)

- Red and scaly bumps that resemble a scar and are shallow in the middle, usually on the face or the arms (but they can appear anywhere on the body)

> **"In people 35 and younger, women have more skin cancers than men.** Evidence supports that sunbathing or tanning beds may contribute to this female predominance."
>
> —SCOTT DINEHART, M.D., PROFESSOR OF DERMATOLOGY AT THE UNIVERSITY OF ARKANSAS COLLEGE OF MEDICINE IN LITTLE ROCK

- Dark spots that are asymmetrical, have irregular borders, have more than one color, and are bigger than the size of a pencil eraser, usually on the legs and trunk (but they can appear anywhere on the body); they may be flat or elevated

You should also see a dermatologist every 3 years for a skin examination. If someone in your family has had melanoma (a potentially deadly form of skin cancer) and you're at risk for skin cancer (you've spent a lot of time in the sun, you've had many sunburns, you have fair skin, or you have many moles), get examined twice a year. If skin cancer runs in your family but you don't have risk factors, get checked once a year.

○ **Tetanus shot** This may seem like stuff for elementary school kids, but everyone needs a tetanus shot every 10 years to stay immune to the rare but fatal disease. Tetanus is caused when bacteria in an open wound attack the central nervous system.

◯ **Blood pressure check** A blood pressure check is usually standard screening every time you see your family doctor or gynecologist. Make sure your blood pressure is checked at least every 2 years or more frequently if it's above 130/85, which is considered a normal reading.

Birth control pills give some women high blood pressure, so have your pressure checked if you start the Pill, and again a few months later.

◯ **Complete blood lipid profile** Today experts are seeing evidence of atherosclerosis (blood vessels with unhealthful deposits of cholesterol and other fats) in teenagers, which is why regular cholesterol checks are so important. With just one blood test, your doctor can measure your total cholesterol, HDL ("good") cholesterol, LDL ("bad") cholesterol, levels of triglycerides, and total/HDL ratio. Get this test done every 5 years, starting at age 20. If the results are abnormal, go every 4 months.

Healthy results are:

- Total cholesterol of 150 or below

- HDL 45 or above

- LDL 130 or below

- Total/HDL ratio of 4 or below

- Triglycerides levels between 100 and 150

◯ **Thyroid-stimulating hormone test** Many doctors don't recommend thyroid screening until age 40 or 50 unless you have risk factors, such as family history of thyroid problems or autoimmune disease, but *Prevention* magazine suggests getting screened at age 20 and every 5 years thereafter. Because 5 to 7 percent of women under age 35 have mild thyroid dysfunction, and because the test is inexpensive and simple, get this screen at the same time you get your cholesterol checked.

Thyroid problems can raise cholesterol levels—which puts you at greater risk for heart disease—or cause conception problems or low birth weight or miscarriages.

◯ **Electrocardiogram (EKG)** This important test identifies injury or damage to the heart, enlargement of the heart, or abnormal rhythms. Get one at age 30 as a baseline. But if you have risk factors for heart disease, such as hypertension or diabetes, and you've never had an EKG, get one no matter what your age, says Elizabeth Ross, M.D., a cardiologist at the Washington Hospital Center in Washington, D.C.

◯ **Fasting glucose test** While the majority of women who develop type 2 diabetes don't do so until they are over 45, the incidence of the disease among younger women is rising. If you're at high risk, get tested now and every 3 years.

Risk factors include:

- A family history

- Being from an at-risk ethnic group, such as African-American, Hispanic, Native American, Asian, or Pacific Islander

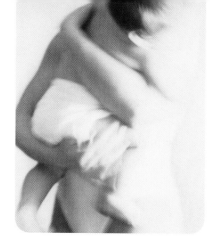

- Being obese

- Having high cholesterol

- Having a history of gestational diabetes

- Having low HDL cholesterol and high triglycerides

○ **Pelvic exam and Pap test** Since 1970, the incidence of and death rate from cervical cancer have gone down by 40 percent, thanks in part to early detection with the Pap test. Starting at age 18—or younger if you are sexually active—visit a gynecologist every year for a pelvic exam and Pap test.

During the pelvic exam, the doctor examines the genitals, vagina, and cervix for infections, rashes, or abnormal growths. The doctor also checks the size and position of the ovaries and uterus to make sure they're not enlarged.

She'll also take a sample of cells from your cervix for the Pap test. This screens for cancer of the cervix, but it may also detect a sexually transmitted disease called human papillomavirus, which causes cervical cancer. This is essential cancer protection since half of all women diagnosed with cervical cancer have never had a Pap test. If you or your partner has multiple sexual partners, you should be tested for other sexually transmitted diseases as well. A Pap test should be given annually or whenever you have an abnormal discharge or pelvic pain or think you have been exposed to someone with an infection.

○ **Clinical breast exam** Most women detect their own breast cancer. That's why you should

"Women should get in the habit at a very young age of not bending over at the waist to pick up anything, especially heavy children.

This helps prevent ruptured disks and back strain

as well as reduce the chance of spinal fractures. Bending at the knees and squatting down strengthens the muscles around the hip, which not only gives you a nice shape but reduces your risk of hip fractures from osteoporosis later in life."

—MARJORIE LUCKEY, M.D., MEDICAL DIRECTOR OF
ST. BARNABAS OSTEOPOROSIS AND METABOLIC BONE DISEASE
CENTER IN LIVINGSTON, NEW JERSEY

give yourself monthly breast self-exams. But get one from your doctor once a year, too. With her expertise, she might be more likely to detect a tumor at an early stage before it spreads.

Symptoms to watch for: breast lumps, thickening, swelling, distortion, tenderness, skin irritation, dimpling, nipple pain, discharge, or scaliness.

AGES 35 to 40

Assuming you've established a healthy lifestyle, now is the time to deal with specific changes that typically occur as women approach midlife.

Some women experience perimenopausal symptoms as early as age 35. During perimenopause, your levels of estrogen and other female hormones drop as your body gets closer to menopause. You might experience irregular menstrual periods, hot flashes, night sweats, insomnia, mood swings, and vaginal dryness.

Under the circumstances, it's harder to become pregnant at this time. In women, fertility gradually wanes after age 35, and the risk of miscarriages increases to about 50 percent by age 45. Women in their forties also have a higher risk of pregnancy complications such as premature labor, stillbirth, and the need for cesarean section.

More than ever, exercise is essential to your muscles and your bones. Beginning in their thirties, women lose 1 to 2 percent of their muscle mass per year, but exercise can reverse the process and keep your metabolism up. Redouble your efforts not to gain weight now because once you reach 40, it won't be as easy to drop 5 or 10 pounds at will.

And along with losing muscle, you could also lose bone if you're not careful. During childhood and puberty, your skeleton built more bone than it broke down. But by the time you reach 35, the process reverses and your body breaks down more bone than it builds. Weight-bearing exercise, such as walking and lifting weights, will strengthen your skeleton and help you avoid osteoporosis.

Your Self-Care Checklist

○ **A fertile weight** Obesity affects ovulation and could make it hard to get pregnant or carry a baby to term. In one study, a group of women who had a 75 percent miscarriage rate lowered that rate to 18 percent after eating a healthy diet, exercising, and losing weight. If you're infertile and overweight, losing weight may help.

On the other hand, being underweight increases your risk for miscarriage, cesarean deliveries, or giving birth to a premature baby. A healthy weight is your best bet for fertility.

○ **Folic acid/folate** Folic acid (the supplement form of folate) is recommended for all women of childbearing age. Once you get pregnant, your doctor may advise you to increase your intake to 600 micrograms. But even if you're not pregnant, getting at least five servings of folate a day from

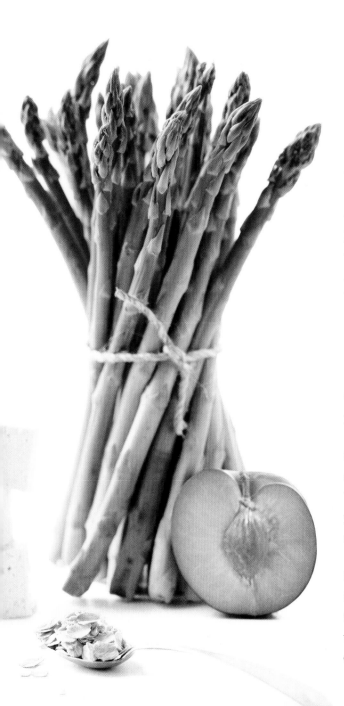

food may decrease your risk of getting colon cancer later on. Folate, which is found in fruits and vegetables such as spinach and legumes, works on your DNA to keep it normal. Your suggested daily intake or DV (Daily Value) is 400 micrograms. If you're deficient in folate, you're more likely to develop the type of DNA damage that can lead to cancer.

◯ **Vegetables and calcium** You should already be exercising and getting enough calcium (DV is 1,000 milligrams) to keep your bones strong, but you also should be eating plenty of vegetables. Research shows that the nutrients in fruits and vegetables—zinc, magnesium, potassium, fiber, and vitamin C—decrease the risk of having low bone mass.

Your Doctor's Office Checklist

◯ **Dental checkups** Schedule them twice a year, or more often at your dentist's advice.

◯ **Eye exams** If you have never had one, schedule an initial comprehensive eye exam. Then see an eye doctor if you notice a change in your vision. Otherwise, you don't need regular exams until you turn 41.

◯ **Serum ferritin test and transferrin saturation test** You should have had a serum ferritin test and a transferrin saturation test when you were 18 to screen for hemochromatosis. If you didn't, do it now, especially if you're frequently fatigued or have liver disease, diabetes, arthritis, or a family history of hemochromatosis. Talk to your physician about the most current recommendations regarding these iron tests.

◯ **Skin exam** Continue getting a skin examination every 3 years if you're not at high risk for skin cancer, every year if your only risk is family history, and twice a year if you're at high risk, as described in the last decade, on page 6.

◯ **Tetanus shot** If it's been 10 years, get another one.

◯ **Blood pressure check** Continue to have it checked at least every 2 years, or more frequently if it's been abnormal.

◯ **Complete blood lipid profile** If your lipids have been normal, you've been getting a complete lipid profile every 5 years. Now's the time to step it up to every 2 years. Abnormal results should be rechecked every 4 months.

◯ **Thyroid-stimulating hormone test** Have this done every 5 years.

◯ **Fasting glucose test** If you're at high risk, as described in the last decade (page 7), get tested now and every 3 years thereafter.

◯ **Pelvic exam, Pap test, and breast exam** Continue getting them every year, and do monthly breast self-exams.

◯ **Mammogram** If two or more close relatives had breast cancer, particularly if they got it before they turned 40, start getting annual mammograms in your thirties.

◯ **Bone-density test** If you're at high risk for osteoporosis because of another illness or a medication, talk to your doctor about getting a baseline bone-density scan prior to menopause. (For example, some medications to treat conditions such as rheumatoid arthritis, endocrine disorders, seizure disorders, and gastrointestinal diseases may damage bone and lead to osteoporosis.) Otherwise, wait until menopause for the test. You're at risk for osteoporosis if:

- You broke a bone after the age of 35 from low trauma (falling from a standing height or less)

- You have a family history of osteoporosis or hip fractures

- You weigh less than 127 pounds, even if you're short

- You smoke cigarettes, or drink excessive amounts of alcohol

- You have taken steroids for 3 months or longer for conditions like asthma

- You have a chronic disease that increases your risk for osteoporosis (both before and after menopause), such as seizure disorders, inflammatory bowel disease, chronic liver disease, kidney disease, or celiac disease

AGES 40 *to* 50

During this time, you might feel a few bumps in the road, particularly as you approach menopause, but paying attention to changes in your body, choosing foods that could lend relief to perimenopausal symptoms, and getting the medical tests you need will help keep you healthy.

Almost all women—85 to 90 percent—experience symptoms of perimenopause, when the ovaries slow down their production of estrogen and hormone levels fluctuate, the most common symptom being irregular periods.

"Anything is possible," says Margery Gass, M.D., professor of obstetrics and gynecology and director of the University Hospital Menopause and Osteoporosis Center at the University of Cincinnati College of Medicine. Your periods could be completely normal and regular up until menopause, or they might move closer together or further apart, skip cycles, or become heavier.

"Although more frequent periods are most common, it's important to stay in touch with your physician to figure out what's normal for you during this time," Dr. Gass says. "Heavy bleeding, irregular bleeding, periods every 2 to 3 weeks, and breakthrough bleeding are always worrisome symptoms that should be checked by your doctor. They could be signs of cancer, polyps, fibroids, infections, or miscarriages."

Other symptoms include:

- Hot flashes, night sweats, and extreme sweating (with or without chills)

- Vaginal dryness

- Changes in sexual desire

- PMS symptoms

- Mood changes

- Frequent urination

- Achy joints

- Difficulty in concentrating

- Headaches

- Insomnia

- Early wakening

Your emotional state also could affect the symptoms. Some life changes that are common during this time include an empty nest, divorce or widowhood, early retirement, anxiety about aging or death, loss of friends and loved ones, loss of financial security, becoming a caregiver to an aging parent, and anxiety about your own health.

Together, the physical and life changes you face might leave you feeling as though you're going through puberty all over again. But there's plenty you can do to ease yourself through the 2 or 3 years it typically takes to make this transition.

Your Self-Care Checklist

○ **Exercise, exercise, exercise** First and foremost, continue to rev up your metabolism with exercise. Researchers have found that women tend to gain about 1 pound a year in their forties, and it's easier to add fat to your abdomen, where it can do the most damage to blood sugar, cholesterol levels, and blood pressure.

It's easy to blame weight gain on your

changing hormones, but recent studies have found that added pounds have nothing to do with menopause or its treatments. Rather, lower physical activity is the culprit. Since women's risk for heart disease goes up after menopause and having more body fat could exacerbate the risk, work on keeping your weight down now by eating healthy and exercising.

○ **Calorie control** With slower metabolism, you might find you're gaining weight even if you haven't changed your eating habits. But training the scale not to budge is as simple as eating one bite less at every meal. That adds up to about 100 fewer calories a day, the number of calories you should cut from your diet each decade.

○ **Hunger signals** "We each have our own unique metabolism, so you're the best judge of food that works best for you," says Jerianne Heimendinger, R.D., Ph.D., a scientist at the AMC Cancer Research Center in Denver who has studied the antioxidant effects of fruit and

vegetables. Listen to your hunger and satiety signals, and pay attention to how food makes you feel by pausing before you start your meal, eating slowly, and chewing more carefully. You'll become more in touch with your body and less likely to overeat.

○ **Fiber** A high-fiber diet of whole grain bread and cereals and fruit and vegetables helps balance your estrogen and could reduce symptoms of perimenopause. Fiber has also been shown to reduce the risk of heart disease, and may help lower your risk for some cancers.

○ **Low-fat dairy** Another great way to stay slim and healthy: Choose low-fat and fat-free cheeses and yogurt. They have all the calcium and other nutrients their high-fat counterparts carry—without the saturated fat.

"They're nutritional powerhouses without the guilt," says Leslie Bonci, M.P.H., R.D., director of nutrition at the Center for Sports Medicine at the University of Pittsburgh and spokesperson for the American Dietetic Association.

○ **Natural foods** Since women need fewer calories as they get older, avoiding processed foods—which are usually low in vitamins, minerals, and fiber and high in fat and sugar—will give you the nutrients you need at a discount: fewer calories.

○ **Vitamin E** Taking about 800 IU of a vitamin E supplement daily not only cools hot flashes but also relieves mood swings and vaginal dryness—three symptoms that result from fluctuating hormones during perimenopause.

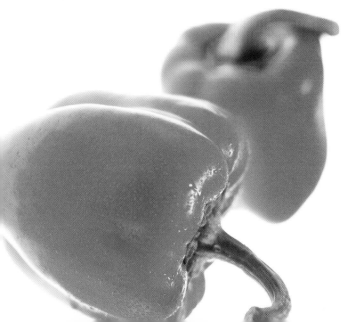

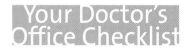

Your Doctor's Office Checklist

◯ **Dental checkup** Continue to go to the dentist every 6 months, unless your dentist advises more trips.

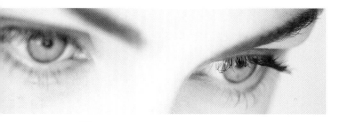

◯ **Eye exams** If you have never had one, schedule an initial comprehensive eye exam now. Then see an eye doctor every 2 to 4 years or sooner if you notice a change in your vision.

◯ **Serum ferritin test and transferrin saturation test** If you're frequently fatigued or have liver disease, diabetes, arthritis, or a family history of hemochromatosis and haven't gotten these tests, get them. Talk to your physician about the most current recommendations regarding these iron tests.

◯ **Skin exams** Until age 40, you've been getting checked every 3 years. Now let your dermatologist look you over annually.

◯ **Tetanus shot** Repeat every 10 years.

◯ **Blood pressure check** The risk of developing hypertension tends to increase as we get older, so get checked at least every 2 years.

◯ **Complete lipid profile** Continue getting this done every 2 years if results are normal, and every 4 months if they're abnormal.

◯ **Thyroid-stimulating hormone test** Get screened every 5 years for an underactive or overactive thyroid.

◯ **Stress-echocardiogram test** If you're 40 or older and at high risk for heart disease (you have high blood pressure, have high cholesterol, have a history of bypass surgery, or have had a heart attack or angioplasty) get a stress-echocardiogram test and an EKG. Also, if you're starting a vigorous exercise program and you haven't been exercising, ask your doctor whether you should first have a stress-echocardiogram test.

◯ **Flu shot** If you have a condition like diabetes, asthma, or other chronic lung or heart problems, get a flu shot in September or October of every year unless you are allergic to eggs or flu vaccines. Even if you're in good health, the flu shot is 70 to 90 percent effective at preventing the fever, cough, sore throat, runny or stuffy nose, headaches, muscle aches, and fatigue the infection is likely to cause.

◯ **Fasting glucose test** All women 45 and older should have their blood sugar tested every 3 years to screen for diabetes. If results are abnormal or if you're at high risk for diabetes, get tested more often.

The signs of diabetes are unexplained weight loss, unusual thirst, frequent desire to urinate, extreme fatigue, extreme hunger, irritability, frequent infections, blurred vision, slow-healing cuts and bruises, tingling or numbness in the hands or feet, or recurring skin, gum, or bladder infections.

○ **Bone-density test** If you're at high risk for osteoporosis, as described in the last decade (page 11)—or at the first signs of menopause—get a bone-density scan.

○ **Pelvic exam and Pap test** It's a fact. Many deaths from cervical cancer could have been prevented through safe sex practices and routine Pap tests. Do yourself a favor and go to your gynecologist each year for this important test.

Also, talk to your doctor if you have questions about signs of perimenopause you might be experiencing. Symptoms to watch for: heavy bleeding, bleeding longer than 7 days (or 2 or more days longer than usual), having fewer than 21 days between periods, spotting between periods, and bleeding after intercourse. They could indicate a hormone imbalance, misuse of birth control pills, pregnancy, fibroids, thyroid dysfunction, abnormalities in the uterine lining, cancer, or bleeding outside the uterus (such as in the vagina or cervix).

○ **Pelvic ultrasound** Women at high risk for ovarian cancer (several family members had breast or ovarian cancer) should have a pelvic ultrasound and a CA-125 test, a blood test that looks for cancer markers in the blood.

Women with BRCA1 and BRCA2 mutations are also at higher risk for ovarian, breast, and some other cancers. If you know you have a gene that could give you cancer, consider getting tested every 6 months.

A new blood test is being studied that could provide more reliable results than the CA-125. It will measure lysophosphatidic acid (LPA), a lipid in the blood. Women with ovarian cancer have high quantities of this acid. This new test could detect the cancer early, when it's most treatable. Some controversy surrounds the testing, as in certain cases it may yield false-negative or false-positive results.

Symptoms to watch for: Enlargement of the abdomen is the most common sign of ovarian cancer, but it's not always present. A large tumor could make you look 5 months pregnant. Another sign is persistent digestive problems, such as unexplained stomach discomfort, gas, and abdominal swelling. In rare cases, abnormal vaginal bleeding will occur.

○ **Mammogram** You've been doing monthly breast self-exams and getting an annual clinical breast exam, but once you reach age 40, it's time to start getting an annual mammogram. A mammogram is a low-intensity x-ray that can confirm whether lumps you or your doctor found are in fact tumors. It can also detect tumors when they're too small to feel with your hand. When tumors are found early, they're easier to treat and could be cured because the cancer hasn't spread to other parts of the body.

Symptoms to watch for: breast lumps, thickening, swelling, distortion, tenderness, skin irritation, nipple pain, scaliness, or dimpling.

AGES 50 *to* 62

From here on in, you can look forward to relief from perimenopausal symptoms. Fluctuating estrogen levels, which have been causing hot flashes, insomnia, headaches, night sweats, vaginal dryness, and mood swings, finally drop off completely. The ovaries no longer produce eggs. Menstruation ceases.

After 12 months without a period, you've reached menopause. It could happen anywhere between the ages of 40 and 58, but the average age is 51. Women who smoke usually go through menopause about a year and a half earlier than women who don't, and women with a higher body mass index (discussed on page 90) or who have had more than one pregnancy usually experience later-than-average menopause. You'll probably reach menopause at the same age your mother did.

For some, menopause may be a day to mourn the loss of fertility. For others, it's a day to celebrate having no more periods, premenstrual symptoms, and fear of pregnancy. In fact, postmenopausal women are the *least* likely of all women to be depressed—due to a sense of well-being.

In the past doctors thought a decline in health after menopause was a normal part of aging. Now we know that a healthy lifestyle can keep women vibrant. Good thing, too, since many women lead at least one-third of their lives after menopause.

Menopause does bring new health challenges, however. Without some form of hormone replacement therapy, women can lose between 2 and 5 percent of bone mass on average per year in the first 3 to 5 years after menopause. Your risk of dying from breast cancer, too, rises with age (although it's still a distant third behind heart disease and lung cancer for women in general). When you were 35, your chance of getting breast cancer was only one in 622. By age 60, the relative risk is one in 24 (although the risk varies greatly from woman to woman). And while estrogen protected you in younger years from heart disease, losing it in menopause raises LDL ("bad") cholesterol levels, and by the time you're 60, your risk will have increased to equal a man's. Estrogen also kept your blood vessels naturally elastic. Without it, the risk of heart disease and stroke increases.

Again, these risks are relative and within your control. That's why a healthy diet and screening are extra important at this age. Calcium and vitamin D help fight bone loss, but if a bone-density scan finds that you have low bone mass, your doctor can put you on protective therapy early to fight it. If a breast tumor is found with a mammogram or breast exam, the earlier it's detected, the easier it is to treat and cure. In the meantime, you can eat food associated with low breast cancer risk. And eating a low-fat diet, getting exercise, and not smoking can lower your odds of getting heart disease.

The scale presents another challenge. It's getting harder and harder to keep your weight down. Increasing your muscle mass with exercise will help you burn calories.

Your Self-Care Checklist

○ **Calorie reduction** To compensate for slower metabolism, cut another 100 calories from your diet daily. Cut down on the size of your meals instead of completely eliminating a food group, such as carbohydrates like bread. To fill your plate without overeating, use a salad plate for dinner, and you won't feel deprived.

○ **Mini-meals** To keep your metabolism going strong, ditch the usual three big meals and eat six smaller ones of about 250 calories each throughout the day. Researchers have found that women who eat larger meals may burn 60 fewer calories per day than women who eat mini-meals—the equivalent of 6 pounds a year.

○ **Portion control** To make sure you're not eating double or triple portions of snacks, crackers, and other packaged foods, check the serving size on food labels, and limit yourself to single servings, not the whole amount provided.

○ **Low-fat, high-fiber diet** A diet low in fat and high in fiber has been associated with a lower risk of both heart disease and colon cancer. Reach for fruit, vegetables, whole grain breads and cereals, legumes, soy foods, and fat-free dairy foods.

○ **Calcium** Postmenopausal women get only half the calcium they need, yet they need more calcium than ever. The loss of estrogen from menopause gives you less protection from bone loss, so increase your daily calcium consumption to 1,200 milligrams.

You don't have to drink three glasses of milk a day if you don't want to. Instead, you may take calcium supplements equal to 700 milligrams toward that Daily Value. *Prevention* magazine recommends that for better absorption you spread

When Calcium Isn't Good

Calcium supplements can help preserve bone density, protecting you from fractures. But did you know that taking calcium just before a bone scan might blur your bone-density test results?

The very best test for measuring bone density in the spine and hip—dual energy x-ray absorptiometry, or DEXA—works by reading how much calcium is present, not only in the bone but also within a cross section of the body. Poorly absorbed calcium can linger in the intestines and mimic dense bone on a spine scan, obscuring telltale signs of thinning bone, says Jeri Nieves, Ph.D., director of bone-density testing at Helen Hayes Hospital in West Haverstraw, New York.

This rarely happens, but it could at least cause inconvenience: If your doctor notices an odd reading, she may suggest a second scan. "Don't quit taking supplements or cancel your DEXA," says Dr. Nieves. Instead, use a calcium supplement labeled "USP"—meaning it's met the U.S. Pharmacopeia's standard for dissolving. And don't take any calcium supplement within an hour of a DEXA, adds Dr. Nieves. ▪

the dose out over the day, and take no more than 500 milligrams at one time. Though you need to take one type, calcium carbonate, with meals, you may take calcium carbonate on an empty stomach. Look for a calcium supplement formula with vitamin D. You may need more D than what your daily multi provides.

◯ **Vitamin B₁₂** Women need only 6 micrograms per day of vitamin B_{12} to fight heart disease, but after age 50 it's harder for us to absorb the vitamin when we get it from food. Take it in a multi supplement—it's well-absorbed.

◯ **Spinach** Lutein and zeaxanthin, antioxidants found in spinach, may protect the retina from age-related macular degeneration. Eat spinach once a day, with olive oil, since fat promotes lutein absorption.

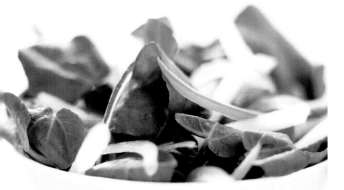

◯ **Fall prevention** As you approach age 60, step up your efforts to prevent falls, to guard against wrist and hip fractures. Keep electrical cords away from through traffic areas of your home, use night-lights, arrange for handrails (and nonskid tape) to be installed in the shower, clean up spills in the kitchen right away, wear sturdy, rubber-soled shoes, and put rubber mats under throw rugs to keep them from sliding under your feet.

Your Doctor's Office Checklist

◯ **Height measurement** You should be getting your height measured every time you're at the doctor's office, or at least once a year. Over your lifetime, a gradual loss of about 1.5 inches is normal. But if you've lost more height than that—or you've lost an inch and a half in 10 years or less—it could indicate vertebral compression fractures as a result of osteoporosis.

◯ **Bone-density test** Get a bone-density measurement if you're in menopause or past menopause and you've never had a test. Out of the 25 million Americans who have osteoporosis, 80 percent are women.

The best measurement for women is a DEXA scan of the spine and the hip, the two places that usually have the most serious fractures. The spine is also where the first bone loss most often occurs after menopause. Some rural areas don't have the machine. In that case, an ultrasound of the heel or a dual or single x-ray of the arm or finger will measure your bone density.

○ **25-hydroxy vitamin D serum level check** If you're older than 49, especially if you're at risk for osteoporosis, have your level of vitamin D checked. Vitamin D helps calcium get absorbed in the body. Your levels should be over 20 nanograms per liter.

○ **Dental checkup** Go to the dentist every 6 months, or more often if you experience pain or other problems.

○ **Eye exams** Go for a comprehensive eye examination, if you have not already done so. You should be getting an eye exam every 2 to 4 years, or sooner if you notice a change in your vision.

○ **Serum ferritin test and transferrin saturation test** You were tested at age 18 for hemochromatosis, an iron overload disease. After menopause is a good time to get tested again. Talk to your physician about the most current recommendations regarding these tests.

○ **Skin exams** Don't let up on those annual skin exams.

○ **Blood pressure check** Get your blood pressure checked at least every 2 years, more often if it's abnormal.

○ **Complete lipid profile** Now more than ever, it's important to have your cholesterol checked at least every 2 years; every 4 months if it's abnormal. Women typically get cardiovascular disease 10 to 15 years later than men, when they experience the postmenopausal loss of estrogen. Also, cholesterol levels change after menopause. "Bad," LDL cholesterol levels go up, while "good," HDL cholesterol levels go down, putting postmenopausal women at greater risk for cardiovascular disease.

○ **Thyroid-stimulating hormone test** Don't forget to get screened every 5 years for an underactive or overactive thyroid.

○ **Pelvic exam, Pap test, and breast exam** Don't stop getting Pap tests when you stop menstruating. The exam could detect cancer. Even if you've had a hysterectomy and your ovaries were taken out, you still need a pelvic exam, says Dr. Gass. This is true even though you may have always had normal Pap test and are monogamous. The pelvic exam can be helpful with other problems, such as incontinence, genital itching, sores, or painful intercourse.

○ **Mammogram** Continue to get an annual mammogram.

○ **Colorectal screening** Colorectal cancer is the third-most-common cancer among American women, but it's almost always curable if found early enough. If everyone started getting regular screenings for colon cancer at age 50, about 25,000 lives a year could be spared from the disease.

Make sure your annual pelvic exam includes a digital rectal exam, starting at age 50. Also, get a colonoscopy at age 50 and every 10 years thereafter—or ask your doctor if you can opt for flexible sigmoidoscopy every 3 to 5 years. In addition, get a yearly fecal occult blood test.

Risk factors for colon cancer include:

- A family history
- A genetic predisposition
- Chronic inflammatory bowel disease
- A previous history of colon polyps or colon cancer

Watch out for rectal bleeding, blood in stool, or a change in bowel habits.

◯ **Low-dose CAT scan** Lung cancer kills more Americans than any other cancer, and it's usually not diagnosed until it's too far along to treat. Annual low-dose CAT scans in women 60 or older who smoke now or smoked in the past may be able to detect tumors while small enough to be treated.

◯ **Flu shot** Everyone over age 50—except those allergic to eggs or the flu vaccine—should get a flu shot each September or October. If you're healthy, the shot can prevent illness, and if you have a chronic medical condition, such as asthma, it can reduce the flu's severity and risk of serious complications.

◯ **Tetanus shot** Two out of three people over age 60 haven't gotten a tetanus shot in the past 10 years, which means they're not immune to tetanus. If you're one of those people, make sure you get the shot.

AGES 62 *and* OLDER

About one in eight Americans has reached the age of 65, and 20.2 million of them are women. By year 2030, one in four Americans will be over 65, most of them women.

There's no doubt about it: we're living longer than ever before—and these years bring unique health concerns.

Screens for colon cancer and mammograms are absolutely necessary now. Almost every time, colon cancer can be cured if screens find the cancer early. And while women over 65 who have had several negative Pap tests don't have to get them anymore, it's still important to see your gynecologist for pelvic exams and clinical breast exams.

Getting exercise should also be high on your list of priorities. Go for walks, garden, dance. Spend 30 minutes three times a week doing this type of weight-bearing aerobic exercise. On the other days, lift weights for 15 or 20 minutes, Dr. Lichtenstein suggests. You'll burn extra calories and strengthen your bones and muscles.

Even if you have low bone mass or osteoporosis, lifting weights is safe if you start with a light weight of no more than 5 pounds and go slowly, he says. You'll build muscle, bone mass, and balance. To avoid injury, give yourself a day to rest between strength-training sessions. Besides keeping you strong, exercise could let you lose weight, which will help you avoid pain in your hips, knees, ankles, and feet.

But your muscles and skeleton shouldn't be

"Studies show that aspirin reduces the growth of polyps that lead to colon cancer. The dose and frequency are not clear, but talk with your doctor about taking either regular or baby aspirin at least every other day. It's probably a good idea if you're not bothered by aspirin's side effects, which can include stomach upsets and gastrointestinal bleeding."

—HAROLD FRUCHT, M.D., DIRECTOR OF GASTROENTEROLOGY
AT FOX CHASE CANCER CENTER IN PHILADELPHIA

the only thing you're exercising, say health experts. Filling up your social calendar, connecting emotionally with friends and family, and staying stimulated also keep you happy and healthy.

"There's no question that people who remain intellectually active and socially engaged in older years do better," says Eugenia Siegler, M.D., associate professor of clinical medicine at Weill Medical College of Cornell University in New York City. Use this time to travel, learn new things, take classes at a local college, volunteer, and connect to friends and family.

Most retired Americans are already active. The proportion of retired American women who are sedentary fell from 44 percent in 1985 to 39 percent in 1995.

Women are challenging themselves by going back to school or work, volunteering, and making use of the Internet. In one survey, 37 percent of older adults said continuing their education was important in retirement. "Learning-in-retirement" programs have even popped up around the United States—some 300 in all, most of which are affiliated with colleges. Also, 44 percent of people who are retired say they work to stay active rather than for the paycheck.

Attitudes toward these years have changed, too. Compared with a generation ago, today fewer Americans over age 65 say poor health, loneliness, few job opportunities, and too little money are problems for people in their age group.

Your Self-Care Checklist

◯ **Nutrient-dense food** Because your caloric needs are still dropping while your nutritional needs are rising, make every calorie count by eating whole grains, beans, low-fat dairy foods, fruits and vegetables, and small amounts of extra-lean meats. Take a multi supplement just to make sure you're getting all your nutrients.

◯ **Antioxidant-rich food** Antioxidants found in fruits, vegetables, and whole grains stimulate your immune system and help you avoid infections like the flu or pneumonia. So polish off your vegetable stir-fry with a bowl of berries.

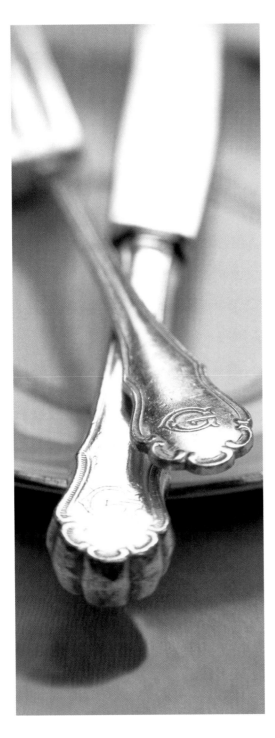

The **average** woman over age 65 **dines out** more than **twice a week**, but avoiding fat and nonnutritious meals at restaurants can be a **challenge**.

○ **Restaurant choices** When ordering fast food, choose salads with fat-free dressing, a plain hamburger, or a grilled chicken sandwich. At sit-down restaurants, look for vegetarian or entrées labeled "light," and ask your server to wrap half your meal in a to-go package before even setting it down in front of you.

Your Doctor's Office Checklist

○ **Flu shot** Continue getting a flu shot in September or October of every year. If you have a chronic medical condition, the shot might not prevent the flu, but it could make your illness less severe if you do get it, and lower your risk of complications.

○ **Pneumococcal vaccine** Get this vaccine for pneumococcal pneumonia at least once after age 64. You'll want to avoid the trip to the hospital or the infections that could result from pneumonia.

○ **Dental checkups** Continue going to the dentist every 6 months, and don't ignore gum pain, swelling, or bleeding.

○ **Eye exams** After you turn 65, start going to the eye doctor every 1 to 2 years if you haven't been already. If you have diabetes, go to the ophthalmologist every year to make sure you don't get diabetic retinopathy, a disease in which tiny blood vessels in the eye weaken and leak, causing blurred vision or even blindness.

○ **Skin exams** This is no time to slack off on skin care, especially if leaving the workforce affords you more time in the outdoors. Continue getting tested annually for skin cancer.

○ **Tetanus shot** Two out of three people over age 60 aren't immune to tetanus, a disease in which bacteria enter an open wound and attack the nervous system, causing muscle spasms, lockjaw, difficulty swallowing, rigid muscles, fever, sweating, and an accelerated heart rate. Get vaccinated every 10 years.

○ **Bone-density test** You should be getting a DEXA scan regularly by now. Nine out of 10 women have osteoporosis by age 75, so being screened regularly is essential.

If your test results are normal, go back for another scan every 3 to 5 years. If you have low bone mass and you're on therapy to treat it, go back in 2 years to track your progress. After that, your doctor will put you on your own screening schedule to see if you're progressing from the therapy.

○ **Blood pressure check** Continue getting your blood pressure checked at least every 2 years, or more often if your readings are abnormal.

○ **Complete lipid profile** Keep getting this test every 2 years if results are normal, and every 4 months if abnormal.

○ **Fasting blood plasma glucose test** Screening for diabetes is still important, so get a fasting blood plasma glucose test every 3 years.

○ **Colon cancer screening** Continue getting a digital rectal exam every year and a colonoscopy every 10 years, along with a yearly fecal occult blood test. If you don't have risk factors for colon cancer, you can get a flexible sigmoidoscopy every 3 to 5 years instead of a colonoscopy.

○ **Thyroid-stimulating hormone test** You should still be getting screened every 5 years for thyroid disease.

○ **Pelvic exam, Pap test, and breast exams** Many women think they don't need regular gynecological exams after menopause, but women's risk for cancers in the reproductive system goes up after menopause, which is why it's so important to keep going every year.

○ **Mammograms** Don't forget your yearly mammogram. If you have trouble remembering, schedule it on your birthday.

WAITING
ROOM

How to Get the Most out of Your Next Doctor's Appointment

For a long time, men and women alike had little access to information about medicine. But in the past few decades, as an increasing number of both general and gender-based health magazines, Web sites, and books have focused on health issues, we have become better informed than ever. Health care has become a partnership between doctors and their patients—and women don't hesitate to ask questions or even suggest their own therapies.

But forming that partnership takes time, and time is a precious commodity in the era of managed care.

Visits with doctors have always been shorter than they should be, and the rise of HMOs has made them even shorter, says Mary Jane Minkin, M.D., clinical professor of obstetrics and gynecology at Yale University School of Medicine. "There's not a heck of a lot you can discuss with somebody in 5 minutes," says Dr. Minkin.

Fortunately, those short visits may be getting slightly longer. An article in the *New England Journal of Medicine* reported that between 1989 and 1998, the time patients spent with doctors increased by a few minutes. Visits with doctors now last up to 22 minutes.

That's still not a lot of time, of course. To make the most of it, women need to plan ahead and communicate effectively. In the following pages, some of our experts and advisors share the same strategies they use when they themselves are the patients.

Your Routine Checkup

This is your chance to discuss recent health problems as well as any physical or emotional changes that have occurred in the past year or 6 months. Routine checkups also give your doctor the opportunity to do comprehensive physical exams. To get the most out of the visit:

Know your family history. Many illnesses (and risk factors for illnesses) are influenced by a woman's family history. Before you arrive for your checkup, take a few minutes to mentally review the health of your parents, siblings, and children. You'll probably be asked to fill out a form and give details about your family's experience with heart disease, diabetes, and other conditions.

Bring medical records. Give your doctor a copy of any medical records that she doesn't already have. These might include reports of mammograms, Pap tests, colonoscopies, or other tests you've had within the past year. If you don't have copies of these reports, you can get them (usually free of charge) from the clinics or hospitals where they were performed.

Make a list of current health concerns. It's easy to forget things when you're in the doctor's office. To make sure nothing gets missed, make a

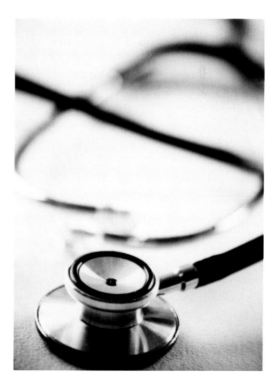

"cheat sheet" that lists symptoms or problems that are worrying you, such as a persistent cough, nagging joint pain, or difficulty sleeping, advises Marianne Legato, M.D., director of Partnership for Women's Health at Columbia University in New York City.

Talk about tests. In the preceding chapter, you learned about health issues that affect women at different stages of life. After reviewing the information, you may want to ask your doctor if you're due for important screening tests, such as a cholesterol test or a mammogram.

Your Annual Pelvic Exam

No one looks forward to it, but the yearly pelvic exam is essential for a woman's long-term health. Here's how to make the most of this important appointment.

Think beyond reproductive health. Your gynecologist needs to know about *all* your health issues, not only those that appear to involve the reproductive organs. Many common symptoms—fatigue, for example—may be linked to a woman's hormones. Your gynecologist can't provide comprehensive care unless she knows about any and all symptoms that may be troubling you, says Dr. Legato.

Don't hold back. It's not uncommon for women to make an appointment to see their gynecologists then neglect to discuss personal or intimate details. Don't let embarrassment hold you back. If you're experiencing low sex drive, for example, tell your doctor. Are you having trouble controlling urine? Talk about it. The issues may be uncomfortable, but this is your chance to find out if something's wrong—and what you can do to resolve it, says Dr. Legato.

Time-Management Tips

doctors and patients agree: There simply isn't enough time in the average visit to get everything done. Here are a few ways to cope with the time crunch.

Find a doctor with time. Every doctor spends different amounts of time with patients. If you're choosing a new doctor, call the office and ask how much time they allot for new-patient visits, annual physicals, and regular doctor visits. One doctor might allow 5 or 10 minutes; another might allow 30.

See other health professionals. Physician's assistants and nurse practitioners are totally qualified to treat most common problems, and they usually spend more time with patients than doctors do, says Dr. Minkin.

Discuss the main topics first. Before walking into your doctor's office, prepare a list of key points you want to bring up—and start with the most important ones. When researchers looked at 264 patient–physician interviews, they found that the doctors tended to interrupt after a patient had been talking for an average of 23 seconds. That doesn't give you a lot of time—so plan on starting with the three or four issues that are most important. ∎

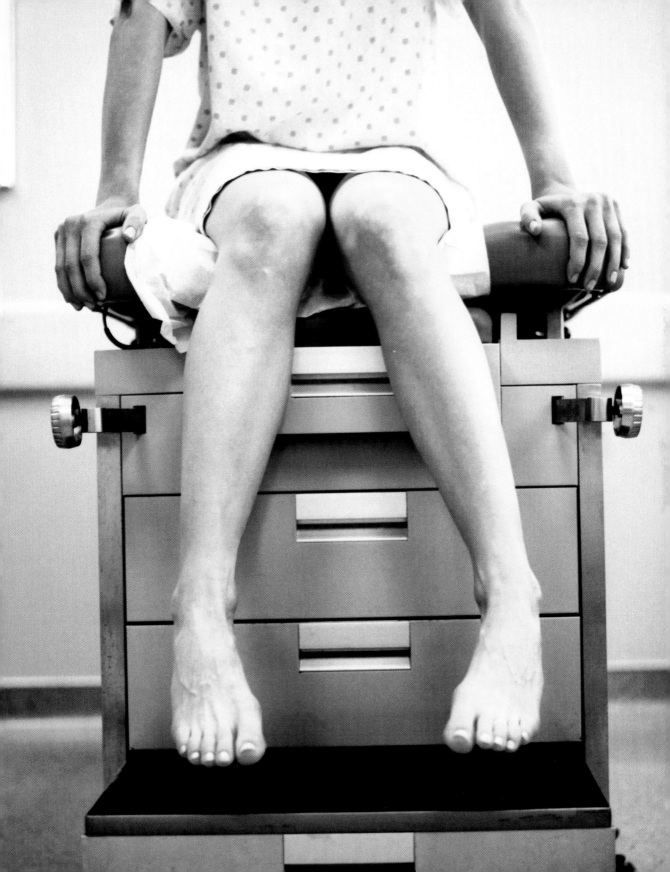

If you're uncomfortable, speak up. No one feels completely comfortable during a pelvic exam, but you shouldn't be in pain. Always let your doctor know if the exam is more uncomfortable than usual. She can probably reduce the discomfort—by using a smaller speculum, for example, or applying less pressure to the abdomen.

> **"Patients have taught me a substantial amount of what's important to me in medicine. The story of a patient's illness as told by an intelligent and sensitive patient is invaluable because it tells you how the disease is experienced."**
>
> —MARIANNE J. LEGATO, M.D., DIRECTOR OF PARTNERSHIP FOR WOMEN'S HEALTH AT COLUMBIA UNIVERSITY IN NEW YORK CITY

When You're Sick

Doctors aren't mind readers. Whether you're seeing your doctor because you have been fatigued, have a persistent discharge, or simply aren't feeling well, she won't know where to begin unless you describe your symptoms clearly.

"In at least 80 percent of cases, we can diagnose the illness before any laboratory testing—if the patient communicates effectively," Dr. Legato says.

To communicate clearly:

Describe your symptoms exactly. If you have pain in a joint in your elbow, don't tell your doctor that you're feeling achy. If you have a cough, tell your doctor if it's "wet" or "dry"—or if it's painful or merely irritating. The more specific you are in describing symptoms, the easier it will be for your doctor to figure out what's going on, says Dr. Legato.

One woman told Dr. Legato that she felt as though blood couldn't get through her right calf. "That happens to be a perfect description of deep-vein thrombosis, which is exactly what she had," Dr. Legato says.

Leave the diagnosis to your doctor. Patients often walk into their doctors' offices and tell them what they think is causing their symptoms. Apart from the fact that a self-diagnosis is unlikely to be accurate, it can waste valuable time by leading your doctor in the wrong direction. You're better off simply telling your doctor your symptoms, says Helen K. Edelberg, M.D., assistant professor in the Brookdale department of geriatrics and adult development at Mount Sinai School of Medicine in New York City.

Give all the details. Your doctor will want to know how long you've had symptoms, what you were doing when the symptoms began, whether you're having other symptoms at the same time, and if anything you do—such as lying down—makes the symptoms go away. The more information you provide, the easier it will be for your doctor to make an accurate diagnosis.

Discuss medications. Both prescription and over-the-counter medications could contribute to your symptoms or affect the treatment your doctor recommends. Before you leave home, make a list of medications you're taking. Remember to write down supplements or herbal treatments as well.

Don't leave without a diagnosis. We often assume that our doctors can figure out everything, but sometimes symptoms don't lend themselves to easy answers. And in some cases doctors simply neglect to explain things clearly. If you're not sure what the diagnosis is, ask your doctor to repeat it. Make sure you also fully understand what your doctor says about test results, future plans, and treatment options. You won't be able to take proper care of yourself if you don't clearly understand what's happening with your health, says Barbara Korsch, M.D., head of general pediatrics at Children's Hospital of Los Angeles and author of *The Intelligent Patient's Guide to the Doctor-Patient Relationship.*

Make sure you understand your instructions. Before leaving your doctor's office, take a moment to repeat everything you were told to do: what medicines to take, the proper dosage, and so on. Doctors often advise men and women alike to bring a notepad so they can jot things down while the information is still fresh.

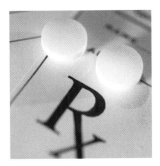

Discussing Treatment Options

More than two-thirds of all doctors' visits end with a prescription's being written, making medication the most common form of intervention.

Whether your doctor is recommending medications, physical therapy, or surgery, you have to be sure that you fully understand the implications

When to Go to the Emergency Room

most illnesses and conditions can wait until you're able to see a doctor—but some symptoms require emergency attention. They include:

- Chest pain that lasts longer than 2 minutes
- Difficulty breathing or shortness of breath
- Any sudden or severe pain that lasts longer than half an hour.

- Uncontrolled bleeding
- Coughing or vomiting blood
- Sudden dizziness, weakness, or a change in vision
- Severe or persistent vomiting or diarrhea to the point of fainting due to dehydration
- Marked changes in mental function, such as confusion ■

of the treatment. Here are some questions everyone should ask.

What are the benefits? People often undergo treatments without really understanding what they stand to gain. Once you know why your doctor has recommended a particular course of action—taking a pill to "thin" the blood, for example, or using physical therapy to relieve pressure on a spinal nerve—you'll be more likely to stick with the plan. It's also important to discuss with your doctor the alternatives to treatment, including the anticipated results if treatment is not initiated. Sometimes people do get well on their own, says Dr. Korsch.

What are the side effects? Doctors are often reluctant to mention a medication's side effects because some people will report anything from itchy teeth to stools that glow in the dark, jokes Dr. Minkin. But you need to know if the medications you'll be taking are likely to cause problems—and you'll be more likely to keep taking them when you're sure that side effects are rare or insignificant, says Dr. Legato.

"My greatest disappointment is when a patient says, 'I didn't fill the prescription because I was afraid of the side effects,'" Dr. Legato adds. "That means I didn't give the patient enough time to express concerns."

How soon will it work? Treatments don't always work right away, and it's important to know what to expect. An antibiotic will relieve symptoms within a day or two, while some antidepressants won't be fully effective for weeks. Physical therapy for back problems may take months. Knowing the time frame ahead of time makes it easier to gauge the effectiveness of treatment, says Dr. Minkin.

Get the Most from Tests

Diagnostic tests are essential for your health. Consider colonoscopy: If everyone—men and women alike—had this test at age 50 and regularly thereafter, there would be 25,000 fewer deaths annually from colon cancer.

No one likes getting mammograms, endometrial biopsies, or other tests. They're uncomfortable and inconvenient. They're also scary because you don't know in advance what the results will be. Don't let that hold you back. When your doctor orders tests, here are a few ways to calm your nerves and get all the information that you need.

Learn the details. Tests are scariest when you don't know in advance what to expect. Ask your doctor to describe the test in detail. Will there be pain? How long will the discomfort last? How long does it take to get results? The more information you get, the less nervous you are likely to be.

Also, don't hesitate to ask other women, including women in the doctor's office, about their experiences with the tests—and what they did to relax and reduce the discomfort.

Know what's normal. When your doctor gives you the results of a test, ask for the normal range. For example, if you're premenopausal and you score a 55 on a follicle-stimulating hormone (FSH) test, your doctor should tell you that you're 25 points above the normal premenopausal score of 30. She'll also explain what this means, and how the numbers affect your long-term health.

Discuss a plan of action. If your test results are normal, your doctor might tell you to keep doing what you're doing. But if they're not, make sure you fully understand what you need to do in the months and years ahead.

How to Ask for Psychological Help

Many women assume that their gynecologists or family doctors are concerned about solely their physical health. But your doctor is also trained to recognize psychological difficulties.

In one study, researchers analyzed the reasons for 537 doctors' visits. They found that 67 percent were at least partly about psychological concerns. Once again, however, your doctor can't know how you're feeling unless you bring it up.

Explain any emotional or psychological changes you have experienced lately. If you're having trouble remembering things, give your doctor specific examples—maybe you've been forgetting where you put things, or you can't remember parts of town that used to be familiar. Tell your doctor if you're crying more than you used to—and how often it happens. If you're having anxiety attacks, describe how they make you feel. Maybe your palms sweat or your heart races. These and other details will provide important clues about the underlying causes of your feelings.

Don't neglect to discuss physical symptoms, even those that appear to be vague or minor. Physical discomfort is a common sign of psychological difficulties, even in people who aren't aware that they're depressed or anxious, says Dr. Edelberg.

> "Doctors' visits are **emotionally charged.** When you're in that type of situation and you're without power, you're not in a state to listen. So one thing I recommend is to **prepare for the visit** so you don't get overwhelmed."
>
> —BARBARA KORSCH, M.D., HEAD OF GENERAL PEDIATRICS AT CHILDREN'S HOSPITAL OF LOS ANGELES AND AUTHOR OF *THE INTELLIGENT PATIENT'S GUIDE TO THE DOCTOR-PATIENT RELATIONSHIP*

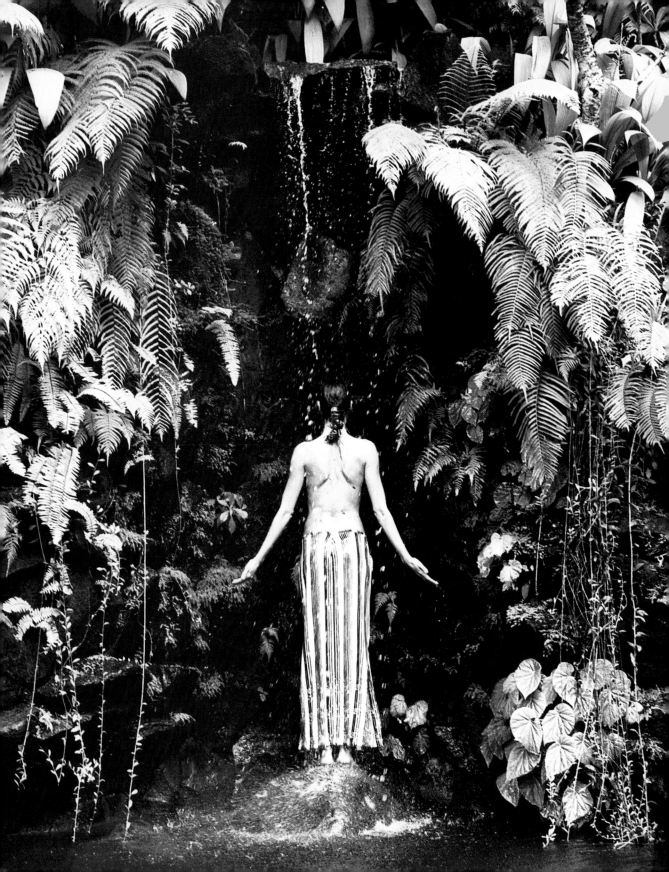

PART
TWO

YOUR STAY WELL,

STAY YOUNG

"TO DO" LIST

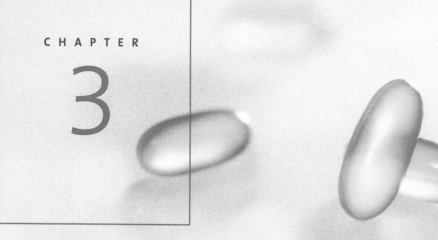

Vitamins, Minerals, and Nutrition: The Complete Plan

Just a few years ago, most health experts felt that women could get all of the vitamins and minerals that they needed from a healthful diet and that supplements were unnecessary. Today, many—including *Prevention* magazine's top advisors—have changed their minds.

Even women who are conscientious about eating a healthful diet will occasionally fall short on essential nutrients. And let's face it: On any given night, most women are more likely to eat pizza and ice cream than baked salmon and a green salad.

"Most women don't meet even conservative recommendations for fruit and vegetable intakes," says Michael Fossel, M.D., Ph.D., clinical professor of medicine at Michigan State University in East Lansing and author of *Reversing Human Aging*. "Even I probably don't eat that many fruits and vegetables, and I know better."

Surveys have shown that only 32 percent of American adults—women included—eat five servings of fruits and vegetables daily. Even if they did, that's probably not enough: Many experts advise that for optimal health protection, women should eat nine daily servings of fruits and vegetables.

Our dietary shortcomings aren't the only reasons that the nutritionists *Prevention* consults advise women to use nutritional supplements. Recent studies have shown that some key nutrients provide the most benefits when they're consumed in amounts greater than it's possible to get from foods alone.

Consider folate. This nutrient has been shown to reduce the risk of heart disease as well as certain birth defects. Unless you eat fortified breakfast cereals, you'd have to eat the equivalent of more than 5 cups of romaine lettuce daily to meet the daily requirement. Taking a 400-microgram folic acid (the synthetic form of folate) supplement makes good sense.

The same is true of vitamin E. Only nuts and vegetable oils have appreciable amounts, which is why women only get about 9 to 12 IU of vitamin E daily. Studies have shown that getting at least 100 IU daily is associated with a reduced risk of heart disease. "There's no way that anyone could get that amount without taking a supplement," says Jane Higdon, R.N., Ph.D., research associate at the Linus Pauling Institute at Oregon State University in Corvallis.

Even though every woman should do everything possible to eat a healthful, balanced diet, adding a multivitamin and a few key nutritional supplements is a reasonable approach for preventing deficiencies and safeguarding your long-term health.

Nutrition: Where to Start

Calories. Calorie needs vary from woman to woman depending on height, weight, age, and body composition. A very muscular woman might need 2,500 calories per day, and a woman with less muscle might only need 1,800 calories. But a good rule of thumb is to eat no less than 10 times your body weight in calories, says Leslie Bonci, M.P.H., R.D., director of nutrition at the Center for Sports Medicine at the University of Pittsburgh and spokesperson for the American Dietetic Association. "And for women who weigh less than 100 pounds, no fewer than 1,500 calories per day," she says.

Carbohydrates. Carbohydrates are the foundation of a healthy diet. Try to get 60 to 65 percent of your calories from carbohydrates, and make three to six of those servings whole grain, such as whole wheat bread and bran cereal.

Whole grains provide all the nutrients from the grain, like fiber, that are taken out of refined products. They're also satisfying. "We feel like we're really eating something, and we feel fuller when we're finished," Bonci says.

To make sure you're eating whole grains, check the label. "Whole wheat" should be listed in the ingredients of bread and crackers, and "100 percent whole grain" should be included on your box of cereal.

Fruit and vegetables. Aim for five servings of vegetables and four servings of fruit a day, and you'll get a good helping of antioxidants, substances that protect your DNA, the genetic information in every cell of your body, from cancer. (For more on antioxidants, see page 42.)

If you're not accustomed to eating so many fruits and veggies, increase the number gradually, Bonci says. Start out by tossing a handful of chopped onions or mushrooms into your spaghetti sauce. Substitute grilled eggplant parmigiana made with low-fat cheese for chicken parmigiana with cheese high in fat. Bake an apple with cinnamon for dessert. Bonci sneaks in two extra servings of vegetables while she makes dinner by snacking on hummus or another bean dip and baby carrots.

You'll be glad you did. Not only are fruit and vegetables good for you, but they also bring crunchiness, sweetness, or a savory taste to your meals.

To get the best health protection, choose from a variety of botanical families. For instance, kiwifruit, blueberries, bananas, apples, oranges, and grapes come from different families. As for vegetables, mushrooms, spinach, endive, sweet potatoes, broccoli, zucchini, corn, lentils, garlic, tomatoes, and carrots come from different families, too. Or look for different colors. There are some exceptions, but fruit and vegetables of different colors usually come from different botanical families. Try to buy two or three fruits and two or three vegetables a week, and try to make them slightly different every trip to the market, says Terri Brownlee, R.D., nutrition director of the Duke University Diet and Fitness Center in Durham, North Carolina.

You'll also benefit from eating the fruit and vegetables themselves rather than taking a supplement, says Jerianne Heimendinger, R.D., Ph.D., a scientist at the AMC Cancer Research Center in Denver who studied the antioxidant effects of fruit and vegetables. "Many of the components of food work synergistically, so it's much better to have the food than it is to isolate one component and give it to people in larger amounts."

Lean protein. Now, and in the years to come, you should be getting 10 to 15 percent of your calories from lean protein, such as beans and peas, nuts, fish, skinless chicken and turkey and lean red meat (if you eat meat), and low-fat milk and eggs (if you eat dairy products).

Don't be fooled by meat labeled "lean," Bonci says. Check the fine print, and take note of how many grams of fat the meat really contains. Don't buy it if it has more than 10 grams of fat per serving.

Dairy. Eat two or three servings of low-fat dairy products a day—or 1,000 milligrams of calcium. Low-fat and fat-free milk, yogurt, and cheese are excellent sources of calcium, which helps keep your bones strong.

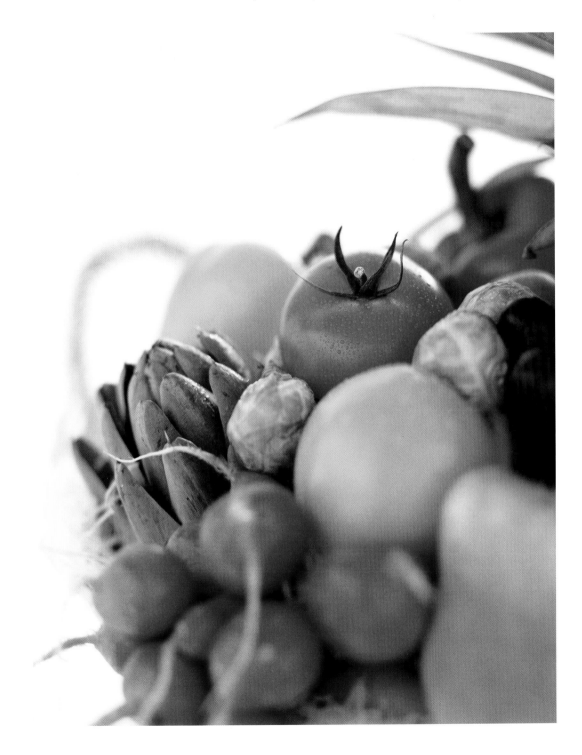

By the time you reach your early thirties, your body begins to lose more bone than it builds. Calcium will help you put bone in the bank, so to speak. The recommended 1,000 milligrams of calcium is the equivalent of about three servings of dairy food: 1 cup of fat-free milk, 8 ounces of yogurt, and 2 ounces of part-skim mozzarella cheese. If you have trouble getting calcium from dairy food, try calcium-fortified food, like orange juice or cereal.

Fat. You probably already know that you're supposed to eat fat and sweets "sparingly." That means no more than 25 percent of your total calories should come from fats. Reach for the healthiest fats and you'll start a habit that will benefit you for the rest of your life. The best choices are monounsaturated: olive oil, canola oil, peanut oil, and avocado. Monounsaturated fats bring down total cholesterol without affecting HDL ("good") cholesterol levels—a strong asset, given that researchers have detected high cholesterol levels even in teens.

Polyunsaturated fats—like safflower, sesame, and sunflower seeds, corn and soybeans, and other nuts and seeds and their oils—are also good choices. These fats bring down all cholesterol levels.

Foods high in saturated fat and trans fatty acids (processed fats that resemble saturated fat) should be eaten sparingly, if at all. Both raise cholesterol levels and contribute to heart disease. Saturated fat is found in animal products, like beef,

Extra Help for Smokers

the smoke from cigarettes does more than damage the lungs. It also triggers the formation of free radicals, which "use up" vitamin C in the body. That's why smokers are advised to get 110 milligrams of vitamin C daily, compared with 75 milligrams for nonsmokers.

There's another reason smokers may need greater amounts of vitamin C and other nutrients. If you smoke, your diet may not be as good as it should be—in part because nicotine suppresses appetite, and also because smokers are more likely to light up than to enjoy nutritious snacks, says Michael Fossel, M.D., Ph.D., clinical professor of medicine at Michigan State University in East Lansing and author of *Reversing Human Aging.*

The best thing, of course, is to quit smoking. But in the meantime, be sure to take a vitamin C supplement daily. You also may want to get extra amounts of vitamin E and selenium, which will lower levels of free radicals in the body. ■

whole milk, and ice cream, as well as in so-called tropical oils: cocoa butter, coconut oil, palm oil, and palm kernel oil. Trans fats are manufactured by adding hydrogen to polyunsaturated fats to make them more solid. Also called hydrogenated oils, they're the primary fat in most vegetable shortenings, crackers, desserts, snacks, chips, and some margarines.

A good rule of thumb, Bonci says, is to choose items with hydrogenated oils listed as far down the ingredients list as possible. Also, look for "trans fatty acid–free" margarine.

Making good choices now could affect your cholesterol all the way through menopause and beyond, when women's risk for heart disease increases. A study found that when women had low cholesterol levels during premenopause, they significantly lowered their risk of heart disease after menopause.

Fish. Eat two servings of salmon, mackerel, herring, or sardines each week, and you'll get 3.5 grams of fish oil omega-3 fatty acids. This type of fat isn't made by the body, but it's necessary for growth and development. It also helps prevent heart disease, hypertension, arthritis, and cancer and reduces inflammation.

Flaxseed. Flaxseed is the vegetable source of omega-3 fatty acids and helps prevent heart disease and possibly cancer.

Add a tablespoon of ground flaxseed to your diet a day in addition to your two servings of fish a week. (Both foods are exceptionally high in omega-3s.) Because the seeds come in hard shells, you'll be able to digest flaxseed better if you grind it in a blender or food processor and store it in the fridge or freezer. Then sprinkle the ground seeds on salad, oatmeal, or muffins. Another option: buy flaxseed oil and use it in place of other oils in your cold dishes. But don't cook with flaxseed oil because heat changes its structure, Brownlee says. Store the oil in the refrigerator as soon as you bring it home.

Fiber. Try to get 25 to 35 grams of fiber a day. Eating high-fiber foods like beans and legumes, whole grain cereal and bread, vegetables, fruit, and nuts also lowers cholesterol and the risk for heart disease.

Garlic. Eating 9 to 10 cloves of garlic a week may protect women against stomach and colorectal cancers. In fact, garlic has killed cancer cells in the test tube. Brush a mixture of olive oil and crushed garlic onto fish, or make your own garlic bread with a spray of olive oil and fresh minced garlic. After you peel and chop garlic, let it sit for 15 minutes before cooking to allow time for the cancer-fighting compounds to develop.

Low sodium. Eating food naturally low in sodium, like fresh fruit and vegetables, and avoiding excessively salty food—like smoked, cured, or processed meat; regular soy sauce; garlic salt; regular canned soup; some frozen meals; and salty crackers, chips, pretzels, popcorn, and nuts—will help lower your blood pressure. Try to get fewer than 800 milligrams of sodium per meal, or 2,400 milligrams a day—the equivalent contained in 1 teaspoon of table salt.

Cinnamon. Cinnamon increases glucose metabolism and lowers your risk of diabetes, which is becoming increasingly prevalent. Doctors who have studied cinnamon's effects recommend stirring a quarter to a full teaspoon of cinnamon into orange juice, coffee, or oatmeal every day.

Carotenoids. Although quitting smoking is the best way to reduce your risk of lung cancer, studies have found that a diet high in phytochemicals called carotenoids is associated with a significantly lower risk of lung cancer for both smokers and nonsmokers.

Carotenoids are found in fruits and vegetables such as sweet potatoes, tomatoes, carrots, spinach, broccoli, cantaloupe, pumpkin, and apricots. Carrots in particular, which are a major source of a carotenoid called alpha-carotene, have been shown to benefit nonsmokers. Tomatoes, which contain a carotenoid called lycopene, have been shown to benefit smokers.

Vanadium. Certain foods containing this trace mineral help keep blood sugar levels normal.

Foods with vanadium include fat-free milk, gelatin, lentils, navy beans, lobster, vegetable oils, radishes, potatoes, turnip greens, squash, lettuce, hazelnuts, buckwheat, rye seed, grains, and cereal.

Potassium. Potassium in fruit and vegetables can help reduce your blood pressure. It's a min-

A Vegetarian's Guide to Supplements

doctors agree that following a vegetarian diet is among the healthiest lifestyle choices a woman can make. But even if you're careful to eat well—ideally a vegetarian diet will include fruits, vegetables, legumes, and whole grains with almost every meal—it may be a challenge to get all the essential nutrients that you need, says Jane Higdon, R.N., Ph.D., research associate at the Linus Pauling Institute in Corvallis, Oregon.

If you're a vegan—one who avoids eggs and dairy as well as meats—you'll have to work harder to get adequate amounts of all vitamins and minerals. Doctors usually advise vegetarians to take a few key supplements, including:

- Iron. Menstruating women who eat meat are advised to get 18 milligrams of iron daily. Women who are vegetarians need almost twice as much—33 milligrams daily—because the iron in plant foods is less easily absorbed. If you're in your childbearing years, choose a multi supplement that contains 18 milligrams of iron. If you're postmenopausal, you may not need supplemental iron unless you are anemic or have a very low dietary intake.

- Vitamin D. It's found mainly in fish and dairy foods. If you're a strict vegetarian, the only way to get enough vitamin D is to use a supplement that contains it, Dr. Higdon says.

- Vitamin B_{12}. Vitamin B_{12} is found in animal products and milk but is not generally found in plant foods. Vegetarian women should make sure they get at least 2.4 micrograms daily by taking a multivitamin.

- Calcium. Even though plant foods contain some calcium, they can't compete with the amounts found in milk, yogurt, or other dairy foods. If you're premenopausal, aim for 1,000 milligrams a day; after menopause try to get 1,200 milligrams per day. Women who don't get that much in their diets, which includes most of us, should make up the rest with a supplement. ■

eral similar to sodium, but it has the opposite effect on the body. Foods high in potassium include acorn squash, green beans, tomato juice, potatoes, spinach, bananas, watermelon, legumes, and avocados.

Blueberries. The dark blue color of blueberries holds antioxidants, which keep free radicals from harming your DNA and causing cancer. With just ½ cup of blueberries, you'll get the antioxidant power of 2½ cups of chopped spinach. You also might slow down the short-term memory loss that comes with age, according to studies done on rats. Blueberries can even help prevent urinary tract infections and improve your night vision and adjustment to bright lights.

Sprinkle the berries on your morning cereal, on a bed of mixed greens and feta cheese, or in frozen yogurt, or pour low-fat milk over them with a little sugar or honey.

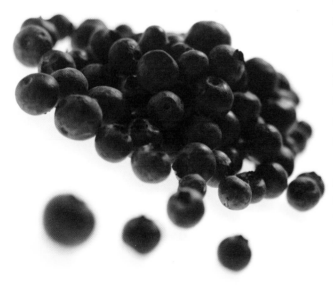

Recycled nutrients. Make your nutrients work harder. After you cook vegetables like broccoli, carrots, or spinach, use the water as a soup broth. You'll get the vitamins, minerals, and nutrients the vegetables had.

Moderate alcohol consumption. For women, having up to three drinks of wine, beer, or distilled liquor a week raises HDL ("good") cholesterol levels, prevents blood clots, and interferes with cell growth in the blood vessels, all factors that lower risk of heart disease. Even better news: The effects are most apparent in people over age 50 or people with risk factors for heart disease. It's best to limit yourself to no more than one drink a day, however. Drinking more than that appears to be a risk factor for cancer and, in susceptible women, could lead to alcohol dependency.

Tea. In animal and some human studies, tea shows antioxidant effects, which lower risk of cardiovascular disease and cancer.

Tea also has protective compounds called isoflavonoids that keep our bones strong, particularly if you add milk to your cup. Researchers think the isoflavonoids' estrogenic effect maintains bone density in women after they go through menopause.

Foods that fight breast cancer. Although research hasn't proven it, several studies suggest that eating some foods could lower the risk of breast cancer. Protection may come from the beta-carotene in carrot juice, lycopene in Spicy Hot V8 vegetable juice, linoleic acid in 1% milk, omega-3 fatty acids in salmon, and antioxidants in grape juice.

The Antioxidant Edge

Vitamins C and E are among the best-known (and best-studied) antioxidants, but many other vitamins and minerals have similar effects. Because antioxidants are so important to your overall health, it's worth taking a moment to explain what these nutrients are and how they protect against dozens (if not hundreds) of illnesses and conditions, including many common among women.

As your cells work, they use oxygen to create energy. But during normal metabolic processes, some oxygen molecules lose an electron and become unstable. These molecules, called free radicals, careen around your body, trying to stabilize themselves by stripping electrons from other molecules. When they succeed, they create still more free radicals—and damage healthy tissues in the process.

Every day, your body faces thousands of assaults from free radicals. Free radical damage is what causes low-density lipoprotein (LDL, the "bad" cholesterol) to stick to artery walls and impede or block the flow of blood. When free radicals damage the DNA in cells, the result can be cell mutations that lead to cancer. Free radicals can damage tissues in the eyes and cause cataracts or macular degeneration, the leading causes of vision loss in the elderly. Many scientists believe that free radicals are the prime force behind aging itself.

There's no way to completely eliminate free radicals. As we've seen, they're a normal byproduct of the body's metabolism. They're also formed by exposure to such things as sunshine, pollution, tobacco smoke, and simple everyday wear and tear.

Nature anticipated the harmful effects of free radicals, and created a number of countermeasures. Just as your body produces free radicals, it also produces antioxidants, enzymes that "voluntarily" give up their own electrons to the marauding molecules. In other words, they essentially come between free radicals and your body's cells, preventing potential damage. These antioxidant enzymes can do only so much, however. In fact, they can easily get overwhelmed by the sheer volume of free radicals.

That's when women need to call in the reserves—the antioxidant nutrients found in foods and many supplements. There are hundreds of natural food compounds with antioxidant properties. The main advantage of these compounds, unlike your body's natural enzymes, is that they're available in inexhaustible quantities. As long as you eat healthful foods and take supplements as necessary, you'll constantly replenish the supply.

In any discussion of antioxidants, you'll come across a lot of references to vitamins C and E, simply because they're the ones that scientists have studied most. But it's worth keeping in mind that they're only a small part of a massive army of protective compounds. For example, the minerals zinc and selenium, which are included in most multi supplements, act as potent antioxidants. So do many of the B vitamins, as well as minerals such as magnesium.

Even though the individual antioxidants are effective on their own, they perform best when they're working together. Vitamin E, for example, is one of the most powerful antioxidants ever discovered, but it's quickly exhausted in the body. When you get vitamin C at the same time, it "recharges" vitamin E and allows it to protect your body longer. This is one reason that health experts encourage people to eat many different healthful foods or to take multivitamins instead of individual nutrients. The greater the variety of antioxidants that you consume, the more protection you'll get.

Vitamins and minerals do much more than fight free radicals, of course. In the following pages, we'll look at the many ways in which the essential nutrients in foods and supplements can prevent and even reverse some of the most serious health threats that women face today.

Menus with the Most

there's nothing wrong with using supplements as extra insurance against nutritional deficiencies, but you don't want to depend on them. Experts agree that you'll get the best nutritional bang for your buck when you get most of your nutrients in their natural form—from deliciously wholesome foods.

"Supplements are like seat belts," says Jeffrey Blumberg, Ph.D., professor of nutrition at Tufts University in Boston. "You don't buckle your seat belt and drive through red lights. You wear one for added security."

Even though supplements can make up for shortfalls in your diet, foods always provide a greater range of health benefits because they provide protein and fiber, along with a host of protective plant chemicals called phytonutrients.

Unfortunately, even women who try to eat a nutritious diet don't always succeed. The average American diet is often deficient in such nutrients as calcium, iron, and vitamins A and C, says Leslie Bonci, M.P.H., R.D., director of nutrition at the Center for Sports Medicine at the University of Pittsburgh and a spokesperson for the American Dietetic Association.

To get the optimal amount of vitamins and minerals from your diet, here's what she advises.

Think plant-based. As long as your diet consists primarily of plant-based foods, such as fruits, vegetables, and whole grains, you'll almost automatically get enough nutrients and fiber.

Color your plate. Foods that are colorful are often the ones that are most nutritious. The colors in plant foods come from phytochemicals, plant-based chemical compounds that are among the most healthful things you can eat. When you have a whole grain cereal, for example, top it with red strawberries or dewy blueberries. Add snow peas to rice dishes, or mustard greens to meat dishes. The more colors you get, the healthier your diet will be.

Give desserts a nutritional kick. There's nothing wrong with enjoying rich desserts on occasion. But why not make them healthier? Topping a slice of chocolate cake with flavorful berries, or adding fruit slices to a bowl of ice cream, will provide important nutrients along with the sweet tastes you crave. ■

Supplements Every Woman Should Take

You may already take vitamin or mineral supplements. A survey of more than 33,000 American men and women found that about 40 percent do. Do doctors disapprove? Not at all. When researchers conducted a survey of 4,500 female physicians, they found that half used vitamin and mineral supplements.

Which supplements do you, as an individual, really need? It's not an easy question to answer because every vitamin and mineral does something different in the body. Many women do the easy thing and take a multi supplement that contains a variety of vitamins and minerals. But this isn't always the solution, either. Some multi supplements contain laughably small amounts of

some key nutrients, and unnecessarily high levels of others.

For example, some multis provide large amounts of vitamin A. If you're pregnant or have a history of liver problems, that can be a problem because doses higher than 10,000 IU of vitamin A in the form of retinol can increase the risk of birth defects or liver damage, says Dr. Higdon. Zinc is another mineral that may cause problems in doses of 50 milligrams or more daily because it interferes with the body's ability to absorb copper.

In addition, supplement manufacturers sometimes try to wow consumers by providing every conceivable nutrient—even those that researchers aren't even sure that people need. When you read supplement labels and see nutrients such as nickel, tin, silicon, or vanadium, you may be

THREE THINGS I TELL EVERY FEMALE PATIENT

JANE HIGDON, R.N., Ph.D., research associate at the Linus Pauling Institute at Oregon State University in Corvallis, appreciates the benefits that come from taking supplements. But to be effective, supplements have to be used wisely. Here's what she advises.

EAT A NUTRITIOUS DIET—AND USE SUPPLEMENTS AS A BACKUP. There's no substitute for eating nutritious foods every day. For most women, increasing their intake of fruits and vegetables is the best way to stay healthy. But when you need a little push in the right direction—for example, getting extra calcium because you don't eat dairy foods—taking a supplement is a good way to go.

SHOP WISELY. Women often spend way too much for multivitamin and mineral supplements. You don't need to buy fancy brands at health food stores. Look for a multivitamin and mineral supplement that contains 100 percent of the Daily Value for most nutrients. Don't worry about phosphorus, pantothenic acid, or potassium, because you easily get adequate amounts from food.

DON'T IGNORE OTHER ASPECTS OF GOOD HEALTH. People who take supplements sometimes feel as though it's acceptable to slack off in other ways. But supplements can't protect you if you don't take care of all aspects of your health—by not smoking, for example, or by getting regular exercise and a good night's sleep. ∎

spending good money for substances that may not be necessary for health, Dr. Higdon says.

Spend a few moments surveying the shelves at the supermarket, pharmacy, or health food store, and you'll see enough different supplements to make your head spin. Many of them are helpful in certain situations, but for most women, the goal should be to get extra amounts of just a few key nutrients. Here are the supplements that *Prevention* magazine recommends.

A multi that contains 100 percent of the Daily Value of all nutrients—but not iron. Except for women who have been diagnosed with low iron levels or iron deficiency anemia, supplemental amounts of this mineral aren't needed and may be harmful.

Vitamin C. *Prevention* magazine recommends a daily dose of 100 to 500 milligrams. A powerful antioxidant, vitamin C may prevent cholesterol buildup in the arteries. It also increases levels of high-density lipoprotein (HDL, the "good" cholesterol), improves blood pressure, and enhances the body's absorption of iron.

A study of more than 11,000 Americans found that all causes of death were lower among those who took up to 300 milligrams of vitamin C daily.

Supplemental vitamin C even appears to help people with mild to moderate hypertension lower their blood pressure. A study of 39 people with high blood pressure found that those who took vitamin C were able to lower their systolic blood pressure from an average of 155 to 142, and their diastolic blood pressure from 87 to 79. These findings have not yet been replicated in larger studies, however. People with high blood pressure who are thinking about taking vitamin C should continue their current therapy (medication, lifestyle changes, and so forth) and follow up with their health care provider.

It's worth mentioning a potential downside to vitamin C. A study presented at an American Heart Association meeting reported that people who took 500 milligrams of vitamin C daily were more likely to develop atherosclerosis, hardening of the arteries, which increases heart disease risk.

The study got a lot of attention by the media and from scientists, but it's important to remember that it's only one study and that it has not yet been published. "Many more studies have found positive results from vitamin C supplementation, so it's important to look at the totality of the studies," Dr. Higdon says.

Vitamin C is easy to get in the diet, Dr. Higdon adds. If you eat five servings of fruits and vegetables daily, for example, you could get at least 200 milligrams of vitamin C. If you do decide to take supplements, follow the advice from *Prevention* and take 100 to 500 milligrams daily.

Vitamin E. Look for a separate supplement that provides 100 to 400 IU. It's especially important for women who have reached menopause, when the risk of heart disease climbs dramatically. As we mentioned earlier, vitamin E helps prevent free radicals from oxidizing, or damaging, cholesterol in the arteries, the process that makes it more likely to cling to artery walls and increase the risk of heart disease or stroke.

Natural forms of vitamin E are easy for the body to absorb, but they tend to be more expensive than synthetic forms. If you use synthetic vitamin E, plan on taking about 50 percent more. For example, to get the equivalent of 400 IU of natural vitamin E, you'll need to take about 600 IU of the synthetic form.

If you're taking blood-thinning medications such as warfarin or regularly taking aspirin, talk to your doctor before supplementing your diet with vitamin E. It inhibits the ability of blood to clot, which can be dangerous in those who are also using clot-inhibiting medications.

Calcium with vitamin D. If you're under age 50, you should be taking a daily calcium supplement that contains 500 milligrams; if you're over 50, take 1,000 milligrams. You may want to choose a calcium supplement that also contains vitamin D, which will help the body absorb cal-

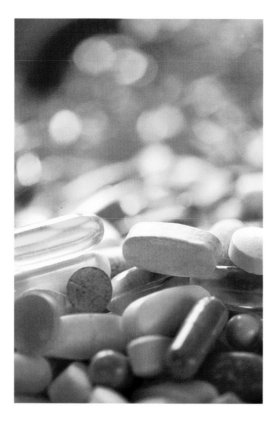

cium and keep the immune system strong. Fortified milk also has vitamin D.

Calcium supplements made with calcium carbonate are the least expensive, but for best absorption you'll want to take them with meals. Calcium citrate costs a little more but can be taken on an empty stomach.

You can absorb only about 500 milligrams of calcium at a time. If you're taking 1,000 milligrams daily, be sure to divide it into two doses.

B vitamins. These help your body turn food into the energy that you need to stay active. Doctors often advise women to take a B-complex supplement that contains vitamins B_6 and B_{12}, folic acid, thiamin, riboflavin, niacin, biotin, and pantothenic acid.

Magnesium. It allows the arteries to relax, which helps control blood pressure. It also plays a role in transmitting electrical signals that keep the heart beating. Most women get about 230 milligrams of magnesium daily—a lot less than the recommended 320 milligrams for women over 30 and 310 milligrams for women under 30.

Those are just a few of the main nutrients that you need every day, but they're among the most important. When they're combined with trace minerals and essential nutrients, such as calcium and vitamins C and E, they'll go a long way toward protecting your long-term health.

Different Women, Different Supplements

The complete nutrition action plan that follows will make it easy for you to eat well at every decade of life. A woman in her twenties who's thinking of getting pregnant, for example, requires different nutrients (and amounts of nutrients) than a woman who's entering menopause. The vitamins and minerals you need to watch for in your thirties and forties aren't necessarily the same ones that you need to focus on in your fifties and sixties.

In Your Twenties

Get relief from PMS. For most women, the bloating, breast tenderness, and other symptoms of premenstrual syndrome tend to get better as the decades pass. But for women in their twenties, PMS can be a real problem. There's some evidence that taking extra amounts of magnesium and vitamin B$_6$ can ease anxiety, premenstrual bloating, and other monthly discomforts.

One study found that women who took 200 milligrams of magnesium daily for 2 months had significantly less fluid retention than women who took a placebo. Other research has shown that taking 400 to 600 milligrams of magnesium can help prevent premenstrual migraines.

"Magnesium is very important, and it's often short in women's diets," says Ann Walker, Ph.D., senior lecturer in human nutrition at the University of Reading in England. Her studies have shown that women who take 200 milligrams of magnesium and 50 milligrams of vitamin B$_6$ will suffer less from premenstrual tension, mood swings, irritability, and anxiety.

Calcium is also helpful for women who experience PMS, she adds. One study found that women who supplemented their diets with 1,200 milligrams of calcium daily for 3 months were able to reduce their symptoms by 45 percent.

Dodge diabetes. There's a good reason to take action against diabetes right away. Women in their teens and twenties are increasingly being diagnosed with type 2 diabetes, which is often triggered by weight gain. In the past, this condition usually affected women after age 45.

Vitamin and mineral supplements are unlikely to prevent diabetes, but they may reduce its severity and potential side effects if you do get it.

After reviewing data collected on almost 10,000 men and women over 20 years, researchers found that people who had the highest levels of vitamin E were the ones who were least likely to develop diabetes. Vitamin E also protects against heart disease, which is important because people with diabetes have a very high risk of getting it. In fact, heart attack and stroke are leading causes of death among those with diabetes. In addition to vitamin E, you may want to be sure that your multi supplement contains chromium and magnesium. Both minerals have been shown to make cells in the body more sensitive to insulin's effects, thereby reducing the risk of developing full-fledged diabetes.

Keep your gums healthy. Young women who don't get enough vitamin C and calcium in their diet are more likely to develop periodontal disease, an infection of the gums and other tissues that support the teeth. Take a multi supplement that contains at least 60 milligrams of vitamin C. For calcium, women in their twenties should take a supplement that provides 500 milligrams daily.

What You Need during Pregnancy

a woman's body changes dramatically during pregnancy. Everything gets larger and more active: The uterus and its supporting muscles enlarge, the joints get more flexible in anticipation of childbirth, and blood volume increases by as much as 60 to 80 percent.

Even if you eat a nutritious diet, it's not always possible to get enough vitamins and minerals to supply your needs as well as those of the baby-to-be. That's why doctors usually advise women to take prenatal supplements during pregnancy, says Bruce K. Young, M.D., professor of obstetrics and gynecology and director of obstetrical services of maternal and fetal medicine at New York University Medical Center in New York City.

Every woman needs different kinds of supplements, depending on her diet, says Dr. Young. A woman who's a vegetarian, for example, may need a supplement with higher-than-usual amounts of iron or vitamin B_{12}. On the other hand, a woman who eats a lot of meat or seafood will want to avoid high-iron supplements because she'll probably get more than enough of this mineral in her diet.

If you're pregnant now or are planning to get pregnant, here are a few nutrients you'll need to pay attention to.

- B vitamins. You don't have to worry about getting too much of the B vitamins during pregnancy because these nutrients do not accumulate in the body. Two B vitamins to focus on are folate and vitamin B_{12}. Folate prevents birth defects called neural tube defects, and vitamin B_{12} aids in fetal metabolism and maintains healthful levels of red blood cells. Foods high in folate include fortified cereals, bread, and legumes. Foods high in vitamin B_{12} are meats and fish. Your doctor may recommend a plasma folate test, which will determine whether you need to supplement your diet with extra folic acid. If you've already had a baby with neural tube defects and you're planning another pregnancy, your doctor may prescribe taking up to 4,000 micrograms of folic acid daily.

- Vitamins A and D. Unlike the B vitamins, your body accumulates vitamins A and D over time. The amount of these nutrients you should get in your prenatal supplement will depend on the amounts you get in your diet. Foods high in vitamin A include squash and carrots; vitamin D–rich foods include fatty fish and fortified milk.

- Calcium. Women who are pregnant often have low levels of calcium, which is essential for strengthening fetal bones.

- Iron. Women who are pregnant are sharing their blood supply with the growing fetus, and they require a large amount of iron in order to keep up with the increased demand for red blood cells. Even if you have a healthful diet, you have a high risk of becoming anemic during pregnancy, says Dr. Young.

Before your doctor gives you a prescription for prenatal nutrients, be sure to mention whether you're eating a lot of iron-rich foods, such as red meat, liver, or green leafy vegetables. This will help your doctor determine how much additional iron you'll need. ■

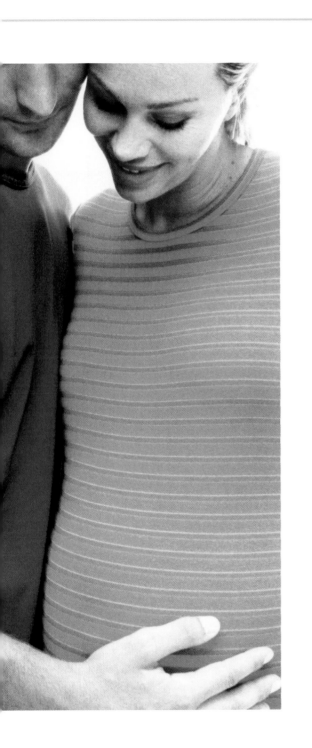

Build strong bones. When women reach menopause, they have a high risk of developing osteoporosis, a bone-thinning condition that's the leading cause of fractures in the elderly. This doesn't mean you can put off thinking about it, however. Keeping your bones strong when you're young will help prevent problems decades down the road. One of the simplest things that you can do is make sure you get enough calcium and vitamin D.

In one study, women who took 500 milligrams of calcium and 700 IU of vitamin D daily for 3 years were able to reduce the loss of supportive bone throughout their bodies. This was impressive enough—but the most important lesson occurred after the study ended. About a third of the participants quit taking the supplements, and within 1 year they lost all of the bone density gains.

If you're in your twenties, plan on taking 500 milligrams of calcium daily. The body can absorb only so much calcium at a time, so it's best to take these supplements between meals, or with meals that don't contain a lot of calcium.

Vitamin C is also important for strong bones. It helps stimulate the body's production of bone and of collagen, a connective tissue. When researchers tested the bone mineral density of 994 postmenopausal women, they found that those who took an average of 745 milligrams of vitamin C daily had bone densities that were about 3 percent higher than those who didn't supplement.

Your regular multivitamin will help, too, as long as it contains the Daily Value of 400 IU of vitamin D. In northern latitudes, like in Boston,

Minneapolis, or Seattle, there is insufficient ultra-violet light available for the body to produce vitamin D. Taking a supplement year-round will ensure a woman has adequate vitamin D stores throughout the year.

Multis also contain vitamin K, which helps with bone formation and reduces bone breakdown. The minerals magnesium and potassium have been shown to help prevent fractures. Magnesium keeps blood calcium at healthful levels, and potassium keeps acid in the blood from pulling calcium from the bones. Look for multis that provide 100 percent of the Daily Value of these nutrients.

In Your Thirties

Kick the common cold. Women in their thirties are often juggling careers and family responsibilities. The nonstop stress makes the body vulner-able to upper respiratory infections—especially when children are always coming home from school with sneezes and runny noses.

On average, Americans get two to six colds a year. Although there is little evidence that vitamin C prevents colds, a number of studies have found that taking at least 1,000 milligrams of vitamin C daily at the first symptoms of a cold reduced the duration of colds by an average of 1 day. This may be due to vitamin C's ability to block the effects of histamines, chemicals in the body that at high levels cause cold symptoms.

It's also a good idea to take zinc every 2 to 3 hours at the start of the cold. A study of 48 men and women found that those who took 80 milligrams of zinc daily when cold symptoms first appeared were able to reduce the duration of the illness by about $3\frac{1}{2}$ days. They also had less severe symptoms.

The vitamin C in multi supplements can also be helpful if you're suffering from low energy. Studies have shown that 20 to 30 percent of American adults get less than the Recommended Daily Allowance of 75 milligrams of vitamin C. This can be a problem because one of the jobs of vitamin C is to move fatty acids into heart and skeletal muscles in order to provide energy.

Protect your heart. One in three women currently under age 40 will eventually develop heart disease. An effective way to protect the heart, apart from getting regular exercise, refraining from smoking, and avoiding saturated fats in the diet, is to get enough antioxidant nutrients in the diet.

We've already discussed how vitamin E prevents free radicals from damaging cholesterol and

WHAT TO DO IF YOU HAVE ONLY 5 MINUTES

Set aside a little time to decide what you can do to improve your health today, suggests Irwin H. Rosenberg, M.D., dean for nutrition sciences at Tufts University in Boston.

Think about the nutritious foods you'll eat at lunch or the exercise you'll get before the day is done, he says. Even if you achieve only part of what you planned, you'll still be on the road to better health.

making it more likely to stick to arteries. Unfortunately, most women don't get anywhere enough of this important vitamin.

The National Health and Nutrition Examination Survey III looked at the vitamin E blood levels of more than 16,000 adults. The researchers found that 27 percent of whites, 41 percent of African-Americans, and 28 percent of Mexican-Americans had blood levels of vitamin E that were low enough to increase the risk for cardiovascular disease.

Vitamin E is important even if you already have blood vessel disease. It relaxes blood vessels and helps prevent the formation of blood-blocking clots. Studies have shown that when people with heart disease take vitamin E supplements, their risk of dying from the disease declines by 40 to 60 percent.

Many doctors advise women to take 100 to 400 IU vitamin E daily. At the same time, it's helpful to take a multi that contains vitamin C. It "recharges" vitamin E in the body, which increases its effectiveness.

The nutrients in your multivitamin and mineral supplement can also protect the heart. For example, selenium, a mineral found in most multis, reduces the amount of cholesterol that's damaged by free radicals. Multis also contain folic acid, vitamin B_6, and vitamin B_{12}. These B vitamins lower blood levels of homocysteine. High homocysteine levels have been linked to heart disease.

In Your Forties

Keep your thyroid healthy. More than one out of five women between ages 40 and 60 don't get enough iodine in the diet. Low levels of iodine can result in goiter, a swelling of the thyroid gland at the front of the throat. Iodine deficiency can also cause a decrease in thyroxine, a thyroid hormone that regulates energy production.

Most of the salt in the United States is iodized (fortified with iodine), but women should also take a multi supplement that provides the Daily Value of 150 micrograms.

Fight cancer with supplements. Studies have clearly shown that women who get an abundance of fruits and vegetables have a lower risk of cancer. Some of the credit for this goes to folate, which is present in fruits, vegetables, and other

---

WHAT WORKS FOR ME

CHRISTINE K. CASSEL, M.D., *chairperson of the Henry L. Schwartz department of geriatrics and adult development at Mount Sinai School of Medicine in New York City, doesn't take a lot of supplements—but there are a few that she makes sure to get every day.*

I take a multivitamin, along with vitamins C and E for their antioxidant protection. I've started taking additional B vitamins, including folate, now that there's some evidence that folate may protect against heart disease by lowering homocysteine levels in the blood. I also take a calcium supplement as insurance against bone loss. ∎

plant foods. Studies suggest that women who don't get enough folate in the diet have a higher risk for developing cancers of the cervix, colon and rectum, lung, esophagus, brain, pancreas, and breast.

The body uses folate to synthesize DNA. If you don't get enough folate in your diet, the DNA becomes more vulnerable to damage, which increases cancer risk. Doctors advise women to get 400 micrograms of folic acid (the synthetic form of folate) daily. In addition, be sure your multi supplement contains vitamin B_{12}. This nutrient is necessary for folate to function in the body.

Another cancer-preventing nutrient is calcium. One study found that people who took 1,200 milligrams of calcium daily were less likely to develop recurring polyps, growths in the colon that often precede the development of cancer.

Vitamin D, too, may help. Scientists have noticed that deaths from colon cancer are more common in parts of the United States that have the lowest amounts of sunshine. Sunshine, you'll recall, triggers the production of vitamin D in the body. This is important because vitamin D has been shown to suppress tumor growth. One study found that women with lower-than-normal levels of vitamin D had an increased risk for colorectal adenoma, damaged areas in the colon that may occur 10 years or more before cancer actually develops.

Selenium, which is included in most multi supplements, is another nutrient that protects against cancer. One study found that people who took 200 micrograms of selenium daily were significantly less likely to die from cancer. The mineral also reduced the incidence of cancers of the lung, colon, and rectum.

Reduce joint pain. By the time women reach their forties, their joints start to rebel against a lifetime of flexing. Osteoarthritis, also known as "wear and tear" arthritis, occurs when tissues in the joints begin to break down over time. One way to prevent this is to take vitamin E, which inhibits the effects of inflammation-causing molecules in the joints. In fact, vitamin E has been shown to relieve arthritis pain better than ibuprofen or other over-the-counter anti-inflammatory drugs. The recommended dosage for easing arthritis is 400 IU vitamin E daily.

Another way to reduce joint damage from arthritis is to take a supplement that provides 400 IU, or 100 percent of the Daily Value for vitamin D.

Vitamin C and calcium also appear to protect the joints. In a study of almost 200 participants, those given a powder supplement that contained vitamin C and calcium reported less pain and stiffness and an improvement in joint function.

Sharpen your eyesight. Studies suggest that people who take supplemental vitamin C when they're young are less likely in their later years to develop cataracts, a common cause of vision loss.

Cataracts occur when proteins in the lenses of the eyes are oxidized, or damaged, by free radicals. When you take vitamin C, the nutrient saturates the tissues of the eye and prevents the oxidation. One study of more than 5,000 women found that those who took vitamin C for 10 years reduced their risk for cataracts by 45 percent.

So far, evidence suggests that taking 150 milligrams of vitamin C daily is enough to provide long-term protection against cataracts.

In Your Fifties

Protect against breast cancer. A woman's risk for breast cancer rises dramatically once she reaches her 50th birthday. It's hardly news that a high-fat diet increases the risk for breast cancer, probably because it increases levels of tumor-promoting lipids in the breast. Eating more fruits and vegetables and reducing fat in the diet are your first lines of defense, but it's also helpful to supplement your diet with calcium and vitamin D. Researchers aren't sure why, but these nutrients appear to inhibit breast changes that can lead to cancer.

If you drink alcohol, be sure to use a multi that contains folic acid. A study of more than 88,000 nurses found that those who had one alcoholic beverage (4 ounces of wine, 12 ounces of beer, or $1\frac{1}{2}$ ounces of liquor) a day had a 24 percent greater risk for breast cancer than those who drank less. Those who supplemented their diet with folic acid were able to cut their risk in half.

Doctors advise taking a multi supplement that contains 400 micrograms of folic acid, the synthetic form. The folate you get from foods such as legumes, fortified juice, spinach, and asparagus will easily take care of the rest.

Maximize your immunity. The immune system becomes less effective over time, which is why older women may be more susceptible to infections as well as cancer. Once again, vitamin E can make a difference. Studies have shown that when older adults take as little as 222 IU vitamin E daily, their immune systems become more active and are better able to fend off infections.

Strengthen your memory. Nearly everyone experiences declines in short-term memory in the latter half of life. Doctors theorize that this may be due in part to the harmful effects of free radicals in the brain. Taking 100 to 400 IU of a vitamin E supplement, which "neutralizes" free radicals, may be one of the best approaches to keeping your memory strong. In fact, a study of almost 5,000 people found that those who had high levels of vitamin E consistently performed better on memory tests than those with lower levels.

Vitamin B_{12}, too, plays a role in memory. It's not uncommon, in fact, for people to go to their doctors because they're experiencing memory loss or other mental declines, only to discover that they aren't getting enough vitamin B_{12} in their diet.

Deficiencies of vitamin B_{12} are common because as people age, their digestive tracts become less efficient at absorbing this nutrient. That's why doctors often advise adults ages 50 and over to take a multi supplement that provides 100 percent of the Daily Value of vitamin B_{12}, which is 6 micrograms.

Say goodbye to kidney stones. If you don't get enough vitamin B_6 in your diet, you may be putting yourself at risk for the agonizing pain of kidney stones. A study of more than 85,000 women found that those with the highest levels of vitamin B_6 in the blood were least likely to develop kidney stones. For protection against stones, doctors advise getting 40 milligrams of vitamin B_6 daily.

In Your Sixties and Beyond

Enhance your hearing and protect your mind. Are you always asking your friends to speak up? It's possible that getting too little vitamin B_{12} and folate is interfering with your hearing. About 24 percent of those ages 65 to 74 have some degree of hearing loss; that number rises to 40 percent after age 75. Your best protection may be to take supplements that contain the Daily Value, or 6 micrograms, of vitamin B_{12} and 400 micrograms of folic acid (the synthetic form of folate).

The same nutrients also appear to play a role in preventing Alzheimer's disease. In one study, researchers looked at 370 people 75 years and older and found that those with low levels of vitamin B_{12} or folate were twice as likely to get Alzheimer's disease as those who had normal levels.

Control aging with copper. Women need only 2 milligrams of copper daily. Unfortunately, most women get half that amount. Over time, low levels of copper can speed up an aging process called protein glycation, which breaks down tissues in the heart, blood vessels, and kidneys. When shopping for a multi supplement, choose one that provides copper sulfate, also called cupric sulfate. Many multis contain a related compound called cupric oxide, which can't be absorbed by the body.

Improve your mood. About 6 percent of Americans 65 years and older experience depression—and studies have shown that about 30 percent of those hospitalized for depression have low levels of vitamin B_{12}. In fact one study found that women over age 65 who were deficient in vitamin B_{12} were twice as likely to suffer from severe depression than those who got enough of this nutrient.

In addition, up to 79 percent of depressed adults are deficient in vitamin B_6. On average, women get only about half as much vitamin B_6 as they should. In addition, birth control pills and other supplemental hormones can interfere with the vitamin's action.

As long as you take a supplement that contains the Daily Value of 2 milligrams for vitamin B_6 and 6 micrograms for B_{12}, you'll have sufficient levels of these nutrients to help protect your long-term mental health.

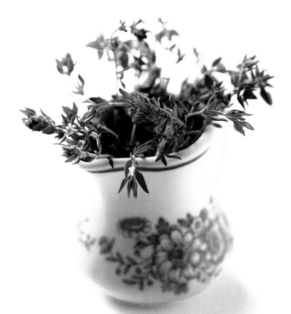

Using Herbs Wisely

From echinacea for colds to black cohosh for menopausal changes and ginkgo for memory problems, women often turn to herbal remedies to solve everyday health problems. And indeed, throughout this book, physicians who practice complementary or alternative medicine offer their female patients herbal solutions to everyday problems.

Women have used herbs as medicine for generations. Long before the development of prescription and over-the-counter drugs, herbs were commonly employed to fight infection, reduce pain, soothe anxiety, and relieve menopausal discomfort.

The ancients knew what they were doing. Scientists have learned that herbs contain dozens or even hundreds of chemically active compounds. In fact, the active ingredients in many of the drugs that you buy at pharmacies are very similar (or even identical) to the chemicals in herbs.

Unfortunately, shopping for medicinal herbs can be a challenge. Herb manufacturers in the United States are prohibited from making health claims on the labels; nor are they allowed to give advice on how to use herbs to treat medical problems. Without medical guidance, it can be difficult to know which herbs are most effective for treating different conditions, or how to use them to get the best results. And because the herb industry isn't strictly regulated, some unscrupulous manufacturers use ingredients that aren't effective or tout herbal combinations that don't work, says Douglas

Schar, Dip.Phyt., an herbalist in London and Washington, D.C.

Used as directed, the herbs suggested in this book can be very effective. When taken correctly, they're often less likely than drugs to cause side effects. They're often milder than drugs, yet still have beneficial effects. But because herbal medicines are sold over the counter, you become the doctor and pharmacist. It's important to have the same respect for herbs that you do for prescription drugs.

In the following pages, you'll find a comprehensive guide to dozens of important medicinal herbs used for women's wellness. The experts at *Prevention* magazine explain which herbs are best for different conditions, tell you how to take the herbs, and offer information on possible side effects or interactions. Schar provides dosage recommendations; the physician or experts that you consult for specific conditions may recommend slightly different amounts.

THREE THINGS I TELL EVERY FEMALE PATIENT

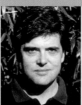

DOUGLAS SCHAR, DIP.PHYT., is an herbalist in London and Washington, D.C., who specializes in preventing disease with herbal medications. He offers this advice to women who use herbs.

1

DON'T ASK THE CLERKS IN HEALTH FOOD STORES FOR ADVICE. They're not medically trained, and they rarely have expertise in the actions (and interactions) of herbal medicines. Instead, consult a professional herbalist, or a physician who incorporates medicinal herbs in his or her practice.

2

READ LABELS CAREFULLY. The best products contain a single herb. Those that contain multiple herbs are less likely to be effective.

3

TRUST YOUR INSTINCTS. When manufacturers make claims that seem too good to be true, they probably are. Does the label "guarantee" you'll lose 20 pounds a month? Save your money. The manufacturer is more interested in marketing the product than in protecting your health. ∎

How Herbs Heal

We have dozens of healing herbs at our disposal, but their active ingredients can all be grouped in a few chemical families. These chemicals, which occur in herbs in varying proportions, are what give herbs their healing powers. They include:

Bitters. As the name suggests, these are bitter-tasting chemical compounds. They stimulate bile flow and digestive juices.

Flavonoids. They're among the most important antioxidants. They protect cells from oxidation, strengthen blood vessel walls, and reduce water retention, inflammation, and muscle spasms.

Volatile oils. They give herbs their unique scents, and they also have a mild antiseptic action. When inhaled, volatile oils relieve stress. They may also enhance appetite, stimulate circulation, and reduce water retention associated with the menstrual cycle.

Alkaloids. They've been shown to fight bacterial and fungal infections.

Gums and resins. They bind to lipids (fats) in the blood. Herbs that contain gums and resins are often used to lower cholesterol.

Mucilage. It's a slippery substance in herbs that helps relieve constipation. Mucilage also soothes irritated mucous membranes in the throat, intestine, and other parts of the body.

Saponins. These have antitussive (cough-relieving) properties. They also regulate women's hormones, reduce stress, and strengthen blood vessels.

Tannins. These promote skin healing. They also help speed the healing of mucous membranes (as with sore throats).

Anthraquinones. They're good for digestion because they stimulate bile production. They're also helpful for strengthening and restoring proper liver function.

Cautions and Caveats

Men and women alike often assume that because herbs are natural, they're inherently safer than synthetic drugs. Nothing could be further from the truth. The chemical compounds in herbs can have powerful effects in the body—including powerful side effects. For the most part, herbs are safe as well as effective, but only when you use them properly. Here's what doctors advise.

Avoid herbs during pregnancy. Very little research has looked at the effects of medicinal herbs taken during pregnancy, Schar says. Your doctor may recommend certain herbs if you're pregnant—but all of the information in the following pages is designed for women who aren't pregnant and aren't nursing.

Don't double dip. Some herbs have similar actions as prescription or over-the-counter drugs. If you elect to take herbs suggested for various ailments discussed in this book, don't combine them with medication. If you're taking a sedative medication such as diazepam (Valium), for example, it might be harmful to combine it with a sedative herb such as kava kava. The same is true of antidepressants: Prozac for example, shouldn't be combined with St. John's wort, an herb commonly taken for depression. We'll talk more about herb–drug interactions in the chart on page 58.

Stick to one herb. Just as it may be harmful to combine herbs and drugs that have similar actions, it can be risky to take two similar herbs.

Know which plant parts you need. The medicinal part of echinacea is the root, but that doesn't stop unscrupulous manufacturers from selling the leaves. In the chart below, we've included information on the parts of herbs that are most effective.

Avoid creative but misleading product names. Products with intentionally misspelled names, such as "Clenze," "Nutra-mune," or "Staminex," are marketing gimmicks; they're unlikely to be effective herbal medicines, Schar says. Also, avoid products that say "pro," "combo," "max," "turbo," or "plus" on the label. Instead, stick to the herbs recommended in this book.

Know when to quit. Herbs act more slowly than drugs, but you should still notice an improvement in your condition within a few weeks to a month. If an herb doesn't seem to be helping, stop taking it and get professional advice, Schar advises.

Your Personal Herb Guide

Allergies

Herb and Standard Doses	What It Does	General Cautions	Drug Interactions
NETTLE (*Urtica dioica*) Three times daily: 20 drops 1:1 tincture or 1 tsp 1:5 tincture. Use only the plant, not the root.	Relieves allergies, allergic skin rashes, hay fever, and seasonal rhinitis.	None.	None known.

Anxiety

Herb and Standard Doses	What It Does	General Cautions	Drug Interactions
AMERICAN GINSENG (*Panax quinquefolius*) Four 500-mg root tablets once daily (use the root only).	Reduces stress.	Don't take if you have high blood pressure. May cause irritability if taken with caffeine or other stimulants.	Insufficient data.
KAVA KAVA (*Piper methysticum*) Two 500-mg dried root bark tablets three times daily (use only the root bark).	Treats nervous anxiety, insomnia, and restlessness. Also calms anxiety due to fluctuating hormones of premenstrual syndrome and menopause.	Don't exceed 300 milligrams of kavalactones per day or take more than the recommended dose. Use caution when driving or operating equipment. Do not take if you have a history of liver disease. Discontinue use if you experience symptoms associated with jaundice, such as nausea, fever, or dark urine.	Do not take with alcohol, prescription, or over-the-counter drugs.

Anxiety *(continued)*

Herb and Standard Doses	What It Does	General Cautions	Drug Interactions
PASSIONFLOWER (*Passiflora incarnata*) Two 500-mg tablets before bed. Use only the flower, leaves, and vine.	Treats insomnia due to anxiety.	None.	Don't take with sedatives, sleeping pills, or anti-anxiety medication.
SKULLCAP (*Scutellaria laterifolia*) 3 cups of tea daily. Use only leaves and flowers.	Treats anxiety, restlessness, and nervousness. Also, reduces premenstrual symptoms and kidney problems.	None.	None known.
VALERIAN (*Valeriana officinalis*) Two 500-mg root tablets 30 minutes before bed. Use only valerian root.	Reduces nervousness and insomnia. Reduces digestive discomfort.	None.	Don't take with sleep-enhancing or mood-regulating medications.

Cancer Protection

Herb and Standard Doses	What It Does	General Cautions	Drug Interactions
GREEN AND BLACK TEAS (*Camellia sinensis*) 1 cup green or black tea three times daily.	Green and black tea act as antioxidants, reducing cell damage that may lead to cancer. Also reduce joint inflammation in those with arthritis.	The caffeine in green and black tea may result in anxiety or insomnia.	None known.
MAITAKE MUSHROOM (*Grifola frondosa*) For prevention, two 350-mg tablets, three times daily. For those with cancer, the recommended dose is six 350-mg tablets three times daily during alternating months. Use only dried maitake supplements.	Improves immune system's ability to recognize or destroy damaged cells. Stimulates production of white blood cells.	None.	None known.

continued

Cardiovascular Disease and High Blood Pressure

Herb and Standard Doses	What It Does	General Cautions	Drug Interactions
ELDERBERRY (*Sambucus nigra*) Three times daily: 1 tsp syrup or 1 tsp 1:5 tincture. Use only the ripe berry and flower.	Acts as a powerful antiviral agent that minimizes coughs, colds, and flu.	None.	None.
GARLIC (*Allium sativum*) One 500-mg tablet three times daily. Use supplements with standardized amounts of alliin or allicin. (Avoid garlic oil gel caps.)	Acts as an antioxidant. Lowers blood pressure, cholesterol, and the risk of cardiovascular disease.	A blood thinner, it should be discontinued 2 to 3 weeks prior to surgery, and for 2 weeks after surgery. Increases stomach acid production in some people.	Do not use if you're on blood-thinning medications.
GUGGUL (*Commiphora mukul*) 500 mg standardized guggul extract twice daily.	Reduces cholesterol levels and eases joint inflammation.	In rare cases, may cause diarrhea, restlessness, apprehension, or hiccups. Avoid this herb if you have hypothyroidism.	None known.
HAWTHORN (*Crataegus oxycantha, C. laevigata, C. monogyna*) Two or three times a day: 20 drops 1:1 tincture; or 1 tsp 1:5 tincture. Use only the berries, flowers, and leaves.	Reduces the risk of cardiovascular disease.	If you already have a cardiovascular condition, don't take without medical supervision. Use with caution if you have low blood pressure—it can lower the pressure even further.	May necessitate lower doses of blood pressure and other medications.

Constipation

Herb and Standard Doses	What It Does	General Cautions	Drug Interactions
FLAXSEED (*Linum usitatissimum*) 2 Tbsp ground flaxseed daily.	Contains soluble fiber to keep you regular.	Take with at least 8 oz water. Don't take flaxseed if you have a bowel obstruction or diverticular disease.	May interfere with the absorption of drugs.

Depression

Herb and Standard Doses	What It Does	General Cautions	Drug Interactions
ST. JOHN'S WORT (*Hypericum perforatum*) Two 500-mg tablets three times daily. Use only the leaves, stems, and flowers.	Improves mood and symptoms of depression. Eases muscle aches; prevents wound infection when applied topically.	May cause sensitivity to light. May cause gastrointestinal symptoms, allergic reactions, and fatigue.	Don't use with antidepressants like Prozac or Paxil, or other prescription medicines. May lower amount of some prescription drugs in your blood.

Endometriosis

Herb and Standard Doses	What It Does	General Cautions	Drug Interactions
EVENING PRIMROSE (*Oenothera biennis*) Two 500-mg tablets once daily. Use oil made from the seeds.	Reduces inflammation and eases pain from endometriosis.	None.	None known.

Fever

Herb and Standard Doses	What It Does	General Cautions	Drug Interactions
CINNAMON (*Cinnamomum zeylanicum*) Pour 1 cup boiling water over 1 tsp powdered; steep covered for 20 minutes. Use only the bark. Drink 3 cups daily.	Reduces inflammation and pain and fever.	None.	None.
GINGER (*Zingiber officinale*) Three times daily: two 500-mg tablets; or 1 tsp 1:5 tincture; or, for tea, grate 1 tsp ginger, cover with 1 cup boiling water, and steep for 10 minutes. (Fresh root is most effective.)	Reduces fever.	Avoid therapeutic amounts of ginger if you have gallstones.	None known.
WILLOW BARK (*Salix alba*) Steep 2 tsp dried bark in 1 cup boiling water for 20 minutes.	Reduces fever.	Can cause stomach irritation. Do not give to children under 16 who have fever or any viral infection, including chickenpox or flu. May contribute to Reye's syndrome, which affects the brain and liver.	Do not take if you need to avoid aspirin, especially if you are taking blood-thinning medication such as warfarin (Coumadin) because its active ingredient is related to aspirin. May interact with barbiturates or sedatives such as aprobarbital (Amytal) or alprazolam (Xanax).

continued

Headaches

Herb and Standard Doses	What It Does	General Cautions	Drug Interactions
FEVERFEW (*Tanacetum parthenium*) One 50-mg tablet every morning. Use only fresh or freeze-dried feverfew leaves. Or take 20 drops 1:5 tincture, or 10 drops 1:1 tincture.	Prevents migraine and cluster headaches.	Chewing fresh leaves can cause mouth sores in some people.	None known.
GINGER (*Zingiber officinale*) Three times daily: two 500-mg tablets; or 1 tsp 1:5 tincture; or, for tea, grate 1 tsp ginger, cover with 1 cup boiling water, and steep for 10 minutes. (Fresh root is most effective.)	Improves circulation and prevents migraines.	Avoid therapeutic amounts of ginger if you have gallstones.	None known.
ROSEMARY (*Rosmarinus officinalis*) Steep 1 tsp dried rosemary in 1 cup boiling water for 10 minutes (use only the leaves). Take 2 cups per day.	Dilates blood vessels and prevents stress-related headaches; acts as digestive aid; may protect against diabetes and artery disease.	None.	None known.

Hepatitis

Herb and Standard Doses	What It Does	General Cautions	Drug Interactions
MAITAKE MUSHROOM (*Grifola frondosa*) 4 to 6 g powder tablets.	Stimulates immune system and may reduce symptoms of hepatitis.	Safe.	None known.

Hives

Herb and Standard Doses	What It Does	General Cautions	Drug Interactions
NETTLE (*Urtica dioica*) One or two capsules freeze-dried nettle leaf extract every 2 to 4 hours until symptoms disappear.	Reduces hives.	None.	None known.

Inflammatory Bowel Disease

Herb and Standard Doses	What It Does	General Cautions	Drug Interactions
CHAMOMILE (*Matricaria recutita*) Pour 1 cup boiling water over 1 to 2 tsp dried herb, cover, and let steep for 10 to 15 minutes. Use only the flowers.	Relaxes muscles in the stomach. Eases indigestion, irritable bowel problems, and colitis.	Causes allergic reactions in rare cases. Those who are allergic to related plants, such as ragweed, asters, and chrysanthemums, should drink the tea with caution.	None known.
PEPPERMINT (*Mentha piperita*) Pour 1 cup boiling water over 1 to 2 tsp dried herb, cover, and let steep for 10 to 15 minutes. Use only the leaves.	Helps ease indigestion, gas, and nausea.	None.	None known.

Irritable Bowel Disease

Herb and Standard Doses	What It Does	General Cautions	Drug Interactions
CHAMOMILE (*Matricaria recutita*) Three times daily: 20 drops 1:1 tincture, or 1 tsp 1:5 tincture. Use only the flowers.	Eases irritable bowel problems and colitis.	Causes allergic reactions in rare cases. Those who are allergic to related plants, such as ragweed, asters, and chrysanthemums, should drink the tea with caution.	None known.
CRAMP BARK (*Viburnum opulus*) Three times daily: 1 g dried-bark capsules, or 20 drops 1:1 tincture, or 1 tsp 1:5 tincture.	Relaxes intestines.	Safe.	None.
PEPPERMINT (*Mentha piperita*) Enteric-coated peppermint oil capsules, 0.2–0.4 ml, twice daily between meals.	May lessen bloating and diarrhea.	None.	None known.

continued

Laryngitis

Herb and Standard Doses	What It Does	General Cautions	Drug Interactions
CINNAMON (*Cinnamomum zeylanicum*) To make tea, pour 1 cup boiling water over 1 tsp powdered; steep covered for 20 minutes. Drink 1 to 3 cups daily.	Reduces inflammation and pain.	None.	None.

Low Energy

Herb and Standard Doses	What It Does	General Cautions	Drug Interactions
ASIAN GINSENG (*Panax ginseng*) Four 500-mg tablets once daily (only tablets that contain the root).	Acts as a mild stimulant and mood enhancer. Also acts as an antioxidant.	Don't take if you have high blood pressure, with caffeine or other stimulants, or when under acute stress. May cause menstrual irregularities or intensify menopause symptoms. May cause headaches, nervousness, and insomnia in women under age 45.	Insufficient data.
SCHISANDRA (*Schisandra chinensis*) Two 500-mg tablets twice daily. Use only tablets that contain the fruit.	Supplies energy by increasing circulation and improving heart function. Protects the liver, improves respiration, speeds reflexes, and reduces symptoms of nervous exhaustion, such as headaches, insomnia, dizziness, and palpitation.	None.	None known.
SIBERIAN GINSENG (*Eleutherococcus senticosus*) Two 500-mg tablets three times daily. Use only the root bark.	Similar properties to Asian ginseng.	None. 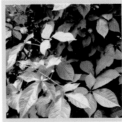	None known.

Low Sexual Desire

Herb and Standard Doses	What It Does	General Cautions	Drug Interactions
SAW PALMETTO (*Serenoa repens*) Two 500-mg berry tablets three times daily. (The berries are the most effective part.)	Increases sex drive in women. Also blocks the effects of androgens, male hormones that can cause excessive hair growth.	May cause stomach problems in rare cases.	None known.

Macular Degeneration

Herb and Standard Doses	What It Does	General Cautions	Drug Interactions
BILBERRY (*Vaccinium myrtillus*) Pour 1 cup hot water over 1 or 2 Tbsp dried whole berries (or 2 or 3 tsp crushed berries). Let tea steep, covered, for 10 minutes, then strain. Drink 1 cup daily. Commercial tea bags are also available.	Improves night vision.	None.	None.
GINKGO (*Ginkgo biloba*) 15 drops extract dropped into a sip of water, once or twice daily for 1 month. 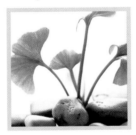	Improves circulation in the eyes.	In very rare cases ginkgo can cause headaches, digestive upset, and skin reactions. Thins blood, so don't take it 2 to 3 weeks before or after surgery. Can cause skin inflammation, diarrhea, and vomiting in doses larger than 240 mg.	Don't take with monoamine oxidase (MAO) inhibitors, such as phenelzine sulfate (Nardil) or tranylcypromine (Parnate); aspirin or other nonsteroidal anti-inflammatory drugs; or blood-thinning drugs, such as warfarin (Coumadin).

continued

Memory

Herb and Standard Doses	What It Does	General Cautions	Drug Interactions
GINKGO (*Ginkgo biloba*) One tablet standardized to 24 percent ginkgo flavone glycosides, three times daily.	Improves memory, concentration, and alertness.	In very rare cases ginkgo can cause headaches, digestive upset, and skin reactions. Thins blood, so don't take it 2 to 3 weeks before or after surgery. Can cause skin inflammation, diarrhea, and vomiting in doses larger than 240 mg.	Don't take with antidepressant monoamine oxidase (MAO) inhibitors, such as phenelzine sulfate (Nardil) or tranylcypromine (Parnate); aspirin or other nonsteroidal anti-inflammatory drugs; or blood-thinning drugs, such as warfarin (Coumadin).

Menstruation and Menopause Problems

Herb and Standard Doses	What It Does	General Cautions	Drug Interactions
ANGELICA (*Angelica sinensis*) Take three times daily: two 500-mg tablets or 20 drops 1:1 tincture or 1 tsp 1:5 tincture. The root is the most effective part.	Relieves hot flashes, increases sex drive, and improves skin. Also stimulates digestion and production and action of immune cells. Binds to free radicals, making them harmless.	Use for short periods of time. Don't take it if you have estrogen-dependent cancer or a bleeding disorder. Increases sun sensitivity.	Don't take if you're on blood-thinning medication or undergoing cancer treatment.
BLACK COHOSH (*Cimicifuga racemosa*) Three times daily: two 500-mg dried root tablets or 20 drops 1:1 tincture. The root is the most effective part.	Relieves menopausal symptoms, such as thin vaginal tissue, vaginal dryness, memory loss, depression, mood swings, and hot flashes.	Don't use longer than 6 months. Avoid this herb if you have estrogen-dependent cancer. May cause occasional gastric discomfort.	Don't use if you're on hormone replacement therapy.
EVENING PRIMROSE (*Oenothera biennis*) 1,000 mg daily. Use oil made from the seeds.	Reduces inflammation and eases pain triggered by surges in prostaglandins during the menstrual cycle.	None. 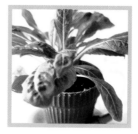	None known.

Menstruation and Menopause Problems *(continued)*

Herb and Standard Doses	What It Does	General Cautions	Drug Interactions
FLAXSEED (*Linum usitatissimum*) 1 Tbsp ground flaxseed daily.	Helps balance shifting hormones at peri-menopause. Contains omega-3 fatty acids, which lower the risk for heart disease. Contains soluble fiber to keep you regular. Also lowers cholesterol and fights breast cancer and depression.	Take with at least 8 oz of water. Don't take flaxseed if you have a bowel obstruction or diverticular disease.	May interfere with the absorption of drugs.
SAGE (*Salvia officinalis*) 4 heaping Tbsp dried leaves steeped 4 hours in 1 cup boiling water. The leaves are the most effective part.	Helps reduce and even eliminate night sweats. May slow progression of Alzheimer's disease; may reduce indigestion, and, when gargled, may soothe throat irritation. Acts as an antioxidant.	None.	Can increase sedative side effects of drugs.
VITEX (ALSO CALLED CHASTEBERRY) (*Vitex agnus-castus*) Twice daily: two 500-mg tablets or 60 drops 1:5 tincture or tablets containing 250 mg 4:1 extract. The seeds (also called the berries) are the most effective part.	Relieves premenstrual symptoms. Helps treat irregular, painful, and heavy periods.	See your gynecologist if you experience bleeding between periods.	May lower the effectiveness of birth control pills.

Pneumonia

Herb and Standard Doses	What It Does	General Cautions	Drug Interactions
THYME (*Thymus vulgaris*) Steep 2 tsp herb in 1 cup water for 10 minutes. (Use the leaves and flowers.) Drink three times daily.	Reduces bronchial spasms and eases coughs.	None.	None known.

continued

Skin Problems

Herb and Standard Doses	What It Does	General Cautions	Drug Interactions
ALOE (*Aloe barbadensis*) Apply three times daily to injured area. Buy pure (clear) aloe gel.	Heals sunburn and minor burns and wounds. Also treats chronic skin disorders such as psoriasis, eczema, and acne.	Don't use on surgical incisions; don't take internally.	None known.
GOTU KOLA (*Centella asiatica*) Apply externally as needed.	Aids wound healing. Eases pain of insect bites, poison ivy, and sunburn. Improves acne, acne rosacea, eczema, and psoriasis.	None.	None known.

Urinary Tract Problems

Herb and Standard Doses	What It Does	General Cautions	Drug Interactions
GOLDENROD (*Solidago virgaurea*) Steep 1 tsp dried herb in 1 cup boiling water; drink 1 cup daily. Use only the flowering tops.	Promotes healthy urinary function.	Don't use if you have a chronic kidney disorder.	None known.

5

The Ultimate Ladder of Fitness

Women weren't officially allowed to run marathons until 1970, largely because of the outdated (and unspoken) perception that we were the weaker sex. But in 1984 Joan Benoit changed that thinking forever. Benoit (now Samuelson) ran in the first women's Olympic marathon—and her time was faster than 11 of the 20 male winners who had run before her.

Is Joan unique? Of course. Elite athletes are in a class by themselves. But every woman, regardless of her current level of fitness, can be athletic—and then notch it up a few levels.

Like many women, perhaps you enjoy walking. You can easily increase the time you walk and the distance you go. Pretty soon, you might be ready to participate in a 5-K walk.

Do you lift weights? It just takes seconds to add more weight or to lift the weights more often. It doesn't matter what physical activities you engage in. Running, hiking, swimming, aerobics, weight lifting—they're all great workouts, and the more you do, the fitter you're going to be.

More is involved than just fitness. Studies have shown that regular exercise lowers anxiety, reduces the risk of heart disease, and even improves the frequency and quality of sex.

Exercise is more important today than it ever was. Researchers have found that the laborsaving inventions of the past 25 years—everything from computers to remote controls—have shaved an average of 800 calories of daily activity from our lives.

That's why *Prevention* magazine experts created the Ultimate Ladder of Fitness—a six-step plan for gaining mobility, burning calories, and trimming inches off your waistline. You'll also discover ways to make exercise a lot more fun, which is the real key to making it part of your life.

Exercise: You Can't Live without It

When it comes to your health, exercise isn't an option—it's a necessity.

We all know that being sedentary increases the risk of heart disease and of other serious health threats. Yet surveys have shown that more than 60 percent of Americans don't get regular physical activity—and women are more likely than men to skip the workouts.

What, exactly, can you gain from exercise? Here's a sampling.

- It reduces your risk of heart attack and stroke. Exercise lowers blood pressure, slows resting heart rate, lowers cholesterol, and burns abdominal fat.

- A number of studies have shown that exercise protects against colon cancer. It may lower the risk of breast and ovarian cancers as well.

- It helps the body secrete insulin, which can reduce the risk of diabetes.

- It boosts immunity and can prevent colds and other infectious diseases.

- It strengthens bones. Older women who are active suffer fewer bone fractures than women who don't exercise.

- It burns fat, builds muscle, and may lower levels of leptin, a hormone that seems to contribute to weight gain.

- It helps you live longer. A study of 14,000 women and men showed that moderate levels of physical fitness increased life span. In fact, walking as little as 2 miles daily could potentially add years to your life.

It's clear that exercise can improve the long-term quality (and quantity) of your life. But what will it do for you right now? Research has shown that women who exercise may have less menstrual discomfort. They're less anxious or de-

WHAT WORKS FOR ME

With work, family, and constant travel vying for their time, exercise experts are every bit as swamped as the rest of us, yet they still manage to work out most days of the week. Here are their secrets for practicing what they preach!

Use your weekends. "I confess, when I'm seeing patients from 7:00 A.M. to 7:00 P.M., I don't exercise. But on weekends (including most Fridays), it's priority number one. I take an hour these days just for me and have a quality run or workout. Then I find a smaller chunk of time 2 more days of the week. The trick is preparation: I always have my gym bag with me. So if I suddenly have 30 minutes free, I'm out the door for a walk or jog!" says Mary Jane Minkin, M.D., clinical professor of obstetrics and gynecology at Yale University School of Medicine and coauthor of *What Every Woman Needs to Know about Menopause*.

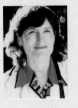

Have a plan B. "I start the day with an exercise plan. But as a doctor, my plans are routinely disrupted. So I have a plan B and plan C. For instance, I always carry exercise bands. If I can't make it to the gym, I can do resistance training at home, in my office, or in my hotel room. I also carry my sneakers. If I have lots of meetings, I take short walks in between to clear my head. Every 5 seconds counts!" says Pamela Peeke, M.D., assistant clinical professor of medicine at the University of Maryland School of Medicine in Baltimore and author of *Fight Fat after 40*.

Make it a family affair. "I have three school-age kids, so my life is out of control. I still exercise at least 4 days a week, but I don't lock myself into a routine. I take advantage of my children's desire to play outside. I run while they bike, I play tennis with my son, or we all play soccer. It's so much better than watching TV," says Miriam Nelson, Ph.D., associate chief in the physiology laboratory at Tufts University in Boston and author of *Strong Women, Strong Bones*.

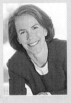

Focus on the benefits. "I practice what I preach: I exercise every day or almost every day. One way I keep myself on track is by focusing on the rewards of my efforts: That time spent exercising will help reduce my risk for heart disease, control my weight, and handle stress more effectively—and I can eat dessert now and then without worrying or feeling guilty!" says James Blumenthal, Ph.D., professor in the department of psychiatry at Duke University in Durham, North Carolina.

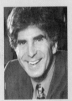

Give it top priority. "It would be easy to put off working out until the house is clean, more writing is done, or I've gone through the mail. But I still put on my shorts and get going. The endless household and work duties will always be there. And if my exercise actually helps me live longer—I'm gaining time," says Christiane Northrup, M.D., cofounder of the Women to Women Health-Care Center in Yarmouth, Maine, and author of *Women's Bodies, Women's Wisdom* and *The Wisdom of Menopause*. ■

pressed. They have less back pain and more self-confidence. They even sleep better.

Convinced? *So let's get started.*

Step 1:
Make the Change

If you haven't exercised regularly in the past, getting started can be a challenge. Your muscles won't be primed for action, and you won't have the force of habit to help you along. But once you get out the door and get moving, it won't be long before exercise feels natural and comfortable. In fact, you may find yourself craving it.

Before you do anything else, get a checkup and let your doctor know about your plans to start exercising. Women who have been sedentary can easily injure themselves if they start out too quickly, says Alan Mikesky, Ph.D., director of the Human Performance and Biomechanics Laboratory at Indiana University–Purdue University Indianapolis.

Look for exercise opportunities. Women often think that physical fitness requires running, biking, swimming, or other vigorous forms of exercise. But anything that gets your body moving counts. It could be walking the dog. Working in the garden. Raking leaves. Even cleaning house can give you a decent workout if you move quickly and your total daily exercise is at least 30 minutes.

"There are many ways to sneak in exercise," says Martha Coopersmith, owner of the Bodysmith Company in New York City. "We all have to go places, so park a couple of blocks away and

walk the rest. Take the stairs instead of the elevator. Or pace while you talk on the phone."

Make it more like play. The problem with formal exercise is that it can easily feel like one more responsibility in an already hectic day. But it shouldn't be like that. Exercise is any physical activity that you enjoy. Coopersmith suggests indulging in some of the activities that you enjoyed when you were young—but with a twist.

Used to climb trees? Try rock climbing—in the wild or on the "rock wall" at a local health club. Are you a dancer? Aerobics might be the ticket. For that matter, swing, salsa, or line dancing can give you quite a workout, Coopersmith says.

Set reasonable goals. One reason so many women start an exercise program and then give it up is that they don't feel they're making progress. Don't set impossible goals for yourself; keep things simple. Try to walk 10 more minutes than you usually do. Do one extra pushup. Lift the weights two more times. Studies have shown that people who believe they can achieve a goal—any goal—are much more likely to stick with the program.

Step 2: Learn to
Stretch Your Muscles

Stretching is an integral part of any fitness plan. It improves your range of motion, helps you stay flexible, improves coordination, and helps prevent muscle strains and other injuries. Start with the stretches that begin on the opposite page, recommended by Carol Espel, M.S., exercise physiologist and general manager at Equinox Fitness Club in Scarsdale, New York.

Learn to
Stretch
Your Muscles

Stretching is most effective when it's done before and after every workout. If that sounds like too much work, it's fine to do your stretches after exercising. Don't stretch when your muscles are cold; you're more likely to get injured. These stretches, recommended by Carol Espel, M.S., exercise physiologist and general manager at Equinox Fitness Club in Scarsdale, New York, hit every major muscle group in the body. For each one, hold the stretch for 10 to 30 seconds, breathing deeply all the time.

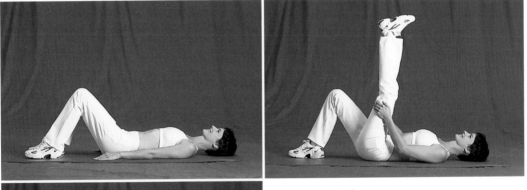

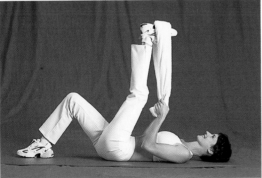

Hamstrings

Lie on your back with your legs bent and both feet on the floor (top left). Straighten and raise your left leg. Gently pull your thigh toward your body and hold (above). If you can't reach your leg, loop a towel under your foot and, with a slight bend at the knee, gently pull your leg toward your chest (bottom left). Repeat with the right leg.

continued

Learn to Stretch Your Muscles

continued

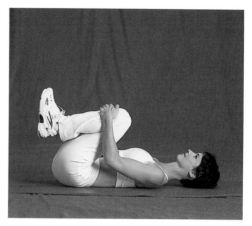

Lower Back

Lie on your back and pull both knees to your chest. Keep your upper body relaxed on the floor.

Calves

Stand facing a wall, with your right foot about 18 inches from wall, and your left foot about 2 feet behind it (below). Place your hands against the wall for support and lean forward while pressing your left heel to the floor. Switch legs.

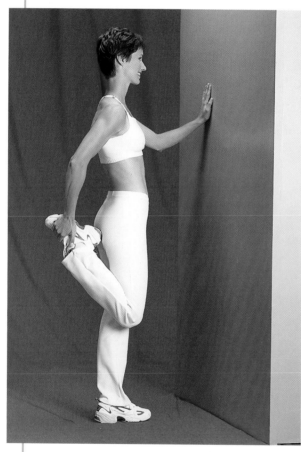

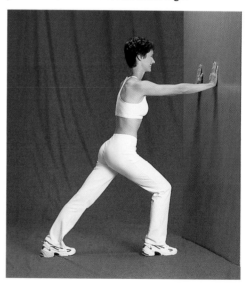

Quadriceps and Hip Flexors

Put your left hand on a wall (above). Bending your right knee, bring your right foot toward your buttocks; hold it in place with your right hand. Keep your knees together and do not arch your back. Repeat with the left leg, putting your right hand on a wall.

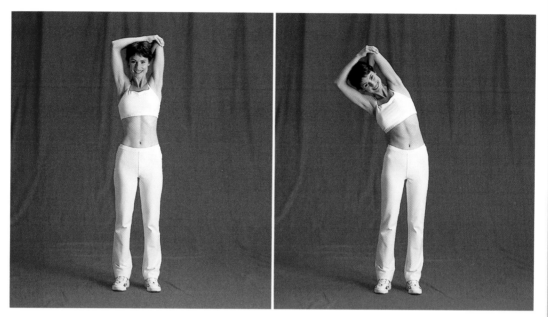

Triceps and Sides

Stand straight and raise your left arm over your head; bend the elbow, and drop the hand toward the middle of your back (left). With your right hand, gently pull your left elbow to the right. Tilt your body to the right (right) to stretch the muscles in your side. Keep your stomach tight. Repeat with your right arm.

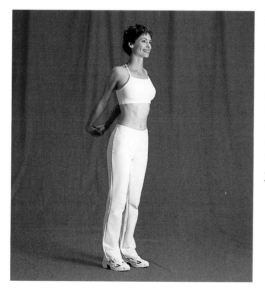

Chest

Stand with your feet shoulder-width apart and knees slightly bent. Clasp your hands behind your back with your palms facing in toward your body. Slowly push your chest forward, keeping your back and abdomen stable. (If this movement is uncomfortable, do the stretch without your hands touching.) You can lean forward slightly, but don't allow yourself to become pitched forward.

continued

Learn to Stretch Your Muscles

continued

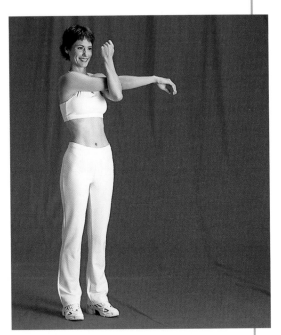

Upper Back and Shoulders

Cross your right arm in front of your chest (right). With the opposite arm, gently pull your right arm toward your body, and hold. Repeat with left arm.

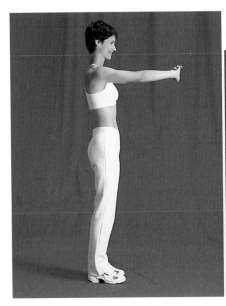

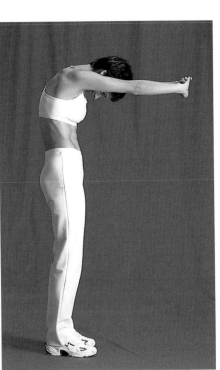

Upper Back

Clasp your hands in front of you with your palms facing away (above). Round your back, drop chin to chest, relax your shoulders, and press your hands forward (right).

Step 3: Work In Regular Aerobic Exercise Four or Five Times a Week

Nearly every health club offers an astonishing variety of aerobic dance classes, and women often confuse "aerobics" with "aerobic dance." They're not the same thing.

Dancing is one form of aerobic exercise, but it's not the only one. Aerobic exercise simply means that you're moving fast enough to increase your heart and respiratory rates. When you exercise aerobically, the heart pumps more blood, and the lungs fill the blood with more oxygen. Aerobic exercise makes the heart work harder, which makes it stronger: It pumps more blood with each beat, which means that it beats less often. In other words, aerobic exercise lowers your resting heart rate. Aerobic exercise can also result in drops in blood pressure because the blood moves more easily through arteries and veins.

You don't have to be an exercise fanatic to get impressive gains from aerobic exercise. *Prevention* magazine recommends that you accumulate 30 minutes of moderate activity most days to stay healthy and fit.

One more point about aerobic exercise: Don't waste time doing something you don't enjoy very much. For years, women felt that they had to run in order to be aerobically fit. But a lot of them hated running, and naturally they didn't do it for very long. You have to do something that you like doing, says Dr. Mikesky. It could be tennis. Bicycling. Climbing the stairclimber. Or even country dancing.

Step 4: Add Strength Training

The next time you go to the health club, take a look at the folks lifting weights. Chances are, most of them are men. That's unfortunate because weight lifting, also called strength training, is among the best workouts for women.

For starters, strength training makes the bones stronger, which is critically important for women. After a woman reaches menopause, she can lose up to 20 percent of her bone strength. Strength training literally adds mass to the bones, which makes them stronger and helps prevent fractures.

Strength training is also among the best ways to keep your figure trim. Muscle tissue is much more active metabolically than fat. When you lift weights and build muscle, you'll automatically burn more calories, even when you aren't exercising.

After age 40, women can lose half a pound of muscle and gain a pound of fat every year. By the time a woman reaches her 65th birthday, she could have lost half of her muscle tissue—and her slower metabolism means she burns 200 to 300 fewer calories daily than when she was younger.

Strength training boosts the metabolism and reverses muscle loss. In fact, women who lift weights or do other forms of strength training twice a week for a few months can replace between 5 and 10 years of "lost" muscle tissue. To make things easy, we've created a customized strength-training plan (see next page) for women.

Strength
Training

Plan on repeating each of the following exercises 8 to 12 times. For those that involve weights, choose weights that are heavy enough so that you can barely complete the set of 12.   To get the most benefits from each exercise, do two or three sets of 12, resting for a few minutes in between. Repeat the exercises two or three times a week, but not on consecutive days, Martha Coopersmith, owner of the Bodysmith Company in New York City, advises. Remember to do your stretches when you're done.

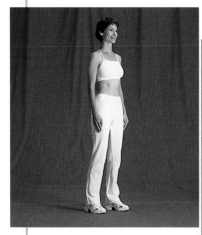

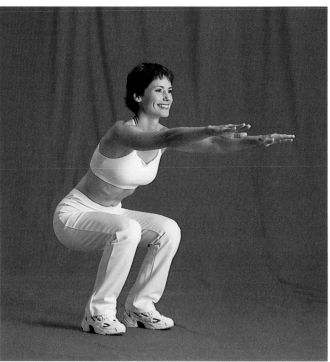

Squat

Stand with your feet shoulder-width apart (above). Bend your knees and squat as though you're sitting; hold your arms in front for balance (right). Make sure that your knees don't extend beyond your toes. Then return to the starting position.

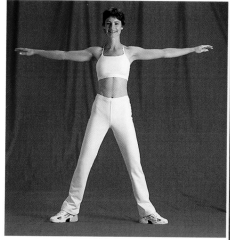

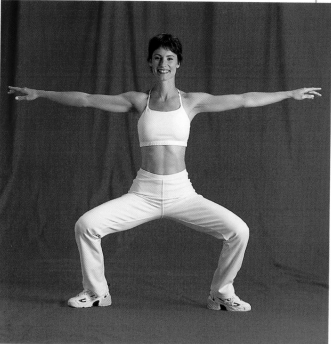

Plié

Stand with your feet about 2 feet apart; your legs should be turned out (above). With your back straight, lower your body (right). Then, as you straighten your legs, squeeze your inner thighs. Your knees should be in line with your ankles. Return to the starting position.

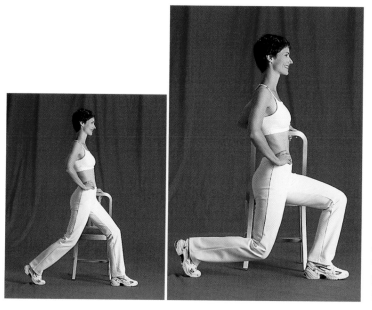

Lunge

Lightly place your left hand on the back of a chair for balance. Step forward with your left foot (far left). Your knee should be above your left foot, not sticking out past your toes. Lower your body by bending your knees and dropping your hips straight toward the floor (near left). Return to the starting position, then repeat with the other leg.

continued

Strength
Training
continued

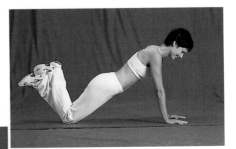

Pushup

Start on hands and knees, hands in line with shoulders. Your hips should be extended so that your body forms a straight line from head to knees. Cross your ankles in the air (left). Push yourself up (above), then return to the starting position. Repeat.

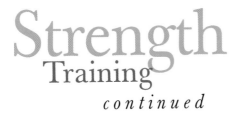

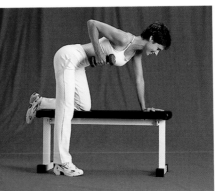

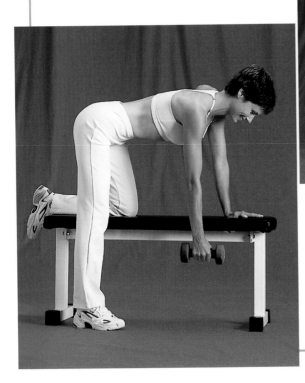

One-Arm Row

Put your left knee and left hand on a bench or a chair, keeping your back flat. Hold a weight in your right hand with your right arm straight and the weight hanging toward the floor, parallel to the bench (left). Raise the weight, keeping it close to your body, until it's even with your waist; your elbow should be pointed toward the ceiling (above).

Military Press

While sitting, hold a weight in each hand. Start with the weights at shoulder height; your palms should be facing forward (near right). Raise the weights above your head without bringing them together or locking your elbows (far right), then bring them back down to your shoulders.

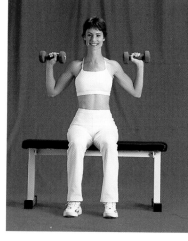
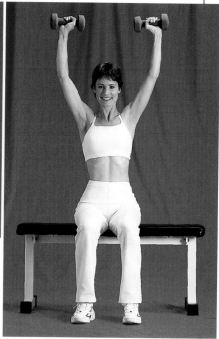

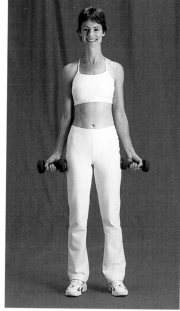
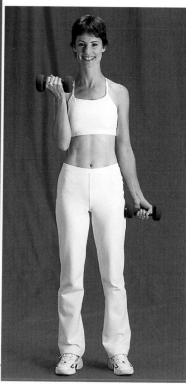

Biceps Curl

Stand straight and hold a weight in each hand, palms facing forward (far left). Keeping your elbow close to your body, bend your right arm and lift the weight toward your shoulder (near left). Return to the starting position, then repeat with the other arm.

continued

Strength
Training
continued

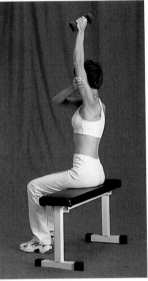

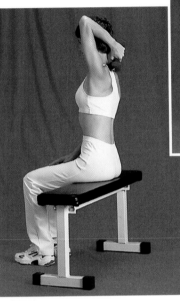

Triceps Extension

Sit on a bench or a chair while holding a weight in your left hand with your palm facing in. Bend your arm and raise it over your shoulder; your elbow will be pointing toward the ceiling, and the weight will be behind your head (near right). Hold your left elbow steady with your right hand, and raise the weight until your arm is straight (far right); return to the starting position.

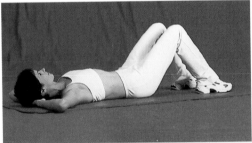

Abdominal

Lie on a mat with your knees bent, your feet flat on the floor and hip-width apart, your hands behind your head, elbows out to the sides (left). Contract your abdominal muscles and raise your shoulder blades off the ground about 30 degrees (below). Return to the starting position.

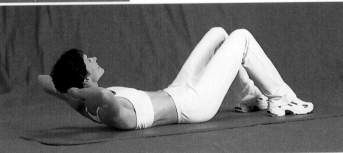

Step 5: Increase the Intensity

When you've being doing the same exercises for a while, you'll find that they get easier. This is because your body has adapted to the workload and is no longer feeling the strain. This is satisfying, in a way, because it means that you've made progress. But it also means that you won't progress further until you push your body a little harder.

To keep your workouts at maximum pitch, increase the intensity. In other words, lift more weight, run faster, and generally exercise harder two or three times a week. The boost in intensity can have substantial health and fitness benefits. One study found that people who regularly pushed their workouts to the limit had higher levels of high-density lipoprotein (HDL, the "good" cholesterol) than those who exercised at lower intensities.

There are a number of ways to boost the intensity of your workouts. They include:

Exercise longer. Suppose you're currently exercising for 30 minutes. To increase the intensity, kick it up to 35 minutes. Keep it at that level for a few weeks, then add another 5 minutes—and then another. Exercising hard for 45 minutes will quickly add up to impressive fitness gains.

Try interval training. Instead of going all-out all the time—or, conversely, coasting along at a comfortable pace—shake things up with interval training. For example, exercise at a moderate pace for 4 minutes, then switch to high intensity for 4 minutes. Interval training will keep your body challenged without exhausting your muscles and lungs, says Wayne Westcott, Ph.D., fitness research director at the South Shore YMCA in Quincy, Massachusetts, and author of 15 books on strength training.

Add new exercises to your workout. Remember the strain you felt when you first started exercising? It's good to repeat the experience periodically because it puts a beneficial load on your whole body. As you challenge different muscles, your heart and lungs will work harder, and that's the cornerstone of boosting overall fitness.

Exercise to music. Sure, it's a good way to make the time go quickly, but music—as long as it has a fast tempo—also promotes impressive fitness gains. In one study, 24 men and women cycled to music. The intensity of their cycling increased when they listened to music with a fast beat. The study's authors think that with the increase in the music's tempo, the participants were distracted from a preoccupation with how tired they felt.

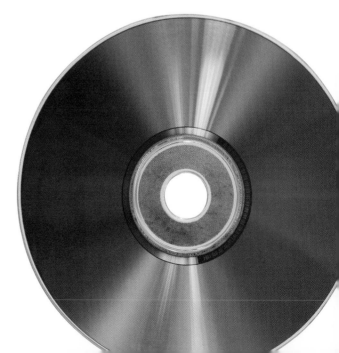

Prevention's
STEP UP
TO FITNESS

If you haven't been active in the past but are getting ready to start, you may be wondering what types of activities you'll enjoy most—and what the fitness benefits will be.

Prevention magazine's Ladder of Fitness makes it easy. You'll find dozens of exercises—from "formal" workouts to recreational activities and hobbies—along with the number of calories that they burn (based on a 140-pound woman who exercises for 15 minutes). You're sure to find some that will satisfy your interests as well as your fitness goals.

The activities at the bottom of the ladder are low intensity. As you go up the rungs, the exercises become more intense.

140
CALORIES

Mountain biking, hiking a moderate-to-difficult grade, snowshoeing in soft snow, running a 10-minute mile, running up stairs, karate or tae kwon do, kickboxing, jumping rope, swimming vigorously, using a stairclimber or a ski machine

120 to 139
CALORIES

Running a 12-minute mile, singles tennis, volleyball on the beach, downhill skiing, rock climbing, swimming laps, water jogging, having a snowball fight

95 to 119
CALORIES

Backpacking, doubles tennis, racewalking, briskly walking uphill, jazz and modern dance, basketball, racquetball, soccer, high-impact aerobics, using a stationary rower, bicycling at a moderate pace, ice-skating, sledding, shoveling snow

70 to 94
CALORIES

Golf (carrying your clubs), downhill skiing on beginners' slopes, gardening, calisthenics, step aerobics, walking at a brisk pace, dancing (country, polka, or disco), playing tag, washing the car, using a snowblower, kayaking, mowing the lawn with a push mower

40 to 69
CALORIES

Lawn and lane bowling, badminton, croquet, dancing (cha-cha or swing), tai chi, golf (using a cart), mowing the lawn on a riding mower, raking leaves, playing catch or Frisbee, walking the dog

Step 6: Keep Yourself Motivated

We've talked about how hard it can be to launch into an exercise program when you haven't been active lately. What's even harder is sticking with it: Researchers have found that many people who take up strength or aerobic training will slack off or stop altogether within a few months.

Men and women alike offer all sorts of reasons for giving up their workouts. Not enough time. Too much work. Family responsibilities. They're all valid reasons, but what about those women with fast-paced careers, growing families, and a lot of outside interests who still find time to exercise?

What it usually boils down to is this: Women quit exercising because they aren't sufficiently motivated, says Dr. Westcott. It's a common problem, which is why creating motivation is an essential part of any training plan. Here are some things you may want to try.

Test yourself often. Dr. Westcott often advises women to keep exercise logs, in which they record how long they exercised, the distance covered, the amount of weight lifted. With every workout, you should try to push yourself just a little bit harder. Setting goals and then reaching them is among the strongest motivators, Dr. Westcott explains.

Show your competitive side. Some women do their best work—and their best workouts—when they're in competition with someone else. You may want to ask a like-minded friend to exercise with you—and keep a friendly competition going to see who improves the most in a certain period of time.

reality *check*

Her Goals Kept Her Motivated

As a lawyer in New York City, Claudia Cohen, 35, knows what it means to be really busy. She spends long days at the office, and for a long time, the idea of getting in a quick workout during the day—or even after work—seemed out of the question.

Her feelings changed, however, when she decided it was finally time to put herself first and lose some weight. So she started exercising—and she did it with a vengeance.

Cohen exercises 5 days a week, for at least an hour each time. Sometimes she rides an exercise bike or uses the treadmill at her health club. Other days, she works out with weights at home with a personal trainer.

Boredom hasn't been a factor, Cohen says, partly because she's always setting goals for herself. When she's doing pushups, for example, she mentally challenges herself to do just one more. Striving for and achieving small goals keeps her focused and motivated, she explains.

Of course, she also wears a smaller dress size than she used to, and few things are more motivating than that. ■

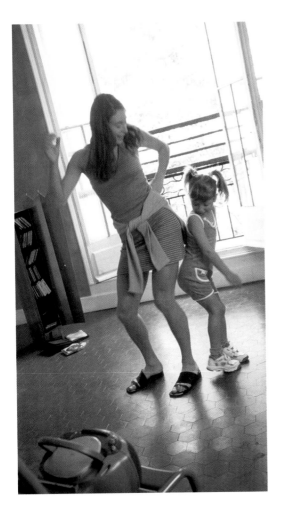

WHAT TO DO IF YOU HAVE ONLY **5 MINUTES**

You don't have to do "formal" exercise to get a great workout: All you have to do is move, says Martha Coopersmith, a certified personal trainer and owner of the Bodysmith Company in New York City.

"Jump rope, walk up stairs, dance, or play tag with the kids," she says. "Just keeping moving—while you wait for a pot of water to boil, for example, or when you're waiting for the laundry to dry."

Push past the doldrums. We all have times when the idea of lifting weights or even going for a walk just seems like too much work. Unfortunately, if you skip one workout, coming back to the routine will be that much harder.

When you find your motivation flagging, mentally force yourself to be active, even if it's only to take a quick walk. Once you get off the couch and start moving, you'll find that you enjoy the way you feel—and you'll probably keep going.

6

Prevention's Guide to Your Perfect Weight

A hundred years ago, only about 10 percent of adults were overweight. Today an estimated 61 percent of Americans are overweight.

Yet we have the same genes as our ancestors. What's changed isn't our genes but our lifestyle.

It took Great-Grandmother hours to make dinner from scratch. She scrubbed clothes clean with her own hands. And without a car, she walked everywhere.

Today we take a whirl through the drive-thru to feed the family. We load the washing machine to clean clothes. And a short car ride takes us to work, the store, or a friend's house.

In the 19th century, machines did 70 percent of the work on farms and factories. Men and women did the rest. Now machines do 99 percent of the work, and many of us earn a living sitting at a desk or computer. Cars have taken the place of walking or cycling. We burn rubber instead of calories. And computers, cell phones, and fax machines only make our society more fast-paced and stressful, which can send added pounds straight to our middles.

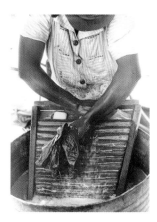

Superimpose stress and inactivity on a world where it's practically impossible not to come face-to-face daily with food that makes us fat, and it's easy to see why so many more women (and men) have a weight problem today than did our ancestors.

That said, a few people genuinely have a genetic disposition toward overweight. Children of obese parents have an 80 percent chance of being obese themselves, while children of normal-weight parents have less than a 10 percent chance. Even adopted children tend to follow their biological parents' weight patterns.

The culprits: metabolism and the hormone leptin.

Some people simply have lower metabolisms than others. That means their bodies burn off fewer calories in the course of eating, breathing, sleeping, and performing other life functions. Metabolic rates seem to vary somewhat from family to family, or ethnic group to ethnic group. A National Institutes of Health study found that African-American women, for example, have lower resting metabolic rates than white women. And when scientists gave sets of twins an extra 1,000 calories a day, some sets of twins gained 30 pounds—while others gained only 10.

We all know women who can eat whatever they want and stay thin, while others seem to gain weight just looking at food. Experts believe that overweight people may be insensitive to leptin, a hormone that turns off appetite once you've had enough to eat. The more fat on the body, the more leptin is produced to keep us from overeating and to increase the amount of energy we expend. Scientists have found that obese people have high levels of the hormone leptin, which suggests that heavy individuals don't respond to leptin. Some compare this to insensitivity to insulin among people with type 2 diabetes.

Does this mean you were born to be fat?

"No, there is no 'fat gene,'" says John P. Foreyt, Ph.D., director of the Behavioral Medicine Research Center at Baylor College of Medicine in Houston and coauthor of *Living without Dieting*. You may have been predisposed to gain weight in a culture of high-fat foods and sedentary jobs. And overweight may run in your family. But ultimately, your behavior determines the number on the scale.

"The only way to gain weight is to eat more than you burn," Dr. Foreyt says. Even if you have a tougher time dropping pounds, that doesn't mean you're doomed to be overweight.

Your Healthy Weight

Reaching or maintaining a healthy weight pays off in many ways. It lowers your risk for heart disease by lowering your blood pressure, cholesterol levels, and triglyceride levels. In fact, weight loss works better than drugs at lowering blood pressure in women with and without hypertension. Losing weight also helps you become more sensitive to insulin, which will help you avoid type 2 diabetes. These effects are especially beneficial to women after menopause, when they're more vulnerable to heart disease.

Because obesity contributes to five of the leading causes of death in the United States—heart disease, stroke, high blood pressure, cancer, and diabetes—losing weight can even help us live longer.

Regardless of the major health benefits, slimming down also improves quality of life. Think about it: Losing extra pounds will help you:

Overweight? Get Your Thyroid Checked

about 11 million people in the United States have hypothyroidism, an underactive thyroid. More than half of all women experienced three or more symptoms of hypothyroidism in the past year. If you're one of them, it could be why you're overweight.

The butterfly-shaped thyroid gland wraps around the front of the windpipe just below the Adam's apple and produces a hormone that regulates metabolism and organ function. It influences every organ, tissue, and cell in the body.

When the thyroid doesn't produce enough of the hormone—often because the immune system creates antibodies that damage or destroy it—you could experience:

- A weight gain of 10 pounds or less of fluid
- Fatigue
- Mood swings
- Dry, coarse skin or hair
- Hoarseness
- Forgetfulness
- Difficulty swallowing
- Intolerance to cold

Women are at higher risk than men for an underactive thyroid. But just being overweight and feeling tired doesn't mean you have thyroid dysfunction.

"I think a lot of us hope that when we gain weight, it's because of our thyroid," says Gay Canaris, M.D., assistant professor of internal medicine at the University of Nebraska College of Medicine in Omaha.

So how do you know if you should get tested? Talk to your doctor about your symptoms. Fatigue could be caused by other disorders, such as anemia, cancer, depression, or sleep disorders. It could also result from too much work.

Even if you don't have symptoms, though, get screened at age 20 and every 5 years thereafter. There are no general screening guidelines for the public, and many doctors recommend screening at age 40 or 50, but since so many women could have dysfunction without knowing it and the test is so inexpensive, it can't hurt to get screened. ■

- Breathe more easily

- Sit more comfortably in movie theaters and airplane seats

- Get into and out of your car with ease

- Wear belted skirts and slacks

- Tie your shoes effortlessly

- Wear a swimsuit and enjoy going to the beach without feeling self-conscious

- Give you the confidence to try new things, like rock climbing

- Live to see your great-grandchildren and great-great-grandchildren

- Improve your sex life and overall energy level

As you slim down, you'll probably discover other, personal benefits of your own.

Here's everything you need to know to lose weight and keep it off, once and for all.

Step 1: Calculate Your Body Mass Index

Successful weight loss begins with setting the right goals.

"So many of the women I work with feel defeated if they don't meet the goal they set for themselves, even if they're within 5 pounds of their ideal weight," says Stephen P. Gullo, Ph.D., president of the Institute for Health and Weight Sciences in New York City and author of *Thin Tastes Better.* "Some only get so far, then throw in the towel."

Others hope to reach whatever weight they were in high school or on their wedding day. But that might not be realistic. A better strategy is to set a goal based on your body mass index (BMI), a ratio of weight to height.

Along with waist circumference (discussed in Step 2), body mass index is a more accurate indication of total body fat than body weight alone.

To calculate your BMI:

1. Multiply your weight in pounds by 703.

2. Divide that number by your height in inches.

3. Divide that number again by your height in inches, and you'll have your BMI.

A BMI of between 18.5 and 25 is considered healthiest. You're considered overweight if your BMI is 25 or over, and you're considered obese if it's 30 or over.

"When someone has a BMI of 25, their risk for disease goes up because their blood pressure, cholesterol, blood sugar, and risk for diabetes may all go up," Dr. Foreyt says. "We've also found that at a BMI of 30, three-fourths of all people have at least one risk factor for heart disease, such as type 2 diabetes or hypertension."

But don't let your BMI go below 18.5—that's too low because it's unhealthy to be that skinny.

Step 2: Measure Your Waistline

Because abdominal fat is associated with a greater health risk than fat carried in the hips, backside, or thighs, your waistline is also a better gauge of your weight than total number of pounds. It's also a good way to double-check your weight if your BMI, measured in Step 1, isn't considered high, but it's obvious that you're heavier than you should be.

There's a right and a wrong way to measure your waist. Hold a measuring tape horizontally around the abdomen at navel level, parallel to the floor. The tape should be snug, but not pulled tight. Breathe out, and note your waist measurement.

For women, a waist circumference of 35 inches or higher is unhealthy.

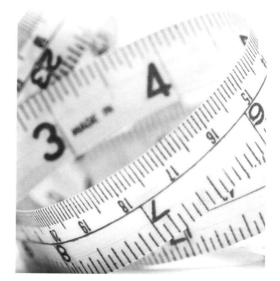

WHAT WORKS FOR ME

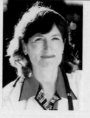

MARY JANE MINKIN, M.D., *clinical professor of obstetrics and gynecology at Yale University School of Medicine, shares her secrets of weight control.*

I love to eat! I've never been skinny, and I've always gained weight easily. I was the first kid on my block whose mother served skim milk; I was drinking a quart of milk a day! Now I eat a sensible, low-fat diet that includes lots of fruits, veggies, and whole grains, and I still love my milk.

My fanaticism about exercise is what saves my life—and my waistline! Three or four times a week, I run 5 miles or do the equivalent on the stairclimbing or rowing machine, or I bike for an hour. This helps me indulge my passion for food but still be able to wear a size 12.

As a child, I was never encouraged by my parents to exercise. It wasn't until I got to medical school that I adopted the exercise habit to relieve stress and get more energy. When I gained 30 pounds during my residency—who had time to work out?—exercise finally helped me to lose it. Now I shoot hoops regularly and play soccer with my kids. I'd like to add strength training to my routine next.

Getting up earlier to exercise in the morning works for me. You don't have to go to a gym, either. I tell women that taking the stairs rather than the elevator and walking short distances frequently during the day all adds up. ∎

Step 3: Set a Starting Date

Once you know where you really stand, weight-wise, your next step is to set your goals and commit yourself to them. If you don't set a starting date, you could fall into the "tomorrow syndrome," Dr. Gullo says.

Make sure you're ready. Before you "X" your calendar, make sure this is really the right time to start a weight-loss program. You might want to wait if other responsibilities consume your life right now, such as a new job or a family illness.

Avoid holidays. You've probably heard that most people gain 5 pounds from November to January. With so many holiday dinners and parties, trying to lose weight during this time is a lofty goal. Instead, try to maintain your weight, and plan to start losing after the holidays.

Mark your calendar. Once you've established the best time to begin, make an appointment with yourself. Use the time from now until your start date to fill your kitchen with healthy foods, find a walking partner, and prepare for an exercise

WHAT TO DO IF YOU COULD CHANGE **ONLY ONE THING**

To jump-start your weight-loss program, eat more fruits and vegetables, says Kristine Clark, R.D., Ph.D., nutrition consultant to the United States women's soccer team. Besides all the nutrients that produce contains, it also plays a role in weight loss. Fruits and vegetables fill you up for a small number of calories.

routine. "There's a reason races have a starting point," Dr. Gullo says. The more you prepare for your goal, the better you'll perform.

Step 4: Determine Your Real Calorie Needs

Eating too much food makes you overweight, but eating too little lowers your metabolism because your body instinctively interprets a dearth of calories as a famine and shifts into low gear to conserve calories. The solution: Balance what you eat with your activity. Here's a point system that makes it easy.

Consider your activity level.

- If your job or lifestyle involves a lot of sitting and you exercise rarely, give yourself 12 points.

- If you get more daily activity than light walking and you exercise aerobically for 45 to 60 minutes three times a week, give yourself 15 points.

- If you get more daily activity than light walking and you get 45 to 60 minutes of aerobic activity at least five times a week, give yourself 18 points.

Multiply your points by your goal weight in pounds to get your daily calories. For example, if you're a 140-pound active woman and you want to lose 10 pounds, multiply 15 by 130 and get 1,950 calories.

To lose fat instead of muscle, you need to eat at least 1,200 calories a day. Problem is, the typical American woman eats an average of 3,800 calories a day—many more calories than she needs. If you eat just 500 extra calories a day— the equivalent of a Snickers bar and a medium Coke—you'll be getting 3,500 *more* calories a week than you need. That adds up to a new pound of fat on the scales.

Step 5: Keep a Food Diary for a Week

People tend to underestimate what they eat by 20 to 50 percent. To take stock of what you're really eating, write down your foods and portions every day for a week. Then review what you've eaten.

Your diary will help you see your eating patterns for workdays and weekends (and holidays) and pinpoint when you tend to overeat. Once you know when those periods of overeating are, you can either make sure you have a healthy snack ready or schedule an activity to keep yourself away from the fridge.

Count what you drink. "A lot of people don't realize how many calories they take in from beverages," says Ellen Albertson, R.D., cohost, with husband Michael Albertson, of *The Cooking Couple* show in Boston. When people drank an extra 450 calories a day in one study (two gin and tonics or a cup of eggnog), they gained weight. But when they ate those extra calories in food, they ate less later in the day and lost weight. Don't sip your weight-loss goals away. Here's how to make your drinks work for you.

Drink water. There's no better thirst quencher. Water has zero calories, it fills you up, and it keeps your metabolism running more efficiently.

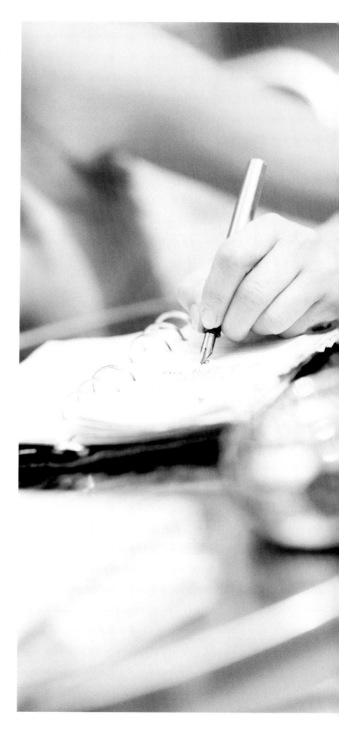

Watch the alcohol. When you choose wine over water, you don't only get extra calories in the drink. In fact, one study found that people ate 200 more calories in food at dinner; when compared with people who drank water, those who drank alcohol ate faster, took longer to feel full, and continued eating after being full.

Even if you don't drink with food, look at how alcohol can stack up the calories.

- 5 ounces of wine: 106 calories

- 12-ounce wine cooler: 220 calories

- 1½-ounce cocktail: 100 to 250 calories

- 3 ounces of sherry or port: 123 calories

- 12 ounces of regular beer: 150 calories

- 12 ounces of light beer: 99 calories

Step 6: Eat More Plant Foods, Fewer Animal Foods

You don't have to count calories if you don't want to. One study found that people who ate a variety of meals based on the dietary guidelines of the USDA lost three times more weight over a year than people on a specific low-fat diet. That's as simple as getting 6 to 11 servings of grains, 2 to 4 servings of fruit, 3 to 5 servings of vegetables, 2 or 3 servings of meat, 2 or 3 servings of dairy products, and a small amount of fat a day. In general, following the food guide pyramid will give you about 2,200 calories a day.

Eat more, weigh less. Four ounces of fried chicken has 250 calories, but the same amount of lean fish, such as sole, has about 100. That's be-

THREE THINGS I TELL EVERY FEMALE PATIENT

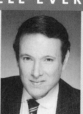

STEPHEN P. GULLO, PH.D., president of the Institute for Health and Weight Sciences in New York City and author of *Thin Tastes Better*, offers this advice to people he counsels about weight loss.

1 KNOW YOUR BEHAVIORS, NOT JUST YOUR CALORIES. If you find that you're constantly regaining weight you've lost by abusing the same types of foods, either stop buying them or find replacements for them, such as a frozen chocolate sorbet instead of a big bag of M&Ms.

REMEMBER THAT WEIGHT LOSS IS ABOUT LIBERATION, NOT DEPRIVATION. It's about a

2 change in perspective. Eat fewer calories and cut down the amount of fat you eat in the spirit of liberating yourself from the discomfort of the pounds that you've been carrying, instead of depriving yourself from certain foods.

DON'T FORGET THAT BEING THIN IS A LIFE MANAGEMENT SKILL. It's normal to experience setbacks and periods of feeling defeated. But in the future, when you turn 40 or 50 or 60 at a healthy weight, it won't be by accident, because aging well is not an accident. It's the gift that those who care deeply give to themselves. It will be because you planned and honed your skills at weight management. **3**

cause less-energy-dense foods like sole are typically low in fat, and high in water and fiber, and carry fewer calories per mouthful so they make satisfying meals.

Foods with low energy density include fruits, vegetables, broth-based soups, potatoes, fish, oatmeal, whole wheat pasta, air-popped popcorn, and bran cereal. Eating them instead of high-energy-density foods like cheesecake could help you eat 20 percent fewer calories.

So push heaps of high-energy meat to the side, and make fruits and vegetables the main attraction. Instead of a sandwich with four slices of meat, crackers, and cookies for lunch, eat just two slices of meat and add sliced tomato, cucumber, and fresh spinach. Follow it with a piece of fresh fruit and a cookie. Instead of ordering veal parmigiana at an Italian restaurant, order a large bowl of minestrone soup, a salad, and half of a portion of pasta with marinara sauce.

In fact, one study found that one particular food—broth-based soup—made women feel so full that they ate 100 fewer calories at a buffet than women who had had an appetizer of chicken rice casserole. If you follow the same logic and start eating broth-based soup before your meals, you could drop 10 pounds in a year.

Eating more fiber, too, could help you lose weight. Your body will quickly absorb the calories from a breakfast made of white flour and sugar, and you'll feel hungry again soon after your meal. But the calories in a bowl of bran cereal with no added sugar are absorbed slower and will keep you full longer. The same is true for fiber in other foods.

"Drink eight glasses of water daily. None of your body parts, from your **brain to your toes**, work well without adequate **hydration."**

—JANE BRODY, HEALTH COLUMNIST FOR *THE NEW YORK TIMES*

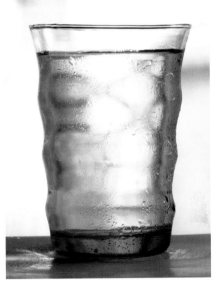

Fiber also helps move other food out of the body before the body has a chance to absorb them. For every gram of fiber you eat, you'll absorb about 4 fewer calories than if you ate simple carbohydrates.

Triple your fiber intake. Most people eat 13 grams of fiber a day. But if you eat about three times that amount—40 grams—you could block the absorption of 160 calories a day.

"Switch to **whole grain** carbohydrates such as **whole wheat bread** and **brown rice.** High intakes of refined carbohydrates and sugar are the main sources of calories in the U.S. diet, and thus a major contribution to being overweight."

—WALTER WILLETT, M.D., CHAIRMAN OF THE NUTRITION DEPARTMENT AT HARVARD SCHOOL OF PUBLIC HEALTH

Start hearty. One study found that people who had eaten high-fiber oatmeal for breakfast ate 30 percent fewer calories at lunch than people who had eaten cornflakes.

Grab beans. Beans are a sure way to get fat-fighting fiber, so add them to salads, soups, chili, and other dishes. Chili has nearly 10 grams of fiber per serving, three-bean salad with balsamic vinegar has 12.5 grams, and red beans and brown rice has a whopping 18 grams.

Eat whole grains. Whole grains, such as brown rice, whole wheat or whole grain bread, whole wheat flour, whole grain and multigrain cereals, oatmeal, oat bran, whole wheat pasta and couscous, and whole wheat, whole grain, and rye crackers not only have fiber but also have more micronutrients, like folate, magnesium, and vitamin E, than their white-flour counterparts.

Aim for nine. Fruits and vegetables are naturally high in fiber, low in fat and calories, and full of healthy nutrients and antioxidant vitamins—like A, C, and E—which are important in preventing heart disease and cancer. You've probably heard advice to eat five a day, but because so many studies link diets high in fruits and vegetables with less cancer, heart disease, diabetes, and osteoporosis, *Prevention* magazine advises nine servings a day. And since they have all the compo-

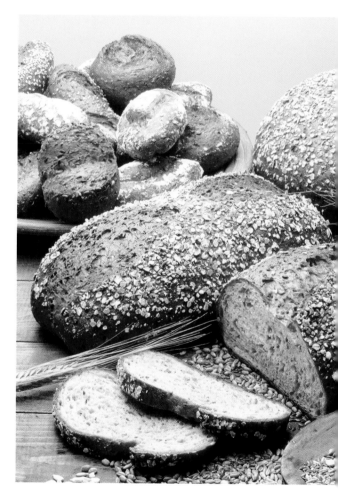

nents to help you lose weight, eating nine a day should be part of your weight-loss program, too.

Step 7: Scale Back Your Fat Intake

Fatty foods are more packed with calories than are low-fat foods. One gram of fat has 9 calories and a gram of carbohydrates has only 4 calories. So with fewer bites of a high-fat food, you'll get a lot more calories.

Fat may also affect the appetites of overweight people. In one study, overweight men who had had a high-fat meal before eating at a buffet ate 56 percent more than lean men who had eaten the same high-fat meal. But when the overweight men had eaten a low-fat meal, they ate the same

> 66 Eliminate all foods containing partially **hydrogenated** oils. There's growing evidence that these **unnatural fats** are not good for us, and avoiding them and the **processed foods** that they come in would be a huge step to improving nutritional health. 99
>
> —ANDREW WEIL, M.D., DIRECTOR OF THE PROGRAM IN INTEGRATIVE MEDICINE AND CLINICAL PROFESSOR OF MEDICINE AT THE UNIVERSITY OF ARIZONA COLLEGE OF MEDICINE IN TUCSON AND AUTHOR OF *EIGHT WEEKS TO OPTIMUM HEALTH*

amount at the buffet as the lean men, who'd also eaten a low-fat meal. It appears that the appetite switch of overweight people is turned off slower from fat because it takes longer for their bodies to detect that fat has been ingested.

To lose weight, try to get 25 percent of your calories from fat. Here are some satisfying ways to do it.

Choose lean meat. Choose meat that's naturally low in fat, such as turkey breast or skinless chicken. And when you're buying any type of meat, make sure it has no more than 10 grams of fat per 3-ounce serving.

Look for low-fat cheese. Another great way to lower your fat consumption is to choose low-fat and fat-free cheeses and yogurt. They carry all the calcium and nutrients of the full-fat varieties.

Bake instead of fry. If you have a recipe that calls for frying—such as potato wedges for french fries—try this instead: coat the potato wedges with nonstick spray and bake in the oven at 450°F to 475°F until they're brown and crisp.

Downsize dessert. Sweet, satisfying desserts don't have to include astronomical grams of fat. Here are some tips on making them healthier.

- Use mini chocolate chips in dough and batters. They'll spread out more, allowing you to use fewer.

- Use at least half of the baking chocolate squares your brownie recipe calls for, and replace the rest with cocoa powder, which is much lower in fat.

- Use phyllo dough instead of puff pastry or strudel dough—it's fat-free. Use nonstick spray, instead of butter, to moisten the sheets.

Step 8: Bone Up on Portion Size

You could count a heaping bowl of spaghetti as one portion, but your body knows how many calories you're eating. Get to know portion sizes, and you'll always have a mental picture of how much you should eat.

- ½ cup of fresh or cooked vegetables, or about a rounded handful

- 1 cup of raw or leafy vegetables, or the size of a baseball

- 1 medium piece of fresh fruit, also the size of a baseball

- ½ cup cooked or canned fruit, about a rounded handful

- 1 slice of bread

- 1 ounce of ready-to-eat cereal could be anywhere from ½ cup to 1¼ cup, so check the nutrition label

- ½ cup cooked cereal, about a rounded handful

- ½ cup cooked rice or pasta, about a rounded handful

- 3 ounces of cooked fish or meat (4 ounces raw), the size of a deck of cards

- ½ cup cooked dried beans, about a rounded handful

- ⅓ cup nuts, about a level handful

- 1½ ounces of cheese (or 2 ounces processed); 1 ounce is the size of four dice

You can also follow the serving size listed on the nutrition label of your food. It should be equivalent to the USDA's standard serving size.

Another tip: Measure out your servings a few times and make a mental note of how much it covers the plate or bowl.

Step 9: Eat All Day

If you plan to skip breakfast to save on calories, your scheme will backfire. One study found that the metabolisms of people who skipped breakfast were about 5 percent lower than those of people who ate three or more meals a day. A 5 percent boost in metabolism could help you lose 10 pounds in a year.

It's also important to keep it up throughout the day. Eating more often—without increasing the amount of food you eat—will keep you full. In two studies, men who had eaten breakfast in small portions throughout the morning had a 27 percent smaller lunch than men who had eaten breakfast as a single meal.

Another good reason to avoid long stretches without food: After 4 hours, blood sugar drops, and you'll crave sweets, instead of healthier foods.

Try these healthy snacks for fewer than 175 calories each.

- Half of a whole grain bagel with jam or low-fat cream cheese

- A handful of baby carrots with a dip of ¼ cup salsa and ¼ cup low-fat sour cream

- A cup of instant bean soup

- ½ cup whole grain cereal

Step 10: Sweat a Little

More than one-third of people who are overweight say they get no physical activity. But working out for 30 to 40 minutes could help you burn between 250 and 500 calories an exercise session. You could also burn as many as 50 or 100 calories more for the rest of the day after exercising.

Working out routinely can change your body's composition. Exercise helps you lose more fat, gain more muscle, and regain less weight. Women who exercise also tend to follow their eating plans more closely than women who don't exercise.

And if you're one of those people with a lagging metabolism, exercise is a great way to speed it up. For more information about establishing a regular exercise program, see chapter 5.

Work it in. So you say you don't have time to exercise. Sandra Adamson Fryhofer, M.D., clinical associate professor of medicine at Emory University in Atlanta and past president of the American College of Physicians in Atlanta, hears that all the time from her patients, but she doesn't accept the excuse. "There's always something you can do," she says. If you watch the morning news before work, do it while you're walking on the treadmill. "Every little bit of exercise helps."

If you take just 15 minutes to walk the dog in the morning, 10 minutes to walk to the deli for lunch, 5 minutes in the afternoon to stretch at your desk, 15 minutes to weed the garden when you get home from work, and 15 minutes after dinner to play tag with the kids, your activity adds up to 1 hour—and 300 extra calories burned that day.

Fidget. For some people, feeling antsy in their chair keeps them thin. Scientists gave 16 normal-weight people 1,000 extra calories a day for 8 weeks, but the amount of weight they gained varied between 3 and 16 pounds. The ones who lost the most weight burned up to 692 calories a

Watch the Sweets, Sugar

eating reasonable amounts of sweets is one thing, but making sugar the main attraction of your eating plan won't help you lose weight.

Sugar may not have fat, but it sure has a lot of calories, and we're not skimping on it. On average, sugar makes up about one-third of women's diets—that's 62 pounds a year and 151,840 calories. But it's more than extra calories that squelch weight-loss efforts: Sugar also makes you hungrier. It's digested faster and its calories are stored quickly, so you'll get hungry again sooner than if you had a high-protein snack.

To get down to the 7 teaspoons of sugar you should be eating a day (rather than the 19 women typically get), try to eliminate or lower your consumption of the five biggest offenders: nondiet soda, baked goods, ice cream, sweetened fruit drinks, and candy. If you have the willpower to cut them out completely, you could save 78,000 calories a year—and lose more than 20 pounds. ■

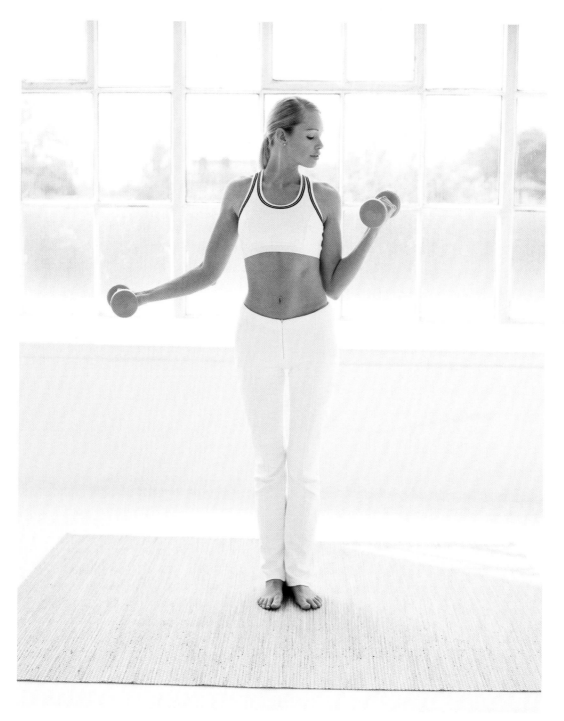

day doing everyday activities, such as walking, climbing stairs, household chores, sitting up straight, standing up straight—and fidgeting. Can you train yourself to be a more active person naturally? "Sure, if you make a conscious attempt at it," Dr. Fryhofer says.

Try adding these habits to your life:

- Stand up to answer to the phone.

- Do a household chore during commercials on television.

- Tap your feet against the floor or rotate your ankles when you're sitting.

- Dance to music as you do the dishes, iron, or fold clothes.

Turn off cravings. While you work out, your body suppresses digestion and releases glucose and fatty acids into the blood for energy. You won't feel the urge to eat until you reach a state of rest and your energy fuels are back in storage. The next time you find yourself hungry out of boredom, get up and take a walk, work in the garden, or do housework. You'll curb your craving and burn some extra calories.

Turn off the TV. If you gave up one television show a day and took a 2-mile walk for 30 minutes instead, you'd burn enough calories to lose 18 pounds in a year.

Don't stop. Once you start an exercise program, you'll probably like it so much you won't want to stop—and that's good news when it comes to weight loss. Research shows that people who manage to maintain weight loss exercise the equivalent of walking 3 to 4 miles a day.

WHAT TO DO IF YOU HAVE ONLY **5 MINUTES**

You can still get in a workout for 5 minutes a day—and see health results. Follow this plan by Glenn A. Gaesser, Ph.D., professor of exercise physiology at the University of Virginia in Charlottesville and author of *The Spark*.

Spend 5 minutes a day doing an exercise, but vary what you do from day to day. One day, walk, go up stairs, or do some other aerobic exercise for 5 minutes. The next, strength train for 5 minutes, with or without weights. And the next, stretch for 5 minutes. (For examples of exercises, see chapter 5.)

If you continue on this exercise schedule—or, better yet, do a little more—you'll probably lose weight, improve your health, and start enjoying exercise.

That was the result of Dr. Gaesser's study of 40 people, mostly women, who didn't like to exercise. They did 15 sessions a week for 10 minutes at a time at least every other day while eating a sensible diet. In 3 weeks they lost 3 pounds, improved their strength and endurance, increased their flexibility, improved their cholesterol levels, and admitted that they actually liked exercising.

You can start out with 5 minutes a day, Dr. Gaesser says. If you find more time for these exercises, you'll benefit even more.

Other Helpful Strategies

If you're doing everything "right" and still not losing weight—or losing it more slowly than suits you—these additional strategies can help get you unstuck.

OUTSMART RESTAURANT FARE

The average American eats four meals a week away from home. Even when you choose the healthy options at family-style restaurants, that's a weekly total of about 3,000 calories and 73 grams of fat.

Calories in restaurant meals stack up quickly because restaurants typically serve more than three times the amount of one serving of food. The Olive Garden serves 25 ounces of pasta with meat sauce, when you really should be eating 8 ounces—and 493 calories less. And Outback Steakhouse serves a 14-ounce steak, more than four times the correct serving of 3 ounces—and 953 more calories.

Restaurants have even increased the size of their standard plate from 10½ to 12 inches to accommodate the excess food, says Melanie Polk, R.D., director of nutrition education at the American Institute for Cancer Research in Washington, D.C.

But you don't have to become a recluse to eat healthy. You can ask for your food at restaurants to be specially cooked with no or less oil, request a nutrition guide from the restaurant ahead of time, or choose healthy foods at a buffet or party.

Wrap it up. According to a survey by the American Institute for Cancer Research, 26 percent of people dining out say they eat everything that's put in front of them. Good reason to have

> "Watch your **portion sizes**. Most of us eat far more food than we really need, and there are many reasons to eat less, including **slowing** the **aging** process."
>
> —KATHLEEN JOHNSON, R.D., DIRECTOR OF THE NUTRITION PROGRAM AT CANYON RANCH HEALTH RESORT IN TUCSON

your waiter wrap up half of your meal before it even makes it to your table.

Share with friends. Since restaurant meals are usually two or three servings anyway, ask your dinner partner if she wants to share an entrée with you.

Get what you want. Don't even open your menu at a restaurant. Instead, think about what you want to eat, such as whole wheat toast and scrambled eggs, and ask the waiter for it. But don't stop there—tell the waiter you don't want sausages or hash browns, or else he might bring it.

Think small. Polk uses an old standby when she's at a buffet. She takes small portions of her favorite foods and refuses to go up for seconds. She takes her time and eats it slowly so she's not left watching everyone else eat when she's finished.

***Really* party.** You don't have to stuff yourself to have fun. Instead of celebrating a birthday or holiday at a restaurant, stay home and shift the emphasis from food to fun, with charades, board games, or music and dancing.

LEARN TO TAKE YOUR TIME

Give yourself plenty of time to eat, rearranging your schedule if you have to. After looking at high-tech images of the brains of 21 adults while they ate, researchers found that their appetite switch turned off 10 minutes after they started their meal. The more time you take to eat, the fewer calories you'll inhale in the first 5 minutes of dinner, so try to spend 20 minutes at the dinner table.

Getting pleasure from your food can actually help you lose weight, says Albertson.

"I find that people gain weight when they're not focusing on their food—when they're at their desks, in their car, or in front of the television," she says. But a great way to lose weight is to make a fantastic dinner and sit down and truly enjoy it. Once you get pleasure from your food this way, you probably won't need so much to feel satisfied.

CHIP AWAY AT STRESS

When you're under stress, your body releases a hormone called cortisol, which sends fat to your abdomen, where it can increase risk for heart disease. It also suppresses growth hormone and testosterone, which protect you against heart disease and gaining abdominal fat. These effects are even more dangerous after menopause, when women's estrogen levels drop.

reality *check* Joining a Church Sent Her Weight Plummeting

When Marilyn Rozsnaki, a 36-year-old homemaker in Sagamore Hills, Ohio, set out to lose 20 pounds, she didn't know going to church would help.

At 5 feet 2 inches and 150 pounds, Marilyn first changed her diet. She started eating less meat and fat, and more vegetables.

In 3 weeks she lost 6 pounds—and then hit a plateau. So she started a walking program—but she wanted to get more active in other ways, too.

Before she started eating better and exercising, lack of energy and insecurity from being overweight kept her from getting more involved with her church. But once the scale slipped down, she had more confidence and energy to spend more time at church. It worked. The time she spent in Bible studies class, at service, and helping out families in need was time she was away from her kitchen—and snacks. She also prayed for the strength to eat well and exercise consistently.

"I knew I couldn't do it alone, so I asked for help," she says.

The spirituality of worship—along with keeping busy—keeps her from worrying about problems that could send her to the cookie jar.

She even found an exercise partner at church. A neighbor who attends her church became interested in Marilyn's weight loss, and now they walk up to 3 miles four or five times a week.

Marilyn's new lifestyle sent her weight plummeting. In 5 months, she had surpassed her 20-pound goal and was 25 pounds thinner.

"Now my 10-year-old son says I look like an 18-year-old chick," she says. ∎

"**Control** your **calorie intake,** get no more than **20 percent** of your calories from fat, and be sure to get **five to nine** servings of fruits and vegetables daily."

—MOSHE SHIKE, M.D., DIRECTOR OF THE CANCER PREVENTION AND WELLNESS PROGRAM AT MEMORIAL SLOAN-KETTERING CANCER CENTER IN NEW YORK CITY

You may find that you eat more when you're under stress. That's because food helps some people to relax. Stress activates your sympathetic nervous system and makes you feel on edge. Eating may activate natural painkillers in your brain, helping you to feel relaxed.

Anxiety can affect your behavior in other ways, too. Stress from financial problems, relationship issues, or just being overworked is often followed by a period of depression. And whenever you're depressed, you're probably going to eat more and be less motivated to exercise, says Dr. Fryhofer. You're also more likely to grab comfort foods, which are usually higher in fat.

A study of 1,300 people found that those who were cynical and had high levels of anxiety had the most abdominal fat. Depression also ranked high among women with the most abdominal fat.

Keeping stress under control should be part of your weight-loss strategy. Here are some ideas on how to do it. (For more on stress, see chapter 7.)

Accept imperfection. The house can't be completely clean, you'll miss a deadline once in a while, and your kids probably won't get straight A's. Trying not to control every aspect of life may help you lose extra flab.

Take care of you. If you make sure you are well-rested, get enough exercise, and eat well, you'll feel better and hold on to positive emotions.

Turn on the radio. Listen to some soothing music, and you may ease your anxiety and even your blood pressure and heart rate under very stressful situations.

Shake, shake, shake. If you get up and dance, you'll burn calories and release endorphins in your brain, which will elevate your mood and erase stress.

Tell a joke. Humor helps ease anxiety. One study found that people who performed a stressful task after watching an episode of *Seinfeld* had lower blood pressure and heart rates than people who hadn't watched the television show.

GET SUPPORT

Pay attention to the small gains you make along the way and congratulate yourself for them. Even if you don't lose weight as fast as you wanted, remind yourself that you can bound up the stairs and not lose your breath or that you cook meals that make you feel good and keep your body healthy. Even if it's 5 pounds, celebrate every step you take to better health.

Lose together. A friend may be the perfect motivator to get out of the house for a brisk walk or to inspire you to eat low-fat meals at restaurants.

Go online. Inspiration may lie on the other side of a Web site link. Some research shows that weight-loss Web sites can help women lose weight. Check out a few chat rooms, calorie counters, and exercise logs to see if this type of support is for you. Look for sites that include food diaries, personal feedback, weekly lessons, and emotional support.

Trade chores. If cleaning the kitchen puts you too close to the cookie jar to avoid temptation, head outside and rake leaves, shovel snow, or garden. Ask your spouse to pick up the indoor chores.

Work together. If you want to join a support group like TOPS (Take Off Pounds Sensibly) or

Forget Fad Diets

the best advice you'll ever get when it comes to dieting: "Quit!"

Whether you're pigging out on pork rinds or living on 800 calories a day, diets that don't include a variety of healthy foods or that severely restrict calories aren't good for long-term weight loss *or* your health. Some fad diets are actually more damaging to your health than obesity.

It's hard to keep up a diet low in calories, for obvious reasons: it's uncomfortable to be hungry. Think of starving as holding your breath underwater—you can do it for only so long before you gulp for air.

"Starving has nothing to do with losing weight," says Stephen P. Gullo, Ph.D., president of the Institute for Health and Weight Sciences in New York City and author of *Thin Tastes Better*. "Hunger pangs are a sign that you're doing something wrong. Succeeding at weight loss doesn't mean you have to give up fine taste in food. It means you have to be a selective gourmet."

When you lose weight from starving, your metabolism may decrease as a result. This means that even though you're eating fewer calories, you're also burning off fewer calories. It also

means that instead of losing weight, you lose muscle. When you go back to eating foods higher in fat or calories, you're more likely to gain fat instead of muscle. With this new efficiency, you may regain weight quicker, and it may take longer to lose weight in the future. Yo-yo dieting also may put your health at risk if you already have health problems. A diet of only 800 calories a day could result in lower immunity, an irregular heartbeat, irregular menstruation, a lower sex drive, lower metabolism, loss of lean body tissue, headaches, fatigue, dry skin, and sleeplessness.

But even when a diet allows you to eat plenty of just a few types of food, your health will suffer. Anytime you eliminate food groups, you lose out on the nutrients they provide, such as the calcium in dairy foods, fiber and vitamin E in grains, carotenoids and phytochemicals in vegetables. And some diets require you to eat foods high in saturated fat, which isn't good for your heart.

Your best bet is to stick to eating plans that include reasonable amounts of a variety of foods and don't allow you to lose more than 2 pounds a week. A satisfying meal of hearty portions of vegetables has fewer calories than some meals recommended by fad diets. ∎

Weight Watchers and your spouse could use a lesson on nutrition, join together and get extra support.

Hide temptation. Don't keep temptation right on the counter. If you're likely to overeat certain snacks, ask a family member to hide them on a high shelf, in the back of the cupboard, in a closet, or somewhere else you won't find them easily.

Lose a Little Weight—At First

If your BMI is 25 or higher, start out by aiming to lose between 5 and 10 percent of your body weight, says Dr. Foreyt. For example, if you're 5 feet 4 inches and weigh 180 pounds, your BMI is 31. To get it down to 25, you'd need to lose 35 pounds. At first, concentrate on losing the first 10 or 15 pounds. Moderate weight loss will give you lower blood pressure, lower lipids, lower blood sugar, and more self-esteem—and it's an easier goal than trying to lose 35 pounds (or more) at once.

Pace yourself. People who lose 5 to 10 pounds in a week lose water, not fat, so try to lose a pound or two a week. Depending on how much you have to lose, it could take as long as 6 months to lose 10 percent of your body weight in a healthy way, but that means you're more likely to maintain your new weight.

Look for other evidence. It may take awhile to see results on the scale, but you'll feel your body getting stronger and healthier immediately after you start to eat well and exercise.

If you lose weight but your body mass index doesn't budge, measure your waist again. Your abdominal fat may disappear—a benefit—even if your total weight or BMI doesn't budge. It will also help keep you motivated when your weight seems to be stuck in the same 5- to 10-pound range despite your efforts to reduce.

Work on maintenance. Once you lose your initial goal of 10 percent, maintaining it for 6 months will continue to improve your health and make it easier to avoid weight regain.

Do it again. If you have more to lose after your first 10 percent, continue to set the same goals until you've reached a healthy BMI.

A Real-Life Guide to Stress Relief

American women have more to do than ever before. At work, we skip lunch and put in overtime. At home, we're in charge of most of the housework and child care. And who takes care of parents and in-laws when they get sick? We do it all.

The result? Women are often overwhelmed and feel out of control. The unrelenting stress disrupts our peace of mind and also damages our health, says Margaret A. Caudill, M.D., Ph.D., professor of stress and pain management at Dartmouth Community College in Manchester, New Hampshire.

Up to 40 percent of American workers—and more women than men—say that they experience high levels of stress on the job. And stress follows women home. Research has found that even American women who are highly satisfied with their jobs have significantly elevated levels of stress hormones during and after work, due to work and home responsibilities.

Stress and the body's reaction to it can be good things. After all, you might not get up in the morning if you didn't have a job to go to. And should you ever face physical danger, your body's stress response could save your life. But when stress becomes chronic, it can damage relationships, steal restful sleep, and even wear out the arteries.

It doesn't have to be this way. Stress isn't the deadline, the traffic jam, or the uncooperative teenager—it's the way you react to things. That's why one woman who sees a long line at the su-

WHAT TO DO IF YOU HAVE ONLY **5 MINUTES**

Find a quiet place to close your eyes. Tune out the rest of the world and rest your mind, says Pamela Peeke, M.D., assistant clinical professor of medicine at the University of Maryland School of Medicine in Baltimore and author of *Fight Fat after 40*. "Or go for a walk around the block if you're a physical type of person."

Even a short break from stress will help you feel better physically as well as emotionally, she explains.

permarket may feel her temper rising out of control, while another simply relaxes and browses through a magazine while she waits.

Your Body on Stress

While we tend to view stress as toxic to our minds, we generally don't consider its potentially harmful effects on the body. But the physical effects of stress are profound.

During times of stress, the nervous system triggers the release of stress hormones: adrenaline, norepinephrine, and cortisol. They stimulate virtually every system in the body. For example, they cause sugars and fats to pour into the bloodstream for quick energy. Blood pressure rises, and the heart beats faster in order to boost circulation to muscles in the arms and legs. Respiration increases, which supplies the muscles with more oxygen. The blood clots more easily as a precaution against injury, and perspiration increases in order to cool the body in this energized state.

The stress response happens very quickly. It's designed to save your life in emergency situations. Once the danger is past, your body gradually returns to its normal state.

Most days, of course, stress isn't a physical threat. Stress is time pressures, traffic, and the weight of responsibilities. But its effects on the body are just as profound, says Dr. Caudill.

Stress affects immunity, which is why people who are under pressure a lot of the time tend to experience more infections, such as colds or flu. One study found that women who cared for relatives with Alzheimer's—which can be an emotionally draining full-time job—had weaker immune responses than those who weren't caregivers.

Depression, which can be a major response to stress, is considered a primary risk factor for cardiovascular disease. Stress raises blood pressure, which damages the linings of blood vessels. At the same time, substances that are released during times of stress, such as fatty acids, are trapped in the damaged areas of the blood vessels. This leads to the development of plaques, fatty deposits that can block bloodflow, increase the risk of clots, and possibly lead to heart attacks.

Fat also heads to your middle during times of stress. Emotional extremes suppress the body's production of testosterone, which helps control abdominal fat.

Researchers have identified dozens of physical symptoms that are associated with stress overload. They include:

- Fatigue
- Frequent headaches or migraines
- Frequent colds or flu
- Asthma or wheezing
- Poor sleep
- Muscle tension and aches
- Nausea
- Reduced sex drive
- Hair loss
- Eating too little or too much

Apart from physical changes, constant stress also affects the emotions. You might notice frequent feelings of:

- Anxiety
- Sadness
- Frustration
- Irritability
- Anger

WHAT WORKS FOR ME

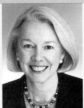

MARGARET A. CAUDILL, M.D., PH.D., *adjunct associate professor of anesthesiology at Dartmouth Medical School and professor of stress and pain management at Dartmouth Community College in Manchester, New Hampshire, has just as much stress in her life as the patients she counsels. Here are her tricks for staying calm.*

I teach stress management, so I have the luxury of doing what I teach. I'm always aware of my comfort and happiness levels. If I find myself saying, "I don't want to do this anymore," I listen closely to the cue, examine what needs to be changed, and take care of it.

I also exercise, even though I've never been an exercise enthusiast. In fact, I hated exercise in the past, so I have to do it on my own terms. I tell myself that I only have to put in 10 or 15 minutes on the treadmill every morning. While I exercise, I listen to books on tape or National Public Radio.

Exercise gives me the energy to face stress later in the day. It also helps me distance myself from problems so I can see them objectively, which gives me new perspectives.

Restoring Sleep

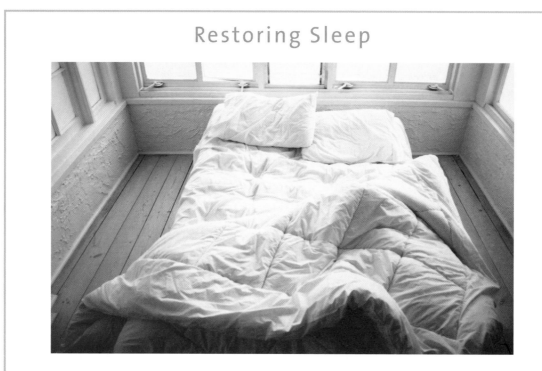

Women are feeling increasingly stressed-out—and they are losing sleep over it.

In a sleep census poll of more than 1,000 Americans, 62 percent said they had a hard time sleeping, and more women than men reported symptoms of insomnia. Americans as a whole lose almost 5 hours of sleep a week because of sleep deprivation. Do that every week, and you'll lose 260 hours by the end of the year—more than a week and a half.

What's behind all this tossing and turning? Stress tops the list.

When you're stressed, your muscles are tense, you have high levels of stress hormones that arouse instead of relax the body, and your mind is full of troubling thoughts.

You might think you can get away with less sleep, but getting fewer than 7 or 8 hours of sleep a night affects your concentration, judgment, reaction time, memory, and physical performance.

Here are a few ways to ensure you get the sleep you need.

Establish relaxation rituals. Every night, take a warm bath. Or read a magazine or watch TV. Everyone should do something relaxing before going to bed. If you do this every night, your body will naturally start preparing for sleep.

Avoid stimulants. The caffeine in coffee, chocolate, soda, tea, diet drugs, and some pain relievers may keep you awake. If you smoke, the nicotine in cigarettes can lead to early-morning awakenings because the body is demanding the next "hit." Now might be a good time to quit smoking—you'll get better sleep if you do.

Stick to your workouts. People who exercise sleep better. But to avoid being too pumped up at bedtime, finish exercising 5 to 6 hours before then.

No matter how much stress you experience, and regardless of the physical or emotional tolls you're currently paying, you can do something about it. Once you identify the causes of stresses in your life and recognize the danger signs, you can start taking steps to reduce them with this six-step action plan.

Step 1: Identify Your Boiling Point

Why do some women get frazzled and irritated when they're stuck in traffic, while others stay cool even during catastrophes? Two things make the difference: the amount of control that you feel you have over your life, and your basic personality.

If you're responsible for the care of your ill mother, on top of being a mom and a full-time employee, you'll understandably be stressed. A lot of things are happening in your life, and you really can't control the outcome.

"Think of Supreme Court justices," says Deborah Belle, Ed.D., associate professor of psychology at Boston University. "They have what seem to be extremely stressful jobs, they have a heavy workload, and they make extremely important decisions."

But they seem to live forever. Why?

"I think it's because they have the best law clerks in the country working for them, they can choose which cases to hear, they have the esteem and admiration of many people, and they can take lavish vacations to recuperate," Dr. Belle says. "On the other hand, their secretaries have a heavy workload without much control. They're probably under much higher levels of stress."

Then there's personality. Women with hostile, type A personalities—they snap at restaurant waiters for making mistakes, tailgate cars on the highway, and blow up at coworkers—have a higher risk of cardiovascular disease due to stress. In a study at the University of Pittsburgh, of 276 healthy men and women, those who were less agreeable had higher blood pressures and levels of stress hormones than those who were calmer and more easygoing.

Other personality types, too, are vulnerable to health damage. In the same study, people who were introverted also tended to have high blood pressure and elevated levels of stress hormones.

Many women share a personality trait that may increase their risk for depression: rumination. Women who are introspective and passive and tend to dwell on their problems—which often makes problems seem worse than they really are—generally experience depression and unnecessary levels of stress.

"All of the complexities that make people human affect the stress response," Dr. Caudill says.

Step 2: Recognize the Triggers

Sometimes the source of stress is obvious: Driving behind a school bus or garbage truck that makes several stops en route is making you late for work, for example. Other times, it's not always clear if your frustration is due to your job, problems with the kids, financial worries, or all of the above.

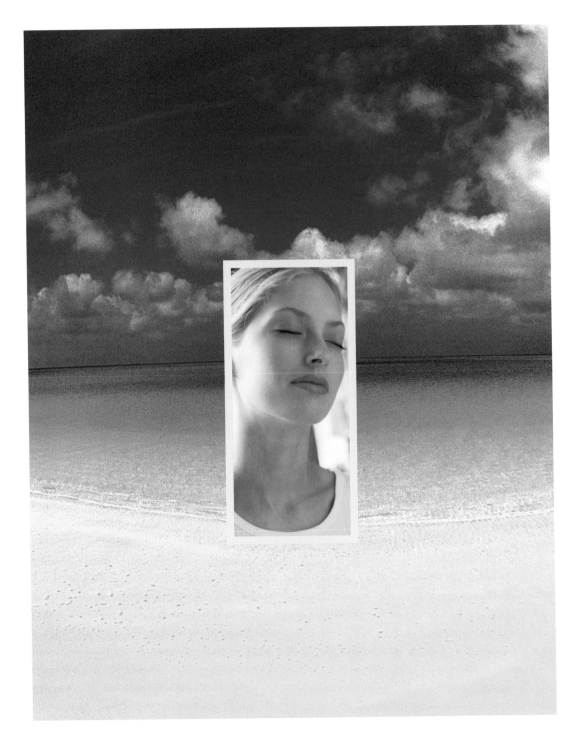

You can't begin to control stress if you're not sure what's behind it. At the first sign that something's wrong, try to get to the bottom of it. One way to do that is by keeping a journal.

Sit down for a few minutes every day to write about issues that concern you. Don't waste time with the little things, like standing in line at the grocery store, says Dr. Caudill. Try to get to the source of what's bothering you. At that point, you can start problem solving. Make a list of some of your options: getting household help, researching a new job, talking to a counselor, and so on.

Once you start identifying your stress triggers and considering solutions, you'll feel a sense of control you didn't have before, and that's one of the best ways to combat stress, says Dr. Caudill.

It's not uncommon for women to feel so tired and burned-out that they can't begin to muster the energy that's required for problem solving, says Dr. Caudill. At that point, it makes sense to see a therapist right away. You'll learn more about yourself and also discover practical ways to bring additional calm to your life.

Step 3: Practice the "Calm Response"

We've already talked about the physical changes that accompany stress. Even though these changes are a necessary part of survival, they can make life really uncomfortable a lot of the time.

Here are a few ways to control the symptoms of stress and bring additional calm into your life.

Breathe deeply. Try to make a fist while taking a deep breath. You probably can't maintain the tension for very long because breathing naturally eases tension, Dr. Caudill says. It's common, however, for people to breathe shallowly when they're experiencing stress—which can make the discomfort even worse.

Doctors often advise women to practice breathing exercises, but simply reminding yourself to breathe deeply now and then can make a difference. It might be helpful to put little cues around the house—sticky notes on the refrigerator or in the car, for example. Every time you see one of the cues, take a moment to drop your shoulders, breathe deeply, and let go of some of the tension, Dr. Caudill advises.

Go to Maui—in 30 seconds. Warm sand beneath your bare feet. A cool breeze against your face. The sound of a crashing ocean in your ears. Your body tenses at the perception of stress, so calm it down by thinking of something serene.

Bend with stress. When life's pressures are getting to you, put your imagination to work. Imagine that you're a strong oak tree. The trunk of the tree is your inner core, and no amount of wind will affect it. "But your branches bend for you," says Pamela Peeke, M.D., assistant clinical professor of medicine at the University of Maryland School of Medicine in Baltimore and author of *Fight Fat after 40*. When you're faced with a traffic jam, for example, tell yourself that your core is strong and sustainable. You don't have to get upset about it.

Get some sun. Even if you don't think you have the time, get outside for a few minutes. Exposure to sunlight increases levels of serotonin, a natural hormone that reduces stress and imparts feelings of calm and well-being.

Take mini-breaks. If you let your mind rest for at least 5 minutes every hour, you'll find it easier to stay calm and focused. Close your eyes and think peaceful thoughts—or stand up and stretch. Better yet, walk briskly for a few moments: It stimulates the release of endorphins, body chemicals that neutralize stress hormones.

Distract yourself. Filling your free time with activities you love will help keep your mind off the stress of tomorrow. "Humans are wonderful at distracting themselves," Dr. Belle says. "And we need to feed our souls this way."

Rewrite the script. When you find yourself believing that a bump in the road is a true catastrophe, take a new perspective. Your roof sprang a leak and the car transmission blew up on the same day? Instead of blowing your lid, laugh at the irony.

"Turn life into a comedy instead of a drama," say Loretta LaRoche, an international stress management consultant in Plymouth, Massachusetts, and author of the audiocassette *Life Is Not a Stress Rehearsal.*

Step 4: Accept What You Can't Change

Stress is never going to go away. Women have to accept that. But remember, stress isn't the issue—how you react to it is. Here are a few ways to unwind, no matter what life throws at you.

Accept the circumstances. Some types of stress, you can't solve. Breathing or taking a mental vacation might help, but nothing will take away the heartache of watching a relative become ill, or the grief over the death of a parent.

"Stay in touch with the complexity of the situation, and do your best to heighten the quality of the days you have," Dr. Belle says.

Be imperfect—and calmer. When you try to achieve the unachievable—as so many women tend to do—you'll feel frustrated, anxious, or depressed. So concentrate on your strengths, instead of obsessing over your flaws. The second a negative thought enters your mind, replace it with "I'm doing the best I can" or "I'm fine and happy and fulfilled."

Acknowledge your mistakes and move on. Because so many people depend on them, women often feel as though they have to make the right decisions every time. It doesn't work that way, of course. Everyone makes mistakes, and the worst thing you can do is berate yourself and dwell on them.

Here's a better approach: Remind yourself that within every mistake is an opportunity for growth and renewal. You can't change what's already happened, but you can take the lessons you learned and apply them to the next challenge that comes along.

Step 5: Stay Socially Engaged

One thing women do well is bond with other women. Some scientists even think that women are hardwired to "tend and befriend," to protect themselves and their children by building a social network that they can rely on for help.

"We're social creatures," Dr. Belle says. "We're healthiest and happiest when we're part of a supportive group."

Talking to friends about what's bothering you might help you see things in a different light. It also helps to get reassurance from friends that you're still loved and supported, despite how crummy you feel, Dr. Belle says.

Step 6: **Practice a Lower-Stress Life**

If you establish certain habits every day, even when you're not under stress, you'll find that you'll naturally be a little calmer when things do get crazy.

Exercise regularly. It's one of the best ways to reduce anxiety, tension, apprehension, depression, and fatigue. Study after study has shown that moderate exercise reduces cortisol, the stress hormone that triggers the runaway stress response.

You don't have to be an athlete to get the benefits of exercise. Walk in the morning and again in the evening. Go the health club three or four times a week. Spend some time weeding the garden or raking leaves. Any kind of physical activity releases "feel good" endorphins, which will help you feel calmer and more relaxed.

Have a plan B. Preparing backup plans is a great way to increase control over your life. Suppose you have to drive your daughter to soccer practice after work—but you always worry that

reality
check She Discovered
Calm in a Life of Chaos

Amy Mitrani of Miami has worked in a notoriously stressful job for years: sales. The phone is always ringing off the hook. Clients are difficult. And the pressure to be "on" all the time takes a toll. Mitrani, who's in her thirties, admits that her stress levels rose out of control.

She didn't want to change careers, but Mitrani knew that she had to bring some calm to her life. So she started taking yoga classes. At the same time, she began keeping a journal, and every morning she repeated the affirmation to herself, "I live in harmony and balance."

They were simple strategies, but they completely changed how Mitrani handled stress. In the past, for example, she would lose confidence when she failed to get a sale. Today she doesn't let it bother her. Her trick, she says, is like "changing the channel on a TV."

When negative thoughts start coming into her mind, she quickly replaces them with positive ones. Sometimes, for example, she'll find she is attacking herself for what she could have done better. Now she turns things around by thinking of what she did that was positive and what she has learned for her next prospect.

Mitrani has more confidence than ever before. She's happier, and she says her newfound calm has made her more successful on the job. ■

you'll get stuck in traffic. Make plans with one of the parents to share driving responsibilities in a pinch. You'll worry less because you'll know that everything is covered "just in case."

Get involved in your church or temple. In one study by the California Department of Health Services, researchers looked at more than 2,600 people over 30 years. They found that those who attended religious services regularly were less likely to suffer from depression. They also engaged in activities that naturally reduce stress, such as attending social gatherings and staying physically active.

Get a pet. Many studies have shown that having a dog, cat, or other pet reduces stress. Pet owners even have lower cholesterol and blood pressure than those without pets.

Put pleasure on your schedule. You can't be a great mother, wife, or friend if you're burned-out and exhausted. So think about what you can do for yourself. Do you want to read the paper on Sunday mornings? Enjoy a long bath in the evenings? Put it on your schedule—actually write it down. It will make you much more likely to actually to keep the "appointment."

Keep healthy finances. Debt—credit card bills in particular—may be linked to high blood pressure, insomnia, and other physical problems. When researchers surveyed more than 1,000 people, they found that those with higher credit card debts were more stressed and had the most health complaints. Get your finances in order now, and you'll enjoy better health.

Keep a low-maintenance house. Dirt won't stress you out if you can't see it. Buy rugs, couches, and chairs in earth tones, which hide stains. Choose easy-to-clean wood or linoleum floors. Put washable gloss or semigloss paint on the walls—they'll be easier to wipe down. And buy low-care plants and shrubbery: Less work in the yard means more time for the things that are important to you.

Spend some time at the playground. If you have young children in the house, spending too much time with them is not good, says Dr. Belle. "Women with kids need time with other adults." She recommends play groups so you have time to socialize with other mothers. You might also consider babysitting for other mothers so everyone gets a break. Women without children often find that it's a real kick to spend time with nieces, nephews, or grandchildren. It's hard to take life too seriously when you're making up rhymes, talking in a silly voice, or pushing a swing. It's a great distraction from life's stress.

Cherish life. A warm breeze in the summer. The beauty of nature. The rush you feel as you ride your bike. If you believe you deserve pleasure from life, you'll be much more likely to achieve all the things that you need to be happy.

A Quit-Smoking Program That Can't Fail

After 27 years of smoking cigarettes, Susannah Hayward crushed her last butt. Once she got over the withdrawal symptoms, she felt reborn.

"Everything smells and tastes better, my skin is pink and healthy, I can run without wheezing, and I have more energy overall," Hayward says. "I'm also more relaxed. I don't feel agitated anymore in a non-smoking environment."

The best part for Hayward? Higher self-esteem.

"If I can give up smoking, I can do anything," she says.

And she did. She wrote a book about quitting smoking, called *Breathe Easy.*

Many women think smoking helps them get through the day.

In reality, smoking makes you cough, lose your breath, and feel *more* stressed when you can't smoke, says Neil Grunberg, Ph.D., professor of medical and clinical psychology at Uniformed Services University in Bethesda, Maryland. Smoking is directly responsible for 87 percent of all lung cancer in the United States, and women's lungs damage more easily than men's. Smoking also can cause heart disease, stroke, and cancer of the larynx, mouth, bladder, cervix, pancreas, and kidneys. Women risk their reproductive health as well.

If scare tactics worked, no one would smoke. The fact is, nicotine is just as addictive as cocaine and heroin.

It's never too late to quit—or to try again. Successfully quitting almost erases the damage of moderate cigarette smoking, if you quit before age 35—which is when the diseases first start appearing in cigarette smokers, such as bronchitis, emphysema, and periodontal disease, and circulatory disorders. Quitting may even extend your life; smokers tend to die 7 years earlier than nonsmokers.

Why Smokers Smoke

Seven to 10 seconds after you inhale, nicotine releases super-normal amounts of norepinephrine and dopamine, brain chemicals that give you pleasure. You'll feel more satisfaction than you do from laughing, watching the sun set, or drinking cool water on a warm day, says Linda Hyder Ferry, M.D., associate professor of preventive and family medicine at Loma Linda University in California.

But after a while, your body depends on nicotine for the release of these chemicals, and it takes more nicotine to feel the same amount of pleasure, says Dr. Hyder Ferry. But on their way to your brain, the components of tobacco smoke *also*:

- Narrow your arteries, some of which are no bigger than a pencil lead, and allow less blood get to your heart. That constriction causes blood to move faster, which traumatizes the lining of vessels.

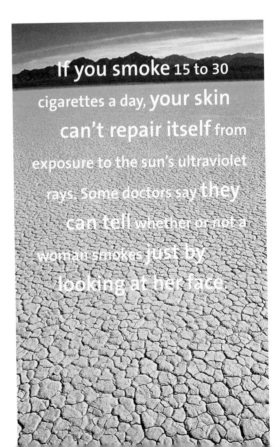

If you smoke 15 to 30 cigarettes a day, your skin can't repair itself from exposure to the sun's ultraviolet rays. Some doctors say they can tell whether or not a woman smokes just by looking at her face

- Rob your heart and blood vessels of oxygen hours or days after you smoke because of the effect of carbon monoxide's attaching to hemoglobin cells, which transport oxygen.

- Lower HDL ("good") cholesterol levels while raising LDL ("bad") cholesterol, which leads to a buildup of plaque and lipids in already damaged arteries.

- Trigger an irregular heart rhythm or heart attack if the heart becomes completely starved of oxygen.

- Interfere with bone rebuilding, contributing to osteoporosis.

- Damage the tiny air sacs in lungs, reducing oxygen exchange.

The effects are immediate. It's hard to breathe, let alone exercise. If you keep it up for 15 or 20 years, you'll lose 40 to 50 percent of your lung function, called chronic obstructive pulmonary disease, and may become short of breath when taking a shower or walking to your car.

Smoking a pack a day also causes 5 to 10 percent bone loss by menopause, a significant loss considering smokers reach menopause up to 4 years earlier than women who don't smoke.

Women Take the Biggest Hit

The 22.3 million American women who smoke experience more wheezing, coughing, breathlessness, and asthma than men who smoke, even if they

● Prevent Bronchitis and Emphysema

If you smoke and you've had a persistent cough for more than 2 years, don't dismiss it as nothing more than "smoker's cough." A consistent cough with mucus could be chronic bronchitis.

While nonsmokers can and do get bronchitis, smoking is by far the most common way to get bronchitis because smoke causes the bronchi to become inflamed and interferes with airflow. But it's also possible to get it from a bacterial or viral infection, air pollution, or industrial dusts and fumes. Bronchitis may lead to or accompany emphysema.

By all means, if you have bronchitis and you smoke, quit. Exercise may also indirectly help by strengthening the heart and body, but because

exercise could make breathing even harder, consult your physician before beginning a new exercise program, recommends Linda Hyder Ferry, M.D., associate professor of preventive and family medicine at Loma Linda University in California.

Like bronchitis, emphysema is accompanied by cough and shortness of breath. If the diseases occur together, they're called chronic obstructive pulmonary disease. And as with bronchitis, smoking is the biggest cause of emphysema. Cigarette smoke damages the air sacs in the lungs so that they have trouble transferring oxygen to the blood. You'll probably notice you can't exercise as well. Even a brief walk could make you lose your breath. Quitting smoking can halt emphysema's progression in its tracks. ■

light up less often, says Jill Siegfried, Ph.D., vice-chairperson of the department of pharmacology at the University of Pittsburgh. Among men, lung cancer is decreasing; for women, it's on the rise.

Researchers don't know exactly why damage is more severe in women, but estrogen may play a role. Researchers think estrogen releases chemicals in the lungs that cause cells to divide. That in turn thickens the airways and stimulates cells with mutations to form tumors, says Dr. Siegfried. Estrogen may also help convert chemicals in cigarette smoke to carcinogens.

Smoking also affects women's reproductive health, causing:

- Lower fertility

- A doubled risk of getting cervical cancer

- Higher risk of low birth weight, sudden infant death syndrome, and stillbirths among pregnant women

- Higher risk of heart disease and stroke while taking the birth control pill

If you quit now, in the years to come you will erase almost all that damage. Your skin will look better and you'll breathe easier. Your risk of cancer will go down, and after 4 years your heart attack risk will dwindle to that of a never smoker, says Dr. Hyder Ferry. When it comes to lung cancer, however, you'll always have higher risk than never smokers. But risk will decrease every year to nearly a nonsmoker's level of risk.

If you've tried to quit before and couldn't, you're not beat yet. On average, it takes five or six

---

reality *check* Once She Quit, She Could Laugh Again

Judy Lin-Eftekhar, a 51-year-old writer and editor in Santa Monica, California, started smoking at 19 to look cool, avoid eating, and feel less anxious. But after 15 years, smoking almost two packs a day made it hard for her to breathe. Then one morning she woke up with the flu, and the thought of lighting a cigarette made her feel even sicker. She knew this was her chance to quit forever, so she did.

Judy made a list of reasons to quit—"to be

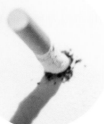

healthy again" and "so my clothes don't stink"— and taped them to her refrigerator. She imagined herself as a happy nonsmoker and exercised every day. She also felt a spiritual awakening and let a higher power guide her.

She realized that she had used cigarettes to suppress negative feelings toward her job and relationship. But instead of going back to smoking, she found a new job and broke off her relationship. Soon Judy felt like a new person. Now she breathes deeper. Her skin looks more vibrant. She's thinner from exercise. And without a cigarette to puff, she laughs more often. ■

tries to quit for good. Today, smokers have more options to quit than ever before. If one strategy didn't work for you in the past, another will. Here's a step-by-step action plan from experts who have studied smoking habits of women.

Step 1: Get Screened for Depression

Researchers estimate that one-fourth to one-third of all smokers experience anxiety or depression. They may self-medicate with cigarettes. Since women are twice as likely as men to experience depression, they're more likely to fall into this group of smokers, claims Dr. Hyder Ferry.

"I screen all my female patients for depression and anxiety before they quit smoking, and I ask them how they are feeling after they quit so they can get treated if they have mood changes," says Dr. Hyder Ferry. (For more on the symptoms of depression, see page 356.)

Step 2: Set a Quit Date

Commit to a quit date that falls sometime in the next 7 to 10 days, and get rid of all your cigarettes and ashtrays by then.

"Like anything, if you don't plan exactly when you're going to do it, it doesn't get done," says Kenneth Perkins, Ph.D., professor of psychiatry at the University of Pittsburgh School of Medicine who has researched smoking cessation.

The worst time to quit is during the second half of your menstrual cycle because premenstrual symptoms could make withdrawal worse. In one study, women who quit in the first 2 weeks after their period and attended group sessions experienced less severe withdrawal symptoms than women who quit smoking later in their menstrual cycle.

Step 3: Choose Your Weapon

Going "cold turkey" is the least effective way to quit—only about 2 to 5 percent of smokers can do so. Most others need help of some kind. If one method doesn't work, try another, recommends Dr. Hyder Ferry. Here are your options, ranked more or less from most to least effective (although this is highly individual).

Phase out cigarettes. Gradually decrease the number of cigarettes you smoke until you're down to five to 10 a day—just enough to keep from going into withdrawal. Then quit completely.

For instance, if you smoke a pack of cigarettes a day, allow yourself to smoke only half of each cigarette for a week. The next week, throw three cigarettes out before you start the pack. Continue to reduce at this pace for 4 to 6 weeks before you quit completely.

Ask your doctor about bupropion. Like nicotine, the prescription compound bupropion (Zyban) is used as an antidepressant and stabilizes the levels of norepinephrine and dopamine, two brain chemicals responsible for feelings of well-being. But while nicotine causes the chemicals to spike and then fall, bupropion releases a smaller, steady stream without causing any addiction. That means withdrawal symptoms won't bother you as much.

You can try combining bupropion with other therapies. When 4,000 people took bupropion with or without nicotine replacement therapy and had professional counseling, 40 to 60 percent of them remained smoke-free for at least a year.

Consider nicotine replacement therapy. Although it's less effective in women than in men, nicotine replacement therapy provides enough nicotine to keep you from going into withdrawal while you break the habit of reaching for a cigarette—which takes about 5 to 10 weeks, says Dr. Hyder Ferry. Nicotine replacement therapy is available over the counter in the form of the patch, which could cause a mild skin rash, and gum. Prescription versions include an inhaler and nasal spray.

If you tried nicotine replacement therapy before and felt miserable, you probably didn't use a high enough dose of nicotine or you stopped using it too soon, Dr. Hyder Ferry says. For best results, talk to your doctor about which therapy and dose is best for you.

Look into acupuncture. Acupuncture is an ancient Chinese health practice that involves puncturing the skin with hair-thin needles at particular locations—usually the ear for nicotine addiction. Although there's little research that proves acupuncture works, some women who try it may experience milder withdrawal symptoms.

To find a certified acupuncturist in your area, call the American Association of Oriental Medicine at (888) 500-7999.

Try hypnosis. Through hypnosis, you might increase your motivation, lower your cravings, and keep from lighting up. To request referrals for

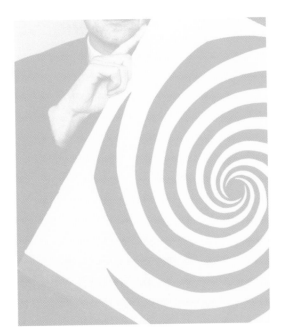

hypnotherapists, send a self-addressed, stamped envelope to the American Society of Clinical Hypnosis at 130 East Elm Court, Suite 201, Roselle, IL 60172.

Step 4: Start an Exercise Routine

The average smoker weighs 6 to 11 pounds less than a nonsmoker but gains that amount of weight after quitting. Ten to 15 percent of women who quit gain more than 28 pounds. That's because nicotine curbs hunger, decreasing between-meal snacking. The elimination of nicotine reverses the weight-suppressing effect, causing women to eat more after quitting.

Research shows it's just too hard to diet *and* quit smoking, but you can exercise. Women who smoked 10 or more cigarettes a day and joined a smoking cessation program that involved weekly behavior modification sessions and about 50 minutes of exercise three times a week gained less weight and were more likely to stay smoke-free than women who didn't exercise.

Even if you do gain weight, you'd have to put on more than 100 pounds to cancel out the benefits to health of quitting, says Dr. Perkins.

Step 5: Quash Cravings

If you eat more to make up for not smoking, your weight will be harder to control. Here's how to deal with those cigarette cravings—during and after therapy.

Change your routine. Cues can make you want a cigarette all day long, and women may be more susceptible than men. The most common cues are the smell of cigarette smoke and drinking coffee. But there are more situations that you may not think about, such as a talking on the phone, opening a beer, or unwinding after work. The solution: change your routine to miss the urge.

Drink tea instead of coffee, take public transportation to work if you have access, and visit a nonsmoking friend instead of talking on the phone. Go for a walk when you feel a craving coming on, and keep hard candy and lollipops handy. If possible, you might want to take a vacation from work the week you quit.

Avoid bars and alcohol. Until you've learned to cope with the craving-inducing sights and smells, and the easy availability of cigarettes, stay away from bars and alcohol. Whenever possible, stay away from people who smoke.

Breathe deeply. Take deep breaths when you get the urge to smoke. It will relax you and help you cope with urges.

Give yourself a 2-minute massage. One study at the University of Miami found that a 2-minute hand or ear massage cut cravings, reduced anxiety, and improved mood. Try these moves.

- Pinch your ear from the top down to your earlobe.

- Gently tug your earlobe.

THREE THINGS I TELL EVERY FEMALE PATIENT

LINDA HYDER FERRY, M.D., associate professor of preventive and family medicine at Loma Linda University in California, says, "Quitting smoking was your first step to minimize aging and slow down the skin wrinkling process."

Here are some other strategies that she emphasizes.

1. Eat a diet high in natural antioxidants, which you'll get from fruits and vegetables.

2. Use a mild cleanser that exfoliates your skin.

3. Wear a UVB/UVA spectrum sunscreen with an SPF of at least 15 every day. ■

- Use your thumb to massage the palm of your hand in a circular motion.
- Use your thumb and index finger to massage each finger from base to fingertip.

Step 6: Join a Smoking Cessation Support Group

Group sessions give you tips and support even if you're using a therapy. After reviewing several studies on smoking cessation, researchers found that people were more successful when they went to group programs that offered behavior techniques and mutual support than when they quit with little or no help. Maybe that's because just when you think you can't go another day without a cigarette, your group knows exactly how you feel. Quality of sessions varies, Dr. Grunberg says, so if you don't like one, try others.

Step 7: Prepare for Withdrawal

Withdrawal symptoms vary from person to person, depending on how much you smoke and your method of quitting, says Dr. Hyder Ferry. Knowing what to expect will help you get through it. Here's a day-to-day guide.

Days 1 and 2. Physically, you'll feel like you have a unique combination of withdrawal symptoms. You might have a headache, increased irritability, or anxiety, and you'll feel uncomfortable. You might also have trouble sleeping at night and concentrating during the day.

Days 3 through 7. Your withdrawal symptoms peak on day 3 and then stabilize. Many give up at this point, but as soon as you get over this hump, you'll feel better—promise.

Days 8 through 13. Your symptoms may begin to improve.

Days 14 through 365. Physically you feel back to normal. For the first several months, you'll probably crave a cigarette occasionally, and you may have trouble sleeping. But studies show that going cigarette-free for a full year increases your chances of staying that way.

Step 8: Give Yourself a Year of Rewards

Make it easier to get to that year mark when cravings subside. Treat yourself to a new book or theater tickets after the first day, the first week, then the first month of no smoking. Be sure to make the reward greater as time goes by.

Not only will your health improve, but your sense of taste and smell will be heightened, you won't have to clean up ashes, your clothes won't smell like smoke, and you'll have more time to spend on other activities or with friends and family (the average cigarette takes 5 to 7 minutes to smoke). In addition to pocketing the cash you would have spent on cigarettes, you'll probably save money on health insurance. Best of all, you won't have to rely on smoking to feel good. And remember: One slip doesn't mean you're a smoker again, so don't quit quitting.

Sun-Proof (And Age-Proof) Your Skin

The sun can do a lot of good. It regulates sleep cycles, stimulates the body's production of vitamin D, and enhances feelings of well-being. But there's also a downside: Exposure to sun can lead to wrinkles, age spots, and skin cancer.

In fact, sunshine is considered the single biggest cause of visible aging. But you don't have to succumb to the damaging rays. Even if you haven't been sun savvy in the past, it's never too late to start protecting your skin, says Darrell S. Rigel, M.D., clinical professor of dermatology at New York University School of Medicine in New York City.

For starters, every woman should eat a diet that's rich in fruits and vegetables. They contain antioxidant compounds, which reduce the damaging effects of sunshine. (Refraining from smoking also makes a difference because cigarette smoke creates huge numbers of skin-damaging molecules.)

But the most important thing you can do is shield your skin from the sun. As long as you use sunscreen, take advantage of shade, and wear the right clothing, you can enjoy your favorite outdoor activities without worrying about the damaging rays.

How Sunshine Makes Skin Look Old

Every time the sun strikes your skin, the skin produces pigment that scatters and absorbs the rays. The resulting tan means your skin is defending itself from harmful radiation.

But a tan can do only so much. Over time, the ultraviolet A (UVA) and ultraviolet B (UVB) radiation in sunshine can weaken the lower layer of skin, known as the dermis, and promote wrinkles, brown spots, and the development of skin cancer.

The most common (and least aggressive) form of skin cancer is basal cell carcinoma. It begins in the top layer of skin, the epidermis, and generally doesn't spread any further. While another form—squamous cell carcinoma—often remains at its original site, it is more likely spread to other parts of the body. Both basal cell and squamous cell carcinomas can be cured if detected early. However, melanoma—a cancer that starts in the skin's pigment cells and readily spreads to other organs—can be deadly. It causes 75 percent of all deaths from skin cancer.

How can you protect yourself from the sun's harmful rays? This four-step action plan will make all the difference.

THREE THINGS I TELL EVERY FEMALE PATIENT

ALAN KLING, M.D., clinical assistant professor of dermatology at Mount Sinai School of Medicine in New York City, offers the following advice for maximal skin protection.

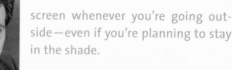

1 CONSIDER THE ALTITUDE. The sun's ultraviolet radiation is strongest at high altitudes. If you live at a high elevation, or if you're hiking or skiing, reapply sunscreen frequently.

MAKE NO EXCEPTIONS. Skin damage can occur even on cloudy days, so apply sunscreen whenever you're going outside—even if you're planning to stay in the shade.

2

3 GET YOUR TAN IN A BOTTLE. If a pale complexion simply rubs you the wrong way, try using self-tanners or bronzers. They're a lot safer than "natural" tans. Just remember that a self-tanner does not protect you from the sun's rays, so be sure to slather on that sunscreen when you're going to be outside. ∎

Step 1: Determine Your Risk Profile

There's no way to accurately predict whose skin is most likely to show premature signs of aging or who is more likely to develop skin cancer, says Dee Anna Glaser, M.D., associate professor of dermatology at St. Louis University School of Medicine.

You should schedule a skin exam with your dermatologist at least once a year after the age of 40. If skin cancer runs in your family, you may want to start earlier than that. In addition, it's important to do self-exams once a month. Signs of trouble include:

- Small pearly white bumps, or sores on the skin that bleed and don't heal.

- Red, scaly bumps that resemble a scar and have a depression in the middle.

- Dark spots that are asymmetrical, have irregular borders, have more than one color, and are bigger than the size of a pencil eraser. These spots may be flat or elevated.

Anyone can get skin cancer, but some people have a much higher risk than others. The risk factors include:

- Fair skin. It doesn't contain as much of the natural pigment called melanin that scatters the sun's rays.

- Multiple moles or "beauty marks." Melanoma cells are more abundant in moles and freckles.

---

reality *check*

She Gets Her Tan from a Bottle

Susan Stern, a 39-year-old public relations consultant in New York City, is light-skinned—but that doesn't mean she shuns the sun. She swims and scuba dives in the summer and takes trips to Florida at least twice a winter.

"As far back as I can remember, I was swimming," Susan says. "I even gave swimming lessons and worked as a lifeguard when I was a teenager."

When she was young, her skin burned at least once a summer. But as she got older, she didn't want the wrinkles and brown spots that she saw on some of her friends' faces. Nor did she want to follow in the footsteps of her sun-loving father, who now has to get suspicious moles removed with some regularity.

To protect her skin while enjoying her favorite activities, she uses a moisturizer with UVA and UVB protection. She wears it every day, even in the winter. Before she gets in the water, she applies an ounce of waterproof sunscreen—and reapplies it every time she comes out of the water. On the beach, she wears a T-shirt and sits under an umbrella.

Susan doesn't mind not having a whole-body tan—but she does want her face and neck to have a sunny glow. Rather than basking in the sun, she applies a dark bronzing powder.

Her precautions have paid off. She looks healthy—and her friends can hardly believe she's almost 40. ∎

The more beauty marks you have, the greater the risk that cancer cells will be present.

- A history of sunburns. Even if you've had only one blistering sunburn in your life, you have a higher risk for developing skin cancer.

- A tropical address. The ozone layer, which blocks ultraviolet light, is thinner in tropical regions. Ultraviolet radiation is stronger in the southern United States than it is in the north.

Step 2: Choose (And Use) the Right Protection

Wearing sunscreen is essential. You should use it every day, especially when you're spending time outdoors. To get the most benefits from sunscreen, here's what Dr. Glaser advises.

Choose products with a high SPF. It stands for "sun protection factor," and it's a measure of how well sunscreen protects your skin.

SPF refers to the length of time that sunscreen protects the skin. Suppose your skin naturally starts to burn in 20 minutes. If you use sunscreen with an SPF of 15, you won't begin to burn for 5 hours—15 times longer. Always use a sunscreen with an SPF of 15 or higher, Dr. Glaser advises.

Apply it often. In real life, sunscreens aren't always as effective as the SPF would indicate, says Dr. Glaser. If you're swimming, sweating a lot, or rubbing your skin with a towel, the sunscreen is going to dissipate. Reapply it every 2 hours—more often if you're swimming or perspiring a lot.

Buy a broad-spectrum sunscreen. These sunscreens will help block UVB and UVA rays.

Treat Psoriasis with Sun — Safely

most people are advised to avoid the sun, but doctors have found that sunshine is among the best treatments for psoriasis, a skin condition that results in itchy red patches or silvery scales on the face, elbows, knees, and other parts of the body. The sun's ultraviolet rays kill T cells, which are a type of white blood cells that trigger the unattractive flare-ups.

To get the benefits of ultraviolet light while minimizing the risks, here's what doctors advise.

Cover unaffected areas. Apply sunscreen to areas that aren't affected by psoriasis. Since your face and hands get an abundance of sunshine naturally, wear gloves and put a towel over your face during "light therapy" sessions, suggests Gerald Kruger, M.D., a dermatologist at the University of Utah in Salt Lake City. Light therapy sessions are prescribed by a dermatologist and involve using a tanning bed or a home ultraviolet light system to treat psoriasis.

Stick to the schedule. Some ultraviolet light is helpful, but excessive amounts can needlessly damage the skin. Your dermatologist will prescribe how much light you should be getting. ■

WHAT TO DO IF YOU HAVE ONLY **5 MINUTES**

Use a moisturizer that provides UVA and UVB protection, advises Alan Kling, M.D., clinical assistant professor of dermatology at Mount Sinai School of Medicine in New York City. It may not block radiation as completely as regular sunscreen, but it provides good protection, and it's fast and convenient to apply. Most cosmetics companies make facial moisturizers with UVA and UVB protection—check the label to be sure.

UVB light is the primary cause of sunburns, and protecting skin against UVA light plays an important role in preventing wrinkling and signs of aging. Choose a product that contains zinc oxide, titanium dioxide, or avobenzone, also known as Parsol 1789.

Apply it with your makeup. If you use moisturizers or other skin products in the morning, it's fine to apply sunscreen at the same time. First, apply topical medications if you use them. Let them dry, then apply alpha hydroxy acid or other anti-aging creams if you use them. Be sure to follow with a moisturizer, especially if you're using alpha hydroxy acids, which may have a drying effect on the skin. Then apply the sunscreen, followed by any makeup you're going to wear.

Give it time to work. In general, sunscreen is most effective when it's absorbed into the skin. Rub it on about 20 minutes before you go outside, says Dr. Glaser.

Use the right amount. It takes about an ounce of sunscreen to cover the average person's body. That's about the amount that would fill a shot glass. "You should feel messy after putting it on," Dr. Glaser says.

Step 3: **Add Extra Protection**

Wearing sunscreen helps to decrease the incidence of wrinkles and prevent the development of skin cancer. But sunscreen isn't enough by itself. Here are some additional ways to protect the skin.

WHAT WORKS FOR ME

TOBY SHAWE, M.D., *a dermatologist at the Philadelphia Institute of Dermatology, knows all too well what happens with excessive sun exposure—which is why she's careful to protect her own skin.*

I always use the best sunscreens I can find. I look for sunscreens that contain transparent zinc oxide, like SkinCeuticals Ultimate UV Defense SPF 30, which contains 7 percent transparent zinc oxide.

When I know I'll be spending some time outside, I wear a sunscreen with an SPF of 30. But when I'm going to be inside most of the day, I use a sunscreen with an SPF of 15. ∎

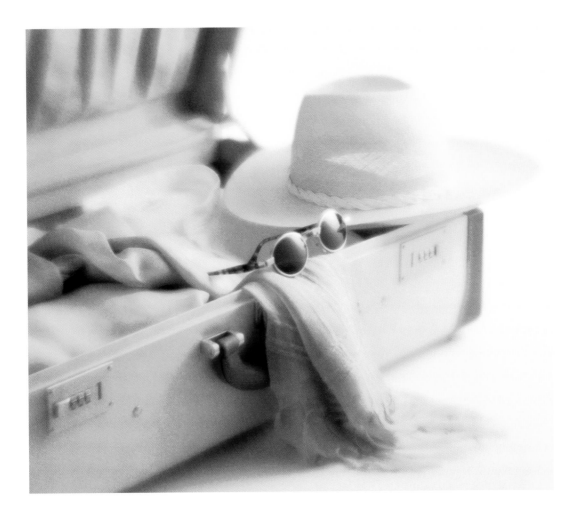

Always wear shades. Sunglasses protect the delicate skin around the eyes from wrinkles. They also help prevent cataracts and macular degeneration, the leading causes of vision loss in the elderly. Wear shades whenever you go outside, even on hazy days, says Phillip Calenda, M.D., an ophthalmologist at Westchester Vision Care in Scarsdale, New York.

The best sunglasses block 99 to 100 percent of UVA and UVB rays—look for ones that have labels claiming 100 percent or total UV protection. Wraparound sunglasses and styles that fit close to the eye are especially good because they prevent the sun's rays from coming in through the sides.

Wear a hat. A tightly woven hat made of canvas, with a 4-inch brim all the way around, helps shade your face, ears, and the back of your neck.

Wear long-sleeve shirts. And wear long pants. They offer the best protection from the sun's burning rays.

Buy clothing with tight-knit weaves. It's best to buy tight-weave clothes, some of which have SPF ratings just like sunscreen. Companies that sell high-SPF clothing include Sun Precautions, Solarveil, and SunGrubbies.com.

Step 4: Protect Yourself Year-Round

Sun protection shouldn't stop at the end of summer. Skiing without protecting your skin can be just as damaging as lying on the beach. To protect your skin in all seasons:

Check the UV index. The National Weather Service and the United States Environmental Protection Agency publish information about the daily UV index—the amount of ultraviolet radiation that is expected to reach the earth's surface when the sun is at its highest point. You'll find the index on the weather page of newspapers and on television or radio news.

Ultraviolet radiation between zero and 2 is considered minimal and between 3 and 4 is low. It's moderate at 5 to 6, and high at 7 to 9. A UV index rating above 10 is considered to be very high. If you can't avoid the sun when the

WHAT TO DO IF YOU COULD CHANGE **ONLY ONE THING**

Women should stop associating a tan with beauty and health, says Dee Anna Glaser, M.D., associate professor of dermatology at St. Louis University School of Medicine. It may take time to become accustomed to a paler complexion—but *not* having a tan means that you're healthier.

index is moderate or higher, be sure to protect your skin.

Avoid midday sun. Whenever possible, stay out of the sun between the hours of 10:00 A.M. and 4:00 P.M., when the rays are strongest.

Stay in the shade. Enjoy the outdoors from underneath a tree or umbrella—and even then, use sunscreen because UV rays bounce around a lot. You can get burned even when you're in the shade.

Forget about tanning booths. For some people, the UVA rays in tanning booths can produce a tan faster than the sun can. That's because the rays are intense—and damaging.

Beauty Products That Rejuvenate

The next time you browse the cosmetics counter at the pharmacy or department store, take a moment to check out some of the "anti-aging" lotions and potions. You'll be amazed at how many there are. Cosmetics companies have developed hundreds of products for protecting and preserving the skin. A few may even reverse some of the visible signs of aging, such as wrinkles and age spots.

Before reaching for specific skin-care products, you should keep in mind that your skin reflects your life.

If you smoke, bake in the sun for a tan, eat junk food, gain too much weight, or experience a lot of stress, your skin will pay for it. If, on the other hand, you relax often, eat healthful meals, and generally maintain positive lifestyle habits—as outlined in chapters throughout this section—you'll be rewarded with skin that's smooth and firm, even in your later years.

Drinking a lot of water—at least eight glasses daily—is especially important because it helps plump the cells of the skin, making them look smoother and younger, says Kathy A. Fields, M.D., clinical instructor of dermatology at the University of California, San Francisco. Equally important to making the skin look plump, she adds, is good humidity in the air around you.

Sunscreen, of course, is essential. It's the only way to prevent future damage because it blocks the sun's ultraviolet radiation. This is important because sun exposure accounts for about 90 percent of all skin cancers. Doctors advise applying sunscreen lavishly after your moisturizer but at least 30 minutes prior to sun exposure and reapply every 2 hours. Choose products that block both UVA and UVB rays and that have a sun protection factor (SPF) of at least 15. (For more information about sunscreens, see chapter 9.)

Wearing sunscreen and generally taking care of your health are just the beginning for healthy-looking skin. The skin naturally breaks down over time, especially after menopause, when declines in estrogen cause the skin to lose elasticity. Genetic factors also play a role: If the men and women in your family have a lot of wrinkles, you have a higher chance of developing them, too.

This doesn't mean that you're at the mercy of time, however. In the past few years, cosmetics companies have created hundreds of rejuvenating products that really can protect the skin, reverse wrinkles, and generally make you look younger.

Some products have been exhaustively tested and proven to work. Others look good in the bottle, and the labels make them *sound* effective, but there's little evidence that they make a difference. The only way to know which products to take seriously is to understand a little bit of the science behind them. To make things easy, we've created an easy-to-follow six-step plan.

You'll learn which products to look for, and how to use them to get the best results.

WHAT TO DO IF YOU HAVE ONLY **5 MINUTES**

Rather than experiment with dozens of anti-wrinkle products, go straight to Renova, which has been proven to work, says Lisa Kates, M.D., a dermatologist at Cook County Hospital and in private practice in Chicago.

Available from dermatologists, Renova is a better moisturizer than Retin-A because it is in an emollient base, and it works just as well at removing fine wrinkles, she says.

Step 1: Start with a Cleanser

The skin needs to be clean to be healthy, so it's important to use cleansers to gently wash away dust, makeup, and surface oils.

Use nonsoap cleansers. They're much less drying than regular soaps. David J. Leffell, M.D., chief of dermatologic surgery at Yale University School of Medicine and author of *Total Skin*, recommends Neutrogena Extra Gentle Cleanser, Aquanil, or Cetaphil.

Exfoliate after age 40. The skin naturally sheds its top layer, uncovering the fresh, youthful-looking layer underneath. In women under age 40, this shedding occurs every 30 days. After age 40, it slows to every 60 days, which makes the skin dry, the pores clogged and enlarged, and the skin dull and sallow. You can, however, speed up the process by using a scrub soap.

Scrub soaps contain tiny polyethylene beads, which gently remove dead cells and moisturize the skin. Don't bother with scrub soaps that contain pits from almonds or walnuts, Dr. Fields advises. They can actually damage the skin.

If you're 40 years or older, you can use gentle scrub soaps every day, says Dr. Fields. If you're under 40, use them only once a week or as needed.

Step 2: Use a Moisturizer

Before using any anti-aging skin product, it's worth giving moisturizers a try, says Dr. Fields. They add moisture and plumpness to cells on the surface, which makes the skin softer.

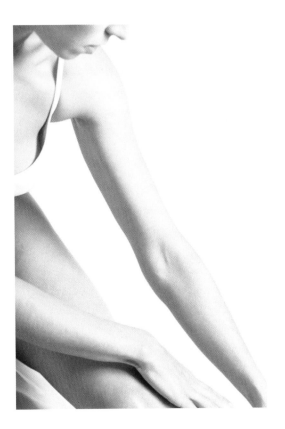

Use oil-free products. They contain an ingredient called dimethicone. It's a type of silicone that gives moisturizers a light feel, Dr. Fields says. A good example would be Oil of Olay.

Keep your moisturizers simple. If you have sensitive skin, avoid moisturizers loaded with fragrances and extracts. Check the label: It should list fewer than 10 ingredients, says Dr. Fields. Cetaphil is a good choice as a moisturizer for sensitive skin, as well as Eucerin and Almay products.

If you still want the luxurious feel of moisturizers made with green tea or other extracts, but you aren't sure how your skin will react, test them on a small area of skin on your neck near the ear.

Apply the moisturizer a few nights in a row. If you don't have any irritation, redness, or itching, it will be fine to use on your entire face.

Moisturize after showers or baths. The moisturizer will form a barrier over the moisture that's already on your skin, which gives it time to be absorbed by the cells, says Dr. Leffell.

Step 3: Fight Wrinkles Naturally

Many anti-aging products claim to "erase" wrinkles and make the skin look years younger. Some of this is marketing hype, but there's good evidence that products that contain natural acids (alpha or beta hydroxy acids) really can erase fine lines or brown spots, at least temporarily. They work by exfoliating the superficial layers of skin and can actually stimulate collagen production, which plumps up the skin and makes it look softer and fresher, says Lisa Kates, M.D., a dermatologist at Cook County Hospital and in private practice in Chicago.

Alpha hydroxy acids come in moisturizers, eye creams, and many other products. Terms to look for on labels include glycolic acid (derived from sugarcane), lactic acid (from milk), tartaric acid (from grapes), citric acid (from citrus fruits), malic acid (from apples), and mandelic acid (from walnuts). You may want to look for products that contain salicylic acid, which is a beta hydroxy acid. In women with sensitive skin, some of these products can be irritating.

Use a mild product first. Over-the-counter (OTC) products can have acid concentrations up to 10 percent, while stronger versions, usually available by prescription only, have concentrations up to 30 percent, says Ira Davis, M.D., assistant professor of dermatology at New York Medical College in Valhalla. The acids can be ir-

---

THREE THINGS I TELL EVERY FEMALE PATIENT

KATHY A. FIELDS, M.D., is a clinical instructor of dermatology at the University of California, San Francisco. She offers women the following advice for achieving fresher and younger-looking skin.

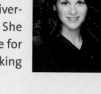

USE AN EXFOLIANT SCRUB. It's fine to use regular soap on your hands, but for your face, use a gentle scrub. Use it once a week or as needed if you are under 40 and every day if you are over 40. It is safe to use daily and makes your skin glow.

2

1 ALWAYS USE SUNSCREEN. Choose a product that blocks both UVA and UVB light. Don't be afraid to use too much. Apply a thick, even layer 30 minutes before you go outside, and reapply every 2 hours if you are in the sun all day.

USE A MOISTURIZER DAILY. It's among the best ways to keep the skin looking healthy. You may want to buy a moisturizer that contains either alpha hydroxy acids, retinol, or kinetin, which will remove old skin cells and brown spots and hydrate the skin. ∎

3

ritating, so it's a good idea to start with a low-concentration product, then move up to something stronger if you need to. Be patient. It may take 6 to 8 weeks to see a difference.

Products with alpha or beta hydroxy acids make the skin more sensitive to sunshine because the top layer of skin is thinned, which allows more ultraviolet radiation to penetrate. Although other factors, such as the amount of melanin, also affect the skin's tendency to reflect or absorb harmful rays, it's essential to use a sunscreen and avoid excessive sun exposure when using these products, says Dr. Davis. Chemical-free sunscreens, such as those containing tita-

nium dioxide or zinc oxide, may be the best choice since other sunscreen ingredients may irritate the skin.

Use furfuryladenine. It's a plant compound that moisturizes the skin, and research suggests it can help improve fine lines or even out skin tone. Look for products that contain N6-furfuryladenine or kinetin (its chemical name), says Dr. Fields. Kinerase and Almay Kinetin are two brands you may find at your local drugstore.

Try something stronger. Over-the-counter aging products usually have such low concentrations of active ingredients that the benefits may

The New Wrinkle Fighter

reducing fine lines and regaining a smoother, younger complexion: Those are the promises of alpha hydroxy acids (AHAs), one of the main ingredients in most age-erasing cosmetics. The downside: These ingredients tend to be harsh on skin.

But you won't find this side effect in products containing the next generation of wrinkle fighters. Researchers say amphoteric hydroxy complexes (AHCs) will give you all the benefits of AHAs, with virtually none of the common side effects, such as stinging, irritation, and redness.

"The stinging associated with AHAs is thought to be caused by the rapid absorption of the acid into the skin," says Barbara Green, R.Ph., who worked on the clinical studies with NeoStrata and Cognis, the companies that first developed AHCs. These new complexes are AHAs combined

with an amino acid that slows the release of the active ingredients into the skin, making them less likely to irritate, explains Green.

"I'm finding that AHCs are great for people with somewhat sensitive skin who have had problems using AHAs in the past," says Linda K. Franks, M.D., assistant clinical professor of dermatology at the New York University School of Medicine in New York City. They can also be great for use on particularly delicate skin, such as the eye area, she says.

This combination of AHAs with amino acids is currently available in Exuviance skin products, available in department stores and salons or by calling (800) 225-9411. They are also available in Nicole Miller Skin Care products, available by calling toll-free (888) 264-2653, or visiting their Web site at www.nicolemiller.com. ∎

be minimal, says Dr. Fields. To change the structure of the skin, you may want to try prescription products that contain tretinoin, such as Renova or Retin-A. These medicines have been studied for more than a decade, and excellent clinical studies have shown that they enhance the structure and function of the skin, says Dr. Fields. They increase collagen production, lighten brown spots, slough off dead skin cells, decrease fine lines, and improve overall texture and tone. Products with tretinoin can dry or irritate the skin, so start slowly, using it just 2 or 3 nights a week, and increase to nightly as tolerated, advises Dr. Fields.

Drugstores carry OTC products with retinol, which is lower in strength than tretinoin and generally well-tolerated. Retinol is converted to active retinoids in the skin and is an excellent start for improvement in texture, tone, and pore size. One of the myths regarding retinol and tretinoin is that they cannot be used if you are trying to tan. Research shows that they are helpful in preventing collagen damage while you're in the sun and therefore can be used daily with good sun protection, says Dr. Fields.

Step 4: Bleaches for Skin Spots

After decades of sun exposure, nearly everyone will develop pigment-related problems, such as age spots or freckles. It isn't always possible to eliminate them completely, but they can almost always be faded to the point of invisibility with bleaching creams.

These products contain active ingredients such as hydroquinone or kojic acid, which interfere with pigment formation, Dr. Kates says. Kojic acid is found in Nu Skin Skin-Brightening Complex and other products. For the most part, it doesn't work as well as hydroquinone. Prescription-strength hydroquinone tends to give better results than over-the-counter products.

Hydroquinone is available in prescription as well as in OTC products, such as Porcelana. It's very effective at fading most age spots and must be used with a good UVA and UVB sunscreen, says Dr. Fields. To get the best results, she advises using prescription hydroquinone in combination with OTC products containing kojic acid. Use daily or twice per day as tolerated and avoid the sun, or the brown spots and age spots will return within hours.

WHAT WORKS FOR ME

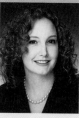

LESLIE BAUMANN, M.D., *is director of cosmetic dermatology at the University of Miami Cosmetic Center. Here's how she keeps her skin looking young.*

I use Retin-A at night, and Eucerin Q_{10} Anti-Wrinkle Sensitive Skin facial moisturizer underneath my sunscreen. Eucerin's active ingredient, coenzyme Q_{10}, is an antioxidant. There haven't been enough solid studies to show whether it offers real benefits topically. Still, I love how it feels as a moisturizer. ▪

Step 5: Freshen Up with Masks or Peels

Over the centuries, women have used an incredible number of natural products to make masks—skin-coating slurries—that remove oils from the skin. Masks leave your face feeling clean and refreshed. Peels are somewhat different. They remove the top layer of skin, as well as lighten some brown spots.

Choose the right mask. When you're shopping for mask products at the cosmetics counter, it's important to find one that matches your skin type. If you have dry skin, buy a hydrating mask. For oily skin, use clay masks or "deep cleansers." For acne, use a sulfur or "purifying" mask.

Make your own. If you enjoy the feel of fresh ingredients on your skin, it's easy to make your own masks. One you may want to try is *Prevention* magazine's Tropical Fruit Masque. It includes pineapple and papaya, natural sources of alpha hydroxy acids.

To make the mask, use a blender or food processor to puree 1 cup of fresh pineapple and ½ cup of slightly green fresh papaya. Add 2 tablespoons of honey, and mix thoroughly.

Test a small amount on your inner arm to be sure you aren't sensitive. Leave it on for 20 minutes. If your skin doesn't get red or itchy, go ahead and apply. Wash your face thoroughly, spread the mixture evenly over your face, avoiding the eye area, and leave it on for 5 minutes. Then rinse with cool water. You can repeat the treatment once a week.

Get a glycolic acid peel. Performed by dermatologists, this is sometimes called the "lunch-

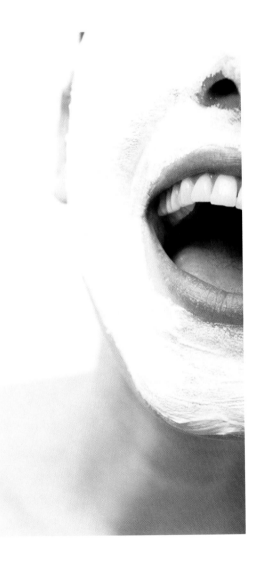

Masks leave your face feeling **clean** and **refreshed**.

time peel" because it works so quickly. The dermatologist will apply glycolic acid to your face, which removes dead cells and quickly uncovers the younger, smoother skin underneath. The peel tingles, but it isn't uncomfortable, says Seth L. Matarasso, M.D., associate clinical professor of dermatology at the University of California, San Francisco, and a dermatologist in San Francisco. Peels cost between $75 and $150, and you can get them as often as once a month.

Try a chemical-free peel (micro-dermabrasion). Your dermatologist will use a very fine brush to exfoliate the top layer of skin. It's very relaxing, takes 10 to 15 minutes, and your skin will look (and feel) younger almost instantly. The cost is usually about $150 to $200, and you can repeat it monthly.

Get longer-lasting results. Many women want to have fresher, younger-looking skin, but they don't want to spend a lot of time on home or professional treatments. One option is to have a peel called the trichloracetic peel. It's performed by a dermatologist or plastic surgeon, and it will improve the appearance of the skin for as long as a year, says James W. Goodnight, M.D., director of the Facial Plastics Center in Teaneck, New Jersey. The procedure takes under an hour.

This is one procedure that you won't want to have done during your lunch break. The skin will burn during the procedure, and it will peel off in large pieces in the days to come. Women who have this treatment usually plan to stay close to home for about a week, until the peeling is complete. It costs between $300 and $600.

Step 6: Say Goodbye to Puffy Eyes

Few things can make you look more tired (or older) than puffy eyes. They're usually caused by such things as fatigue, water retention, allergies, or even a reaction to eye makeup. To quickly tighten the skin and help your eyes look younger, here's what doctors advise.

Try grape seed extract. It's found in Caudalie's products, jO_2 Firming Lotion, and Napa Valley Spa products. Some people report good results from their personal experience, and preliminary studies suggest that applying grape seed extract to the skin can reduce eye puffiness caused by water retention or poor circulation. As a bonus, it helps smooth the complexion and may protect against the sun's harmful rays. It can be used nightly.

Reduce puffiness with tea bags. Brew a cup of tea using two tea bags. Set the bags aside until they're cool, then place them on the puffy areas of your eyes for a few minutes. The cool moisture can reduce swelling for up to 24 hours. In addition, tea contains tannins, compounds that reduce eye inflammation, says Dr. Matarasso.

You can get similar effects by placing cool cucumber slices or even cooled spoons on the puffy areas, Dr. Matarasso adds.

Balancing Your Emotions

Imagine a time when you felt at peace. Relaxed. Content. Free of worry. Now imagine that you could feel that way every day.

Sounds impossible? It's not. You can balance your emotions.

Although psychologists have different views of what constitutes emotional balance, they agree that it involves spending more time at peace than blowing up in anger, writhing with jealousy, or being dragged down by sadness.

"Internally, we all have a central home base," says Terry Murphy, Psy.D., assistant clinical professor in the department of community health and aging at Temple University in Philadelphia. "It's a state of normal calm and contentment."

No one spends all their time in that peaceful zone, of course. Life is full of conflicts. But a reasonable goal—one that any woman can achieve—is to return to that soothing home base after a setback, such as a clash with a coworker or a disagreement with your husband.

You'll feel better immediately, but that's not the only benefit. You'll also enjoy better health. Negative emotions such as anger and anxiety can weaken the immune system and leave you vulnerable to illness. Stress and tension also increase the risk of high blood pressure, heart disease, and dozens of other serious conditions.

Experts don't suggest that women should never get mad, jealous, or sad. What you can do is minimize the amount of time that you spend experiencing these or other negative emotions. In just six steps, you can strengthen your ability to handle any situation with calm and confidence.

Step 1: Take an Emotional Inventory

Before you start working on your emotional skills, it's helpful to know just how balanced you already are. Start with a quiz.

1. **How often do you feel physically healthy, energetic, and well-rested?**

   A. Almost every day

   B. About 50 percent of the time

   C. Rarely

2. **How often do you experience the gamut of emotions: sadness, guilt, fear, joy, love, and excitement?**

   A. Every week

   B. Every month

   C. I can't remember the last time I felt some of those emotions

3. **How often do you express your emotions to other people?**

   A. Only when I think it's appropriate

   B. Only when the emotions are strong

   C. All the time

4. **How often do you feel physically or emotionally numb after an activity, such as watching television, exercising, working, browsing the Internet, or reading a book?**

   A. Hardly ever

   B. Once in a while

   C. Every day

5. **When you're sad, what are you most likely to do?**

   A. I look for people to be with

   B. I spend time with others, if it's convenient

   C. I'd rather stay home when I'm sad

6. **How often do you find yourself struggling to do things that were easy in the past, such as balancing the checkbook or completing projects on time?**

   A. Only when stress is very high

   B. Once in a while, but not regularly

   C. Regularly

7. **Do your spouse, family, children, and close friends support you?**

   A. Every day

   B. Only when I really need them

   C. Not enough

8. **How often do you ask friends and family for help?**

   A. Daily or weekly

   B. Monthly

   C. Only when I'm desperate

9. **Do you have hobbies?**

   A. Yes, and I do them regularly

   B. One or two, which I tend to neglect

   C. There's no time for hobbies

Step 2: Identify Your Emotional Strengths and Weaknesses

If you answered all of the quiz questions honestly, you'll have a pretty good sense of how good a job you're doing staying balanced. If most of your answers were A, congratulations: You're on the right track. If most of the answers were B, you could use a little work—and this chapter will help. If most of your answers were C, you're going to have to try harder to find your emotional center.

Let's take a moment to look at each of the quiz questions to see how they measure emotional health and wellness.

Question 1. Negative emotions frequently result in physical symptoms. It's normal, for example, for people to feel tired or lethargic before they actually feel the underlying emotions, such as anger or rage. When you're feeling physically "off" and there's no good reason for it, it's likely that your emotions are out of balance.

Question 2. Many people don't feel comfortable with certain emotions, such as anger or jealousy. These feelings still have to come out, however. What people often do is transfer their energy to another emotion, such as guilt, says Vivien D. Wolsk, Ph.D., a clinical psychologist and dean of faculty of the Gestalt Center for Psychotherapy and Training in New York City. Soon guilt will overwhelm you because it's the only emotion you allow yourself to feel.

Question 3. Expressing emotions to others is important. This doesn't mean blowing your temper at the slightest provocation, of course. Nor does it mean you should always say exactly what's on your mind. In healthy human relations, emotions have to be expressed appropriately, says Dr. Murphy. Suppose, for example, that your husband says something that annoys you. If it's a minor issue, the healthy thing would be to respond to it as if it *is* a minor issue. If you overreact and go into a rage, your emotional balance is a little off, and your relationships are going to suffer.

Question 4. Most people have ways of coping with emotional troughs. A common strategy is to numb negative emotions, such as guilt or anger, by engaging in routine activities—watching television, working extra-long hours, or even exercising long past the point you'd normally quit, says Lisa Firestone, Ph.D., a clinical psychologist and education and program director at the Glendon Association in Santa Barbara, California. When you're in this defensive state, you push away the people who can help you through rough times.

Question 5. Negative thoughts become more powerful when you're alone. And the more powerful the thoughts become, the less likely you are to seek out human contact. That's why therapists advise people who are feeling blue to spend time with others. Even if you decide not to talk about your problems, the simple human contact will boost your mind and even relieve mild depression.

Question 6. When you're emotionally out of balance, concentration and focus diminish. Tasks that should be easy become increasingly difficult and fatiguing.

Question 7. Women are responsible for a lot these days. They keep the house clean. Take care

A Quick Course in Anger Management

In the traditional view, women aren't supposed to get mad. Maybe that's why women often cry instead of confronting the person who is pushing their buttons. Why they're nice to people who have insulted them. Or, in some cases, why they blow their tops at the slightest provocation—because the pent-up anger just has to come out.

Whether you express your anger or suppress it, there are a number of ways to understand it and keep it at healthful levels.

Use anger as a signal. Rather than push anger away, figure out what it's telling you, says Vivien D. Wolsk, Ph.D., a clinical psychologist and dean of faculty at the Gestalt Center for Psychotherapy and Training in New York City. Say to

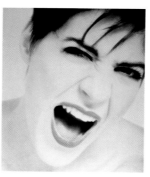

yourself, "I'm angry because something's wrong here." It will help you figure out what needs fixing.

Think before you act. Feeling the emotion isn't the same as acting on it. When you're boiling with rage, ask yourself if this is the time and place to express it. You may want to go to a private place to vent. Or take a long walk to think things over.

Confront the source. There's nothing wrong with confronting people who have made you angry, says Dr. Wolsk. Wait until you cool off. Then explain how their words or actions made you feel. As long as you approach people calmly and with a genuine desire to work things out, they'll usually work with you to find a solution. ■

of children. Do the shopping. And all this is often on top of working at jobs outside the home. If you aren't getting a lot of support in your life, your emotions—and your health—are going to suffer.

Question 8. "Women expect themselves to be able to handle everything," Dr. Murphy says. "They haven't given themselves permission to ask for help."

Feeling uncomfortable with or overwhelmed by your workload is a red flag. Not only does it mean that your physical and emotional resilience is needlessly being sapped, but it also means that you're not taking responsibility for getting the help you need.

Question 9. Hobbies—such as collecting antiques, bird-watching, or writing short stories—are a great way to incorporate downtime into your life. If you don't have a few hobbies that you enjoy, there's a good chance that you're spending too much time working, caring for others, or generally assuming the burdens of the world.

Step 3: Keep a Journal

If you completed the quiz above, you have a pretty good sense of your emotional strengths and weaknesses. But that's just the beginning. Inside everyone are vast, subterranean networks of emotions. These emotions guide everything you do—and everything you think and feel. To find and maintain your emotional balance, it's essential to understand what's happening deep inside—and keeping a journal is a great place to start.

Studies have shown, for example, that people who write in journals, especially about the traumas in their lives, report feeling better about themselves. An increasing number of psychologists and psychiatrists have begun incorporating journal writing into their practices as a treatment for depression and anxiety disorders.

There are no formal rules for keeping a journal. In fact, the opposite is true—your personality and desire for creativity should be your guides. To get started:

Please your personality. Your journal can be leather-bound or made of recycled paper. It might have leopard-print designs or flower petals on the pages. It can be as simple as a spiral notebook. Everyone has different tastes—and this is your chance to indulge them.

Write as much or as little as you like. You don't have to write in a journal every day to achieve emotional balance. There isn't a prescribed number of words you should write. Keeping a journal is simply a tool, and it's up to you decide how it works best for you, says Susan Heitler, Ph.D., a clinical psychologist and author of the book *From Conflict to Resolution* and the audiotape *Anxiety: Friend or Foe.*

On one day, for example, you might sit down to write—and realize that you don't have a lot to say, maybe only a sentence or two. That's fine. On another day, especially one with a lot of emotional challenges, you might find yourself writing page after page as you think about what happened, what people said, and how you reacted to everything.

Put it on your schedule. While it's best to avoid feeling obligated to write in a journal, it's often helpful to set aside certain times when

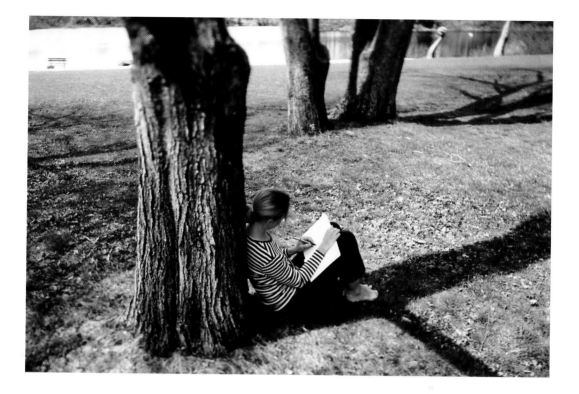

THREE THINGS I TELL EVERY FEMALE PATIENT

LISA FIRESTONE, Ph.D., a clinical psychologist and education and program director at the Glendon Association in Santa Barbara, California, offers this advice for achieving emotional balance.

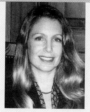

1 **ACCEPT ALL YOUR EMOTIONS, THE GOOD AND THE BAD.** Nobody chooses to feel a certain way, she says. Allow yourself to experience all of your feelings—including emotions typically labeled as negative, such as hostility and anger. Accept all of your emotions, but know that you choose your behavior in response to them.

2 **MOVE BEYOND NEGATIVE THOUGHTS.** Everyone is self-critical at times. Pay attention to how you criticize yourself, and expose these thoughts to a more rational evaluation. Write them down or tell them to a friend. It is important to act in your own self-interest, not on negative self-critical thoughts. Taking action in your own self-interest can help combat these thoughts.

3 **MAKE A LIST OF THE ACTIVITIES AND PEOPLE THAT BRING YOU JOY.** Then make a list of those that bring negative emotions. Look at the lists daily—and do everything you can to embrace the "good" and avoid the "bad." ∎

you're going to write—first thing in the morning, for example, or right after dinner. If you miss an "appointment," fine—but setting a schedule will make it easier to keep at it.

Date the pages. Some journals have the dates already on the pages. If yours doesn't, jot down the dates, including the year, you're writing. When you review your journal entries months or even years later, the dates will provide fascinating insights into what you were thinking or feeling at different stages of your life.

Write anything. Nearly everyone experiences writer's block when they first start keeping a journal, says Dr. Heitler. This might be the time to remind yourself that you're not trying to create literature for the ages but only trying to explore and understand your innermost feelings.

Still blocked? Dr. Heitler suggests that you close your eyes for a moment and imagine a stressful situation in your life. That's your topic: Describe the situation in as few or as many words as you wish. Once you start, you'll probably find that the words will flow faster than you can write them down.

Step 4: Create Pockets of Tranquillity throughout the Day

In today's busy world, it's easy to get so caught up in responsibilities that you never set aside quiet times for yourself. Women who don't take time to recharge their physical and emotional batteries will experience ever-escalating amounts of stress and tension.

Getting a Grip on Guilt

guilt is what you feel when you've done something wrong or when you are toying with the idea of doing something wrong. It's what you feel when you call in sick at work to go shopping with a friend or fantasize about having an affair with an attractive man.

Women suffer from guilt to a disproportionate degree, says Karen Clark-Schock, Psy.D., a licensed psychologist, board-certified art therapist, and associate professor and director of the art therapy program at the University of the Arts in Philadelphia. "I think that it comes from feeling as though they can never do enough."

Women are raised to be caretakers, Dr. Clark-Schock explains. As a result, women focus on the needs of others. And when the other person isn't happy, for whatever reason, women can feel responsible, thinking either that they caused the unhappiness or that they must fix it or solve it—or both.

As with many emotions, guilt can easily take on a life of its own, especially if you don't talk about it. One of the best ways to come to terms with guilt and to shrink it to a manageable size is to discuss your feelings with others, be it a friend, family member, or therapist, advises Dr. Clark-Schock. The guilt that looms so large in your own mind will probably appear pretty small to others. Plus, your friends can share their own guilty secrets—which will put your own in perspective. ■

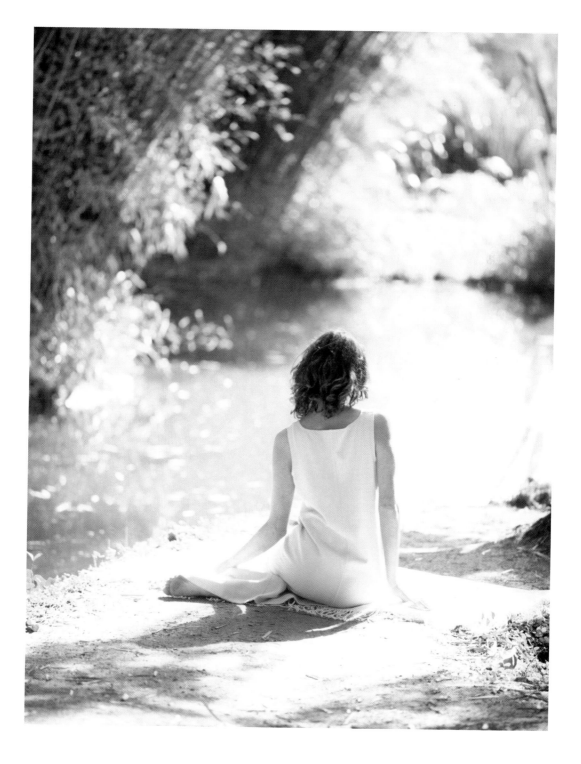

It may feel like an indulgence to give yourself some daily quiet time, but it's not: It's as important for good health as eating nutritious foods or getting a good night's sleep. Here are some places to start.

Take the time to breathe deeply. According to a proverb, "He who half breathes, half lives." It's extremely common for women to briefly hold their breath when they're under stress—or to breathe shallowly throughout the day. Apart from the fact that shallow breathing doesn't supply the body and brain with the necessary oxygen, doing so also makes it more difficult to experience emotions fully, says Dr. Wolsk.

She advises women to set aside a few minutes each day to do nothing but breathe deeply. Breathe in through your nose, and keep taking in air until your abdomen swells. Hold the breath for just a moment, then slowly exhale through your mouth. This technique, called diaphragmatic breathing, floods the tissues with oxygen and makes it possible to get in touch with your emotional life, she explains.

Find a safe place. When you're overwhelmed with a negative emotion, it helps to have a private room or place to let the emotion out. When you're feeling sad or depressed at home, for example, you might want to retreat to the bathroom and have a long, hot shower. At work, people often retreat for a few moments to an empty of-

New Help for Bipolar Disorder

We all experience emotional ups and down—feelings of elation followed by troughs of sadness. For most of us, these emotional swings are triggered by real-life events: getting a raise at work or a compliment from a supervisor might be followed by finding out a roof needs repair. We deal with the emotions, then get on with our lives.

For people with bipolar disorder, however, the emotional swings come out of the blue—and the emotions may be so extreme that it's almost impossible for people to function normally without medical help, says Francis Mark Mondimore, M.D., assistant professor in the department of psychiatry and behavioral science at Johns Hopkins University School of Medicine in Baltimore and author of *Bipolar Disorder: A Guide for Patients and Families.*

People with bipolar disorder—an estimated 1 percent of Americans have this condition—may go from being profoundly depressed to being wildly elated, or manic. During the depressive stage, they may lose their appetite and have little interest in their normal activities. When they're manic, they almost seethe with energy. They can't keep up with their own thoughts, they have little need for sleep, and they may have hallucinations.

A generation ago, there weren't a lot of treatments for bipolar disorder. Today, with a combination of medications and lifestyle changes—such as avoiding alcohol, getting enough sleep, and exercising regularly—many people with this condition are able to keep it under control, says Dr. Mondimore. ■

WHAT TO DO IF YOU HAVE ONLY **5 MINUTES**

Set aside at least 5 minutes every day to meditate and get away from the distractions of the world, says Lucy Papillon, Ph.D., a clinical psychologist, author of *When Hope Can Kill: Reclaiming Your Soul in a Romantic Relationship*, and director of the Center of Light in Beverly Hills, California.

Find a quiet place that's free of distractions, she advises. Close your eyes, or maybe look at the flame of a candle. Allow your thoughts to float through your mind, but don't dwell on them. If you practice this regularly, you'll find that you'll be able to disregard self-critical thoughts and self-destructive emotions, no matter where they come from or when they arrive.

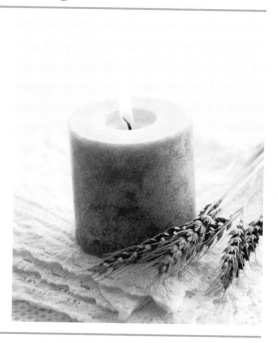

fice or even to their car. Giving yourself the time to escape makes it possible to release negative emotions as they accumulate, rather than allowing them to build and surge throughout the day, says Dr. Wolsk.

Move your body. Any kind of exercise— walking up and down stairs, raking a few leaves, jogging in place—increases your breathing rate and triggers the release of endorphins, chemicals in the brain that help regulate mood.

Don't wait until you're stressed to start moving. Women who get aerobic exercise four or more times a week will feel physically and emotionally stronger, says Dr. Wolsk.

Give yourself positive messages. Everyone deals with a lot of negativity throughout the day, and it's normal to feel overwhelmed and frustrated. Over time, however, these negative feelings can begin to take over—which is why it's so important to remind yourself of how strong and special you really are," says Lucy Papillon, Ph.D., a clinical psychologist, author of *When Hope Can Kill: Reclaiming Your Soul in a Romantic Relationship*, and director of the Center of Light in Beverly Hills, California. "It could end up being a self-fulfilling prophecy," she says.

"When you're having a tough time, tell yourself, 'This is hard, but I have the strength to get through it,'" she advises.

Step 5: Plan and Conquer

Emotional stress and negative emotions come in infinite forms, and they're often unpredictable. But that doesn't mean you can't anticipate them—and plan ahead for how you're going to deal with them.

Imagine, for example, that you're blindsided at work—by a difficult coworker, for example, or an unexpected problem with a supervisor. On top of the challenge of working things out, you'll also have to deal with the rush of adrenaline and other stress hormones that are released when the unexpected hits. Multiply this by a few dozen times a day, and it's easy to see why so many women feel embattled and exhausted.

You can't anticipate all the specific problems you're likely to face every day, but you probably have a few emotional hot buttons in your life—things that consistently sap your strength and batter your emotions. If you take a few minutes to plan your coping strategies ahead of time, you'll be less likely to be taken by surprise—and you may be able to circumvent the problems altogether. Whatever the issue is, plan ahead for it by identifying at least three alternative ways to approach it.

Put the Brakes on Anxiety

anxiety is a normal reaction to threatening situations. For some women, however, the emotion is so intense or frequent that they find it difficult to go about their lives.

Doctors estimate that 19 million Americans, a majority of them women, suffer from anxiety disorders. These can result in panic attacks, a racing heart, nausea, chest pain, dizziness, and other symptoms. The attacks can be so severe that people rush to emergency rooms because they think they're having a heart attack.

A full-fledged anxiety disorder is a serious problem that requires medical attention. In most cases, however, women can control mild-to-moderate anxiety with a few simple steps.

Prepare yourself. Some things in life, like job interviews or talking to groups of people, are especially likely to provoke anticipation anxiety. One of the best ways to control it is to be as prepared as possible—by rehearsing a presentation ahead of time, for example, or by learning more about the company you're applying to, says Susan Heitler, Ph.D., a clinical psychologist and author of the book *From Conflict to Resolution* and the audiotape *Anxiety: Friend or Foe*.

Take some deep breaths. It's one of the best ways to reduce shortness of breath, a speeding heart, or other anxiety symptoms, says Brenda Wiederhold, Ph.D., executive director of the Virtual Reality Medical Center in San Diego.

Stop irrational thoughts. People often feel anxious because of what experts call "catastrophic thinking"—the belief that the worst is about to happen.

When this is happening to you, imagine a red flashing light—and mentally yell "Stop!" advises Dr. Wiederhold. At the same time, distract yourself—by counting backward from 100, for example. Your mind will find it difficult to return to the same troublesome thoughts, she explains. ∎

When you plan your options, you'll be much more likely to achieve your goals—and you'll also feel stronger and more confident, she explains.

Plan your words. Confrontation is a fact of life. Hardly a day goes by when you don't have to deal with uncomfortable situations: a mail-order package that didn't arrive when it was supposed to; a friend who always says something inappropriate; a neighbor who plays loud music late at night. Just thinking about it gets you upset—and the tension keeps building.

Plan ahead of time what you'll say. You'll be less likely to respond in the heat of the moment (which can make a bad situation worse), and you'll also feel more confident about your ability to handle it.

You can't eliminate confrontation, but as long as you plan for it and give yourself choices, you'll always feel you are in charge—and that's an essential part of keeping your emotions in a healthy balance.

Step 6: Practice the Art of Acceptance

Women who achieve a sense of control in their lives are often amazed by how much stronger and confident they feel. Unfortunately, there are thousands of things we all wish we could control—everything from dress size to the behavior of teenagers—but can't. Sometimes you just have to accept that some things are out of your hands.

Allow yourself to feel your emotions. Emotions are going to come and go whether you want them to or not. Instead of pushing uncomfortable emotions away, be honest and allow yourself to feel them. Cry when you're sad. Don't automatically say "fine" when someone asks how you're doing. Admit it when you're depressed or anxious.

"People believe that if they feel an emotion, it will take over," Dr. Firestone says. But being aroused emotionally can last only so long. The sooner you allow yourself to feel an emotion, the sooner it will go on its way.

Be good to yourself. And say it with words. Every morning, look in the mirror and say something positive: "I appreciate you" or "I love you." Saying things out loud helps them become real, says Dr. Wolsk.

Remember the anchors in your life. When things feel like they're spinning out of control, take an inventory of all the things that you know are solid and reliable: Your child is safe on the bus; your car will get you to work on time; your computer will turn on and work. When you realize how much in your life is dependable, you'll have more trust in your ability to work through life's problems, says Dr. Murphy.

Healthy Sex at Any Age

Sex therapists say that most women— whether they're young or old, single or married—have one thing in common: They want to be more in touch with their sexuality.

Sex helps women feel intimacy. Intimacy creates passion, and passion is sexually satisfying.

Sex also helps women feel more feminine, more attractive, and closer to their partners.

"For many women, living without an intimate sexual relationship is like living without chocolate or their favorite meal," says Bonnie Saks, M.D., clinical associate professor of psychiatry at the University of South Florida in Tampa.

After reviewing research on women's sexuality, including a survey of more than 2,600 women, researchers concluded that women in general are sexually satisfied. Although women and men tend to have sex less often as they get older, sex and intimacy remain just as important in their lives.

Low energy, menopausal discomfort, and side effects from medications are just a few of the factors that may get in the way of good sex—but they don't have to. Here's a three-step plan that will help keep your passion at healthy and satisfying levels.

Step 1: Accept Your Sexuality

Some women were raised to think of sex as something "forbidden" or improper. Some feel that it's inappropriate for a woman to express her full range of sexual desires—or even to admit them to herself. These and other emotional barriers may prevent women from fully exploring—and enjoying—their sexuality.

Open your mind to possibilities. Sexuality is a natural part of who you are. You may choose how much or how little sex you have, but the feelings will always be there, says Marian Dunn, Ph.D., director of the Center for Human Sexu-

Drug "Cocktails" Are the Closest Thing to a Cure

It's hard to imagine that until about 20 years ago, no one had ever heard of AIDS. Although scientists first identified the human immunodeficiency virus (HIV, the virus that causes AIDS) in 1959, it wasn't until the late 1970s that it made its appearance in the United States.

Today more than 750,000 Americans have AIDS. People continue to think of AIDS as a "male" disease, but the rate of infection in women has increased steadily. In 1985, women accounted for 7 percent of AIDS cases; in 1999, they accounted for 23 percent. Ten percent of women infected with the AIDS virus are 45 years or older.

Most women get the virus from having sex with men who are infected or from injecting drugs with a contaminated syringe. Women who have other sexually transmitted diseases have a higher risk of being infected with the AIDS virus.

HIV can survive in the body for years without causing symptoms. In the early stages, the only way for a woman to know she's been exposed to the virus is to have a blood test.

Scientists have made tremendous progress in understanding the AIDS virus, but there still isn't a cure. However, it's often possible to dramatically reduce levels of the virus in the body by giving people a combination of antiviral drugs. There are many medications to choose from, so when one combination doesn't work, another probably will.

Until doctors find a way to beat the virus, the best strategy by far is prevention. For women who aren't in long-term, committed relationships, this means always using a condom during sex. Sex with a condom isn't as spontaneous as some women would like, but it's among the best ways to stay healthy and infection-free. ■

ality at State University of New York Downstate Medical Center in Brooklyn.

Millions of Americans—men and women alike—aren't entirely comfortable with their sexuality, she adds. One solution is to browse your favorite bookstore or online catalog. There are literally hundreds (if not thousands) of informative books that explore all aspects of female sexuality. You'll discover many emotional and physical possibilities that you may want to explore for yourself.

Love your body. Research has shown that body perceptions, positive as well as negative, strongly affect sexual satisfaction.

Few women are completely satisfied with their bodies—but don't let this hold you back. When you're with your partner, focus on the parts of your body that you feel good about, suggests Dr. Saks. It might be your soft skin or delicate hands, or the gentle curve of your neck. When you think about the things that please you most, you'll feel

Dealing with Herpes

When a woman diagnosed with herpes first learns that she's infected with the virus, she'll probably assume two things: that she'll suffer from frequent and painful outbreaks and that her current partner hasn't been faithful.

Neither is necessarily true. Although there isn't a cure for herpes, many women can live most of their lives free of outbreaks. And it's not uncommon for men and women to unknowingly harbor the virus for years or even decades without having symptoms, says Marian Dunn, Ph.D., director of the Center for Human Sexuality at State University of New York Downstate Medical Center in Brooklyn.

The herpesvirus often lives silently in the mouth or genitals. When an outbreak starts, a woman may experience itching or burning, pain in the legs or buttocks, or a feeling of pressure in the abdomen. After a few days, she may develop small, painful sores—either on the mouth or on the genitals, depending on the type of herpes she's infected with.

The first outbreak usually lasts for 2 to 3 weeks, but future episodes tend to be less severe. However, the virus is highly contagious during the active phase. A woman who has sex without a condom at that time could very well pass the virus to her partner.

Here are a few ways to ease the discomfort—and possibly prevent the outbreaks from occurring.

- The prescription drug acyclovir (Zovirax) can reduce the discomfort of outbreaks and shorten their duration. A prescription drug called famciclovir (Famvir) also treats herpes outbreaks, and may help prevent future attacks.

- Try aspirin. Taking 125 milligrams of aspirin at the first sign of cold sores (caused by the herpesvirus) may speed their healing time.

- Take soothing baths. Or gently dab the sores with a warm, moist towel. Applying moist heat is one of the best ways to reduce irritation. ■

more attractive, and feeling attractive will make you more confident and assured.

Conquer old memories. Negative feelings about sex are often caused by early experiences. For some women, it was sexual abuse; for others it was the outcome of having sex before they were fully ready. As a result, they see sex more as a service than as a means to self-fulfillment, says Dr. Saks.

One way to overcome these feelings is to let your partner know that you want more control in the bedroom. This might mean that you'll be the one to initiate sex, and you'll also take charge of setting the pace. Limit touch to only what is comfortable for you. As you gain a greater sense of control, your enjoyment will also increase, says Dr. Saks.

Step 2: Keep Your Body Healthy

It's hardly a coincidence that the line "Not tonight, I have a headache" has become a catchall cliché for avoiding sex. If you don't feel good physically, you aren't going to want to have sex—and you probably won't enjoy it very much when you do.

How do you maintain or improve your "sexual fitness"? By doing the things that promote your health overall.

Eat a healthful diet. Apart from preventing illnesses and improving energy, a diet that's high in essential nutrients and low in fat will make you feel better—and maybe sexier—overall, says Lily A. Arya, M.D., assistant professor of urogynecology at the University of Pennsylvania in Philadelphia.

THREE THINGS I TELL EVERY FEMALE PATIENT

MICHAEL PLAUT, Ph.D., is associate professor of psychiatry at the University of Maryland School of Medicine in Baltimore and past president of the Society for Sex Therapy and Research. Here's what he advises women who want to explore and renew their sexuality.

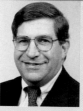

ALLOW INTIMACY TO HAPPEN. It's easy to get so caught up in life's responsibilities—overdue bills, looming deadlines, problems with the children—that you never really let yourself go. During intimate moments, try to focus entirely on the moment at hand. Deal with the responsibilities later.

2

1

COMMUNICATE WITH YOUR PARTNER. Men aren't mind readers. The only way your mate will know what pleases you—and what you don't like—is if you're honest and forthright about your preferences.

BE OPEN TO NEW THINGS. The sex that you enjoyed when you were 20 may not be what you enjoy today. Men and women are constantly changing, and there's no reason for sex and intimacy to stay the same. ■

3

Stay physically active. Regular exercise will relieve stress, improve your mood, and help you feel great about your body, says Yula Ponticas, Ph.D., a clinical psychologist in the Sexual Behaviors Consultation Unit at Johns Hopkins University School of Medicine in Baltimore. When researchers looked at women 50 years and older, they found that those with the highest levels of physical fitness were also the ones who enjoyed intimacy more often.

Protect yourself. Nothing dampens ardor faster than the thought of sexually transmitted diseases. Your best move: Always use a latex condom, whether or not you use other forms of birth control, says Michael Plaut, Ph.D., associate professor of psychiatry at the University of Mary-

The Pill versus Libido

When researchers from the Kinsey Institute for Research in Sex, Gender, and Reproduction, located in Bloomington, Indiana, followed 79 women who took birth control pills for a year, they found a life-altering side effect that women and their doctors usually don't mention: lowered libido and less sex.

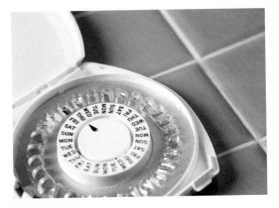

"There's currently no way to predict which women will experience adverse sexual or emotional side effects or which pills are more likely to cause them. We each have our own individual chemistry," says Stephanie Sanders, Ph.D., associate director of the institute and associate professor of gender studies at Indiana University, also in Bloomington. "The important message is this: If you like the convenience and reliability of oral contraceptives, you can usually work with your doctor to find a pill that's right for you—if you let her know what it is that's bothering you."

Here's how to preserve your sex life without discontinuing the Pill.

Discuss your symptoms with your doctor. Research shows that health professionals rarely discuss the emotional and sexual side effects of the Pill with their patients. Speak up.

Don't skip a dose. In addition to the obvious—an unplanned pregnancy—missed doses or irregular timing may cause hormonal fluctuations that could dampen your mood and sex drive.

Consider a switch. There are more than 45 different types of birth control pills sold in the United States. If one pill causes side effects, try another with a different type or amount of progestin. ∎

land School of Medicine in Baltimore and past president of the Society for Sex Therapy and Research. If you're in a long-term, committed relationship, of course, condoms probably aren't necessary unless you're using them for birth control or if one of you already has a chronic condition, such as herpes, that is transmitted through sexual contact.

Step 3: Give Nature an Assist

Lack of desire is the most common sexual problem for women. This may be caused by issues in the relationship, but it can also result from physical changes or underlying health problems.

When women approach menopause, the body's levels of estrogen begin to decline. This can result in vaginal dryness and more irritation. It can also result in hot flashes, insomnia, or other physical factors that can lower libido.

Start with lubrication. The vagina naturally produces less lubrication as menopause approaches; women who take low-dose birth control pills also may be too dry for comfort. Don't let this slow you down. Pharmacies stock a variety of water-based lubricants, which are safe and comfortable to use, says Dr. Saks.

Look into side effects. A number of medications—including some antidepressants, birth control pills, and drugs for controlling blood pressure—may inhibit sex drive in some women. If you've noticed a dip in your libido, ask your doctor if switching to a different prescription would be helpful, says Dr. Saks.

Ask about hormone tests. If your thyroid gland is underactive, you may have decreased levels of androgens, hormones that fuel the sex drive. Conversely, high levels of prolactin, a female hormone, also can cause libido to diminish. Your doctor can check hormone levels with a simple blood test—and if they're lower (or higher) than they should be, you may need medications to restore the proper balance.

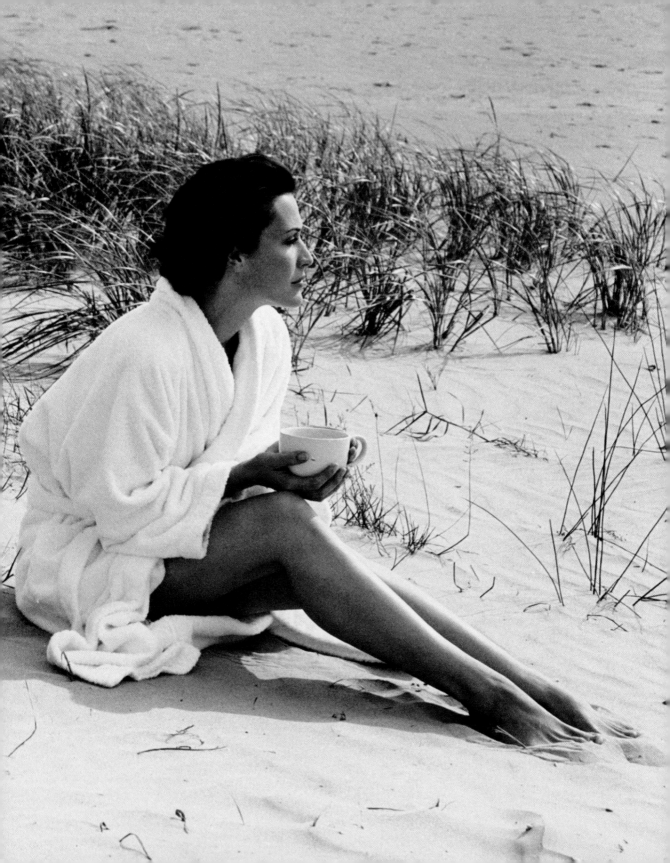

PRIMARY CARE:

ESSENTIAL

PROTECTION

AGAINST MAJOR

HEALTH THREATS

13

Heart Disease

If cancer tops your list of health worries, you're not alone. Studies have shown that women tend to overestimate their chances of getting cancer, and they fail to think enough about a much more serious health threat: heart disease.

More than one in two women will die from a stroke, heart attack, or other forms of cardiovascular disease. Cancer deserves serious attention, but it's a distant second to cardiovascular disease, which plagues about one in five women.

Even though heart disease threatens more American women (and men) than any other health condition, it's nearly always preventable. Studies have shown that women who follow a healthy lifestyle—refraining from smoking, exercising regularly, eating healthful foods, and so on—can slash their risk of heart disease by 82 percent.

Even if you're premenopausal, don't put off taking care of your heart. More than one in five women who have heart attacks are under age 65.

It's true that a woman's risk of heart disease increases as she gets older. After menopause, when the body's production of estrogen declines, there's an increase in atherosclerosis—the accumulation of fatty deposits in the arteries that can reduce blood-

flow and increase the risk of heart-damaging clots. But atherosclerosis actually starts much earlier.

"We see the beginnings of it in teenagers," says Rose Marie Robertson, M.D., professor of medicine and director of the Women's Heart Institute at Vanderbilt University Medical Center in Nashville. "Many women have the sense that they don't need to worry about heart disease until after menopause. But they may be ignoring risk factors that could be treated, such as high blood pressure or high cholesterol, because they don't think they have to worry about them yet."

Here's what the country's leading cardiologists say women should be doing, right now, to protect their hearts.

Lifestyle Strategies

Maintain a healthful weight. Many of us gain a little weight over time, but those extra pounds can substantially boost your risk for developing heart disease. Women who are overweight are much more likely to develop diabetes—and diabetes is one of the main risk factors for heart disease. Obesity also increases cholesterol and puts more strain on the heart.

Most women who are overweight know it. However, while the *amount* of extra weight is important, the way it's distributed on your frame also makes a difference. Doctors often use a guide called body mass index (BMI) to determine how close you are to your ideal weight. You'll find a detailed guide to calculating BMI on page 90. For now, just remember that your BMI should fall somewhere between 18.5 and 24.9, and your waist should measure less than 35 inches. If your waistline is larger than that and if your BMI is above 25, it's time to get serious about losing weight.

If you follow the guidelines in chapter 6, you'll find that losing weight doesn't have to be an all-consuming chore—and the more you lose, the healthier your heart will be.

Get serious about exercise. Every woman knows that exercise is important for health, but people don't always realize just how damaging a sedentary lifestyle can be, says Lori J. Mosca, M.D., Ph.D., associate professor of medicine and director of preventive cardiology at New York Presbyterian Hospital of Columbia University in New York City. Women who are sedentary have about twice the risk of heart disease as those who are physically active. Put another way, not getting regular exercise is potentially as harmful as smoking or having high cholesterol.

Obviously, vigorous activity is great for your heart—but what if you're not a serious athlete? Studies have shown that even modest levels of ac-

Angina: Heed This Warning Sign

about 4 million women suffer from angina, a condition that may cause chest pain or other symptoms that occur when narrowed blood vessels prevent the heart from getting all the blood and oxygen that it needs. Women are nearly twice as likely as men to get angina. In a way, angina may be a good thing because it's often a clue that a woman is developing heart disease.

"Often there's not actually a sensation you would call 'pain' with angina, but rather a deep discomfort or tightness under the breastbone that can radiate up to the shoulder or jaw," says Rose Marie Robertson, M.D., director of the Women's Heart Institute at Vanderbilt University Medical Center in Nashville and former president of the American Heart Association. The lack of

sufficient bloodflow to the heart, which causes angina symptoms, can also result in fatigue or shortness of breath. It usually comes on when women are doing something physical and subsides when they're at rest. "Hopefully, angina will lead a woman to seek medical attention before things become worse," she notes.

If you experience any of the pain or other symptoms associated with angina and they last for more than 5 minutes, call 911—you could be having a heart attack and need medical attention right away.

Angina doesn't always mean that surgery or angioplasty is needed, Dr. Robertson adds. It can often be treated with medications, although some women may need surgery to improve bloodflow to the heart. ∎

tivity can make a real difference. Women who walk, ride a bike, or exercise at the gym for 30 minutes most days of the week can achieve nearly the same health benefits as those who go all out, says Dr. Robertson.

In fact, you don't even have to get the exercise all at once. While one longer daily walk of 30 minutes is preferable, women who exercise three times daily for 10 minutes each time will get measurable cardiovascular benefits, too.

You don't even have to do "formal" exercise to protect your heart. "Vacuuming can be exercise if you do it vigorously," says Dr. Robertson. So can gardening, doing dishes, or making the beds. "Look for opportunities to exercise throughout the day," she adds. This might involve walking around the perimeter of your office building on your lunch hour, taking stairs instead of elevators, and walking to the corner store instead of hopping in the car and driving. "Taking a dog for a walk is great, too, whether you have a dog or not," Dr. Robertson suggests.

If you smoke, do your best to quit. The risk of heart disease in smokers is two to four times higher than in nonsmokers. As every ex-smoker knows, quitting is hard—it may be the hardest thing you've ever done. But the payoff is dramatic. If you haven't been able to quit smoking on your own, talk to your doctor about starting a stop-smoking program. (For more information on getting cigarettes out of your life, see chapter 8.)

Consider aspirin. Studies have shown that this over-the-counter painkiller "thins" the blood and reduces the risk of heart-damaging blood clots. In a recent study, Italian researchers looked at nearly 4,500 men and women. Those who took 100 milligrams of aspirin daily were 44 percent less likely to die of heart disease.

The one problem with aspirin is that it may cause stomach upset and increase the risk of

Good News for Chocolate Lovers

Who says heart-healthy eating has to be dull? Researchers have found that chocolate contains chemical compounds called antioxidants, which prevent harmful oxygen molecules in the body from damaging cholesterol—the process that makes it more likely to stick to artery walls.

Chocolate is so effective, in fact, that it blocks free radicals better than green tea, grape juice, or blueberries—all of which are potent antioxidants. As a bonus, the active compounds in chocolate, called flavonoids, make the blood "thinner" and may reduce the risk of harmful clots in the arteries.

Of course, chocolate is high in calories as well as fat. While it may have some benefits for women, it's hardly as nutritious as fresh vegetables, legumes, or other wholesome foods.

"The key is moderation," says Carl L. Keen, Ph.D., professor of nutrition and internal medicine at the University of California, Davis. "For the average person who's physically fit, having an occasional cup of cocoa or a bar of chocolate can be part of a healthy diet." ■

bleeding. Researchers have found that enteric aspirin—coated to protect the digestive tract—dissolves in the small intestine instead of in the stomach and is less likely to cause side effects than regular aspirin.

While the dosage of aspirin used in the Italian study was different from the dosages commonly available in the United States, doctors often recommend taking an 81-milligram dose—the amount found in baby aspirin—once daily, particularly if you have already experienced a heart attack or have other risk factors. Of course, consult with your physician before beginning any aspirin regimen.

Nutritional Treatments

Eat lots of fruits and vegetables each day. Women who follow this simple advice can dramatically reduce their risk for heart disease.

What makes fruits and vegetables so powerful? They're packed with antioxidants—powerful plant chemicals that block the effects of free radicals, harmful oxygen molecules in the body that make cholesterol more likely to stick to artery walls. Fruits and vegetables are high in fiber, which helps remove cholesterol from the body. They're also filling, which means that women will be less likely to fill up on other, less healthy foods.

WHAT WORKS FOR ME

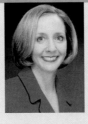

LORI J. MOSCA, M.D., PH.D., *associate professor of medicine and director of preventive cardiology at New York Presbyterian Hospital of Columbia University in New York City, has seen too many women suffering, unnecessarily, from heart disease. In her own life, she does everything possible to keep her heart and arteries healthy.*

I definitely practice what I preach in terms of heart health. No matter how busy the family gets, we have a couple of priorities. We sit down every night and eat well together—and we exercise together, too.

We always cook meals that are heart healthy. The meals might include salad, soup, and a main course—something like a stir-fry made with garlic, olives, capers, broccoli, and chicken, served over pasta.

One trick I've learned is to do a lot of cooking on Sundays. I make things like soup or pasta sauce and store them in plastic containers. That way, if we're stretched for time during the week, we don't have to cook hamburgers. We can take something out of the freezer, make a quick salad, and have a nutritious meal.

I always find time to exercise. I work out in the mornings before I wake my two boys. As a competitive Ironman triathlete, I do 20 minutes of swimming, 20 minutes of biking, and 30 to 40 minutes on the treadmill. One day a week, I do strength training, and another day I take a stretching class. I also swim with my kids regularly, and I ride a bike with my husband.

Exercise helps me unwind, too. Sometimes I run through the nature center near our home and listen to the frogs and birds. It's so serene. I love the feeling of the sun on my back and the wind through my hair. ■

WHEN BAD THINGS HAPPEN TO HEALTHY WOMEN

She Woke Up with a Heart Attack, Not the Flu

Nancy Loving woke up early one morning because she was nauseated, lightheaded, and achy. She figured it was the flu and tried to get back to sleep. But the symptoms kept getting worse, so she decided to go to the emergency room—and that's what saved her life.

"The next thing I knew, a doctor was leaning over me, telling me I was having a heart attack," says Loving, executive director of WomenHeart: The National Coalition for Women with Heart Disease in Washington, D.C. "I was 48 years old and never had any symptoms. I didn't even know that women had heart attacks."

While she was in the hospital, Loving learned that her cholesterol was a frightening 313 milligrams per deciliter. Obviously, she had suffered from high cholesterol for years, but none of her doctors had ever discussed her cholesterol or her risk for heart disease—despite the fact that she had been a smoker and that her father and three uncles had all died young of heart attacks.

For 3 years after the heart attack, Loving was terrified of what might happen next. She was, she admits, a "basket case." "The doctors offered no counseling or support groups," she says.

Loving finally took charge of her recovery. She quit her high-powered job as a public relations executive and set up a small agency in her home. She now swims 4 or 5 days a week, and she tries to walk for 30 minutes every day.

"I was a driven, type A workaholic before the heart attack," she says. "Now I'm a lot more careful about how I spend my time, and I try to keep the stress levels down. I take bubble baths, listen to music, and read. I give myself permission to put my health first." ■

According to the American Heart Association, women should eat at least five servings each of fruits and vegetables daily. "It's so simple, it's unbelievable," says Dr. Mosca.

Cut back on fat. This includes cooking oils, butter, and lard, as well as fatty foods such as red meats, fast foods, and rich desserts and snacks. The fats in foods—especially saturated fats and trans fatty acids—raise blood cholesterol levels and increase the risk of heart disease.

Women should limit total fat intake to 25 percent of total calories—20 percent is even better. In addition, do everything you can to restrict your intake of saturated fat—the kind found in red meat, regular milk, and other animal foods—to no more than 7 percent of total calories.

Study after study has shown that women who limit their consumption of animal foods and fill up on fruits and vegetables can dramatically lower the risk of heart disease, says C. Noel Bairey Merz, M.D., director of the Cedars-Sinai Preventive and Rehabilitative Cardiac Center in Los Angeles.

Follow the Mediterranean example. Even though people in Italy, Greece, and other Mediterranean countries consume more fat than Americans, their rates of heart disease are a fraction of what they are in this country. What are they doing differently?

For one thing, they consume very little saturated fat. They enjoy meat, but they have much smaller portions than Americans do. Much of the fat in their diets comes from olive oil, which contains heart-healthy monounsaturated fats. They also eat large amounts of whole grains, fresh fruits and vegetables, and other plant foods. As a result, the Mediterranean diet is among the healthiest in the world, says Stephen T. Sinatra, M.D., a cardiologist at New England Heart Center in Manchester, Connecticut, and assistant clinical professor at the University of Connecticut School of Medicine in Farmington.

Sip a little wine with meals. Or pour a glass of grape juice. They contain chemical compounds called flavonoids, which have been shown to reduce fatty buildups in the arteries and reduce the risk of heart disease.

Sprinkle some flaxseed on your cereal. This nutty-tasting grain is rich in alpha linolenic acid, which helps to prevent blood-blocking buildups in the arteries. Dr. Sinatra advises women to have at least 2 tablespoons of ground flaxseed daily.

Eat more fish. It's among the most powerful strategies for preventing heart disease. One study

The Couples Connection

marriage is about sharing—everything from tackling the daily chores and caring for the children to making the monthly mortgage payment.

Now there's some evidence that sharing may go further than anyone imagined. If your husband has heart disease, there's a good chance that your risk for getting it is also high.

In one study, researchers surveyed 177 couples in Oklahoma and Washington 2 months after the husband had either had a heart attack or undergone open-heart surgery. They found that even though spouses didn't share the same physical risk factors as their husbands—they were unlikely to have high cholesterol or elevated blood pressure, for example—they often shared unhealthy lifestyle habits, such as smoking or being overweight.

In some cases, the wives had even greater risks than their husbands after the initial hospitalization because they didn't always join their husbands in adopting heart-healthy habits. After the hospitalizations, in fact, the women were twice as likely as the men to continue smoking.

Of course, just as couples may share bad habits, they can also work together as a team to reverse them, says Lynn C. Macken, M.S.N., R.N., coordinator of cardiac and pulmonary rehabilitation in Scottsbluff, Nebraska, and one of the study researchers.

"It's not easy to change these kinds of risky behaviors, but when couples work together, it's probably easier to do," Macken says. ■

found that men who ate mackerel, herring, salmon, or other fish several times a week were 34 percent less likely to die from heart disease than those who ate less. The results are assumed to apply to women as well.

Prevention magazine recommends that women eat fish twice a week. If you don't care for fish, it's fine to take fish oil supplements. Look for products that contain docosahexaenoic acid, or DHA. The recommended dose is 300 milligrams daily.

Take heart-healthy nutrients. Women who eat a nutritious diet will get most of the nutrients that they need for long-term heart health—but supplements can provide extra insurance, says Dr. Sinatra. He advises women to take the following:

- Vitamin E. Take 200 IU daily. If you have a high risk for heart disease—you're a smoker, for example, or have a family history of heart disease—take 400 IU. Vitamin E helps prevent cholesterol from sticking to artery walls.

- Vitamin C. Take 500 milligrams daily. Like vitamin E, it helps prevent fatty accumulations in the arteries. It also lowers levels of Lp(a), a type of blood fat that's harmful for the heart. If you are on cholesterol-lowering medications, check with your doctor before taking vitamin C supplements.

- B vitamins. They help lower levels of homocysteine, an amino acid that increases the risk of high cholesterol and artery disease. Dr. Sinatra advises taking 800 micrograms of folic acid daily; 20 micrograms of vitamin B_{12}; and 20 milligrams of vitamin B_6.

- Coenzyme Q_{10}. It boosts the heart's pumping ability—but a number of medications, including antidepressants and cholesterol-lowering drugs, can deplete coenzyme Q_{10} from the body. Whether or not you're using other medications, it's a good idea to take 100 milligrams of coenzyme Q_{10} daily, Dr. Sinatra advises.

WHAT WORKS FOR ME

ALICE H. LICHTENSTEIN, Sc.D., *nutrition professor at Jean Mayer USDA Human Nutrition Research Center on Aging at Tufts University in Boston and a spokesperson for the American Heart Association, believes that you don't have to make dramatic changes in your eating and exercise habits to keep your heart healthy.*

Make small changes by eating a little less and exercising a little more.

When preparing dinner, and at other times when hunger's likely to strike, I keep clemen-

tines, carrots, and raw snow peas on hand. That way, I'm less tempted to eat high-fat, high-calorie fare. I cook with small portions of lean cuts of meat, and I choose fat-free milk, reduced-fat cheese, and fat-free yogurt. And I skip butter and other spreads altogether.

To get more exercise, I make it a point to always use the stairs, and I take the stairs to and from my fifth-floor office several times every workday. ∎

Mind-Body Techniques

Keep stress under control. Studies have shown that women with high levels of stress in their lives may have a higher risk of heart disease, says Dr. Bairey Merz.

You can't eliminate stress, of course, but you can take steps to keep it under control—by exercising, practicing yoga or meditation, or simply taking some deep breaths at the end of the day.

Accept what you can't change. Stress itself doesn't necessarily increase the risk of heart disease—it's how you respond to stress, says Dr.

Robertson. "Many of the things we get stressed out about just aren't that important. You have to step back and ask yourself, 'Am I going to let this bother me or not?'"

Take a vacation. A recent study showed that men who took annual vacations were less likely to die of heart disease than those who kept their noses to the grindstone. The same applies to women. It makes sense because few things reduce stress more quickly than taking a vacation. In addition, vacations are a good time to spend quality time with family and friends, and studies have shown that maintaining social connections

Prayers for the Heart

prayer may have the power to heal your heart, according to a preliminary study by researchers at Duke University and Durham Veterans Administration Medical Center, both in Durham, North Carolina.

In the study, patients who were undergoing angioplasty, a procedure to open clogged coronary arteries, were divided into five groups. Patients in one group were treated with standard medical therapies only. Those in the other four groups also received standard treatments, plus one additional therapy: touch therapy, music relaxation therapy, guided imagery, or directed prayer from religious groups around the world, including Carmelite nuns outside Baltimore, a Moravian prayer group in North Carolina, Buddhist monks in Paris and Nepal, and others.

Compared with people who received only standard therapy, those who were prayed for by the religious groups experienced 50 to 100 percent fewer complications, including heart attacks or death. Patients who received the other relaxation therapies had about 30 percent fewer complications than did those in the standard treatment group.

"When people are hurt and fighting for their lives, or when a loved one is sick, people often intuitively say a prayer," says lead researcher Mitchell W. Krucoff, M.D., associate professor of cardiology at Duke University Medical Center and director of the Cardiovascular Laboratories at Durham Veterans Administration Medical Center. It's not clear from the study why people who were prayed for—who weren't even aware of the prayers—did so much better, says Dr. Krucoff. The study was too small to make statistically meaningful conclusions, he adds. A follow-up study is under way at eight medical centers around the nation. ■

is an important strategy for keeping the heart healthy.

Let go of anger. The same goes for hostility and irritability. If you're always on edge and ready to snap at people or overreact to difficult situations, your heart may be paying the price.

"Studies show that the less angry and hostile you are, the less your blood pressure responds when you're provoked," says Dr. Robertson. "Having a positive, optimistic view of the world is clearly good for you."

Get in touch with your spiritual side. Research has shown that people who are spiritual have a lower risk of heart disease than those who don't practice a religion or cultivate spiritual beliefs.

"Spirituality provides important support in many ways," says Dr. Robertson. "It allows you to take a bad event and put it in a different perspective. It allows you to have less fear and anxiety, and it provides solace. Going to church also performs a very important social function by providing a sense of community."

Medical Options

Rx Many of the things that increase the risk of heart disease, such as smoking, gaining weight, or not getting enough exercise, are easy for women to recognize—and reverse— on their own. But other types of risk factors are "silent"—you won't know you have them unless you work with your doctor.

"The first step in taking action against heart disease is to identify all your risk factors, but many women have nowhere near the awareness that they need," says Dr. Mosca.

Some risk factors, you can't change, of course. If you have a family history of heart disease, there's not much you can do about it. But other risk factors can be controlled—if you know you have them. That's why it's important to discuss your concerns about heart disease with your doctor.

Don't wait for your doctor to bring it up, Dr. Mosca adds. Many doctors aren't aware that women, including premenopausal women, can have a high risk for heart disease. "Women need

Vitamin Alert!

If you take a statin and niacin, don't also take antioxidants over and above the amount in your multivitamin. (Antioxidants prevent harmful oxygen molecules in the body from damaging artery walls.)

In a new study, taking high-dose antioxidants reduced to zero the benefits of taking the cholesterol drugs simvastatin and niacin for raising the type of HDL that actually clears your arteries, called HDL2. But subjects taking the same drugs without antioxidants showed a healthy gain in levels of beneficial HDL2 of 42 percent. High doses of antioxidants in this study were 1,000 milligrams of vitamin C, 800 IU of vitamin E, 100 micrograms of selenium, and 25 milligrams of beta-carotene. ■

to ask questions," says Dr. Mosca. "Always ask your doctor what your risk factors are and what you can do about them."

Women are often amazed to learn that they have heart disease, but it can often be predicted years or even decades before it occurs, adds Dr. Bairey Merz. "But if you don't know you have high cholesterol or high blood pressure, you'll have missed the opportunity to prevent future problems."

Get regular blood pressure checks. High blood pressure has been called a "silent" disease because it doesn't cause symptoms at first. By the time it does cause symptoms, damage to the arteries has already occurred. It's essential to get your blood pressure checked regularly because high blood pressure boosts the heart's workload and greatly increases the risk of heart disease and other cardiovascular problems.

You want your blood pressure to be under 140/80. A reading of 120/80 (or lower) is even better.

If your blood pressure has climbed to 140/90 or higher, it's essential to take fast action—by exercising, limiting salt intake, losing weight if you need to, or taking medications.

Keep an eye on cholesterol. If you were to do only a few things to protect your heart, maintaining healthful levels of cholesterol would certainly be near the top of the list.

Cholesterol, also known as lipids, enters the bloodstream every time you eat. Over time, the fatty molecules are taken up into artery walls, where they restrict bloodflow, promote the development of blood clots, and greatly increase the risk of heart attack and other cardiovascular conditions.

According to the latest guidelines from the American Heart Association, here's what you should strive for.

- Total cholesterol: Keep it under 200 milligrams per deciliter. Women whose cholesterol is between 200 and 239 milligrams per deciliter are considered to have borderline high cholesterol; those whose cholesterol is above 240 are putting their hearts at serious risk. Keep in mind that a total cholesterol reading over 200 may not be a bad thing if your HDLs are high.

- LDL: It stands for low-density lipoprotein, the "bad" cholesterol. Ideally, your LDL should be below 100 milligrams per deciliter, but any reading below 130 milligrams per deciliter is pretty good.

when to see a doctor

 If you experience chest pain, or if you have fullness or tightness in your chest, are suddenly dizzy, fatigued, or nauseated, or if you're having trouble breathing or are cold and clammy, call 911 immediately. These are the most common signs of a heart attack in men and women, says Rose Marie Robertson, M.D., director of the Women's Heart Institute at Vanderbilt University Medical Center in Nashville. "Women are more likely than men to have less typical symptoms, such as fatigue or shortness of breath alone," says Dr. Robertson.

- HDL: Shoot for keeping your high-density lipoprotein, the "good" cholesterol, at 50 milligrams per deciliter or above. Levels under 40 put you at considerable risk for heart disease.

- Triglycerides: Keep them under 150 milligrams per deciliter.

Many doctors believe that the ratio of total cholesterol to HDL is more accurate than total cholesterol alone as a marker for heart disease. To determine your ratio, divide your total cholesterol reading by your HDL number. The Framingham Cardiovascular Institute recommends a total cholesterol/HDL ratio below 4.

Keep in mind that these guidelines are variable, depending on other risk factors you may have. If your doctor says your risk for heart disease is low to moderate, for example, it may be acceptable to have an LDL reading of up to 160. If you have multiple risk factors for heart disease, on the other hand, you'll want to keep LDL below 100.

These days, there's no reason for most people to have high cholesterol. Apart from lifestyle changes, such as lowering your intake of saturated fat, there are a number of very effective cholesterol-lowering drugs that can bring the numbers down to a healthy level.

Ask your doctor for a blood protein test. Scientists have identified a number of proteins in the body that can increase (or decrease) your risk for heart disease. One type of protein, called apolipoprotein B (apoB), causes cholesterol and other fatty substances to stick to artery walls. Another protein, apolipoprotein A (apoA-1), scavenges fat and cholesterol from the blood and transports it to the liver for disposal.

In a study of more than 1,000 people who had suffered a heart attack, those with low levels of apoA and high levels of apoB were four times more likely to have a second heart attack than those with a healthier protein balance. If test results indicate you have a low apoA-1 level or a high apoB level, a low-fat diet, regular exercise, and cholesterol-lowering medications can help.

Think twice about hormone replacement therapy (HRT). "In healthy women, we don't recommend HRT solely for the purpose of preventing heart disease, but there are many other reasons to take it," Dr. Mosca says. Supplemental hormones can reduce the risk of osteoporosis, the bone-thinning condition that's the leading cause of fractures in older women. Hormone therapy also can prevent hot flashes and other types of menopausal discomfort. It's best to discuss the pros and cons of HRT with your doctor.

High Blood Pressure and Stroke

The frightening thing about high blood pressure, or hypertension, is that it doesn't cause any symptoms in the early stages. Even when the numbers reach potentially dangerous levels, you probably won't feel different than you did before.

But even in the absence of symptoms, the force of blood roiling through the arteries will be doing serious damage. Unless high blood pressure is diagnosed and treated early, it can lead to a host of cardiovascular conditions, including stroke and heart disease, says Debra R. Judelson, M.D., a cardiologist and medical director of the Women's Heart Institute at the Cardiovascular Medical Group of Southern California in Beverly Hills.

About one in four Americans has high blood pressure, and more than a third of them don't know it. One in every five adult women in the United States has high blood pressure, and more than 60 percent of all deaths from stroke are women. Women often enjoy healthy blood pressure levels until they reach menopause. Then, when their estrogen levels decline, blood pressure starts creeping upward—and the women won't even suspect there's a problem.

Understanding the Numbers

Blood pressure measures the force with which blood travels through blood vessels. The numbers typically start to rise when artery walls thicken, constrict, or lose their elasticity, which makes it harder for blood to push through them. In the majority of cases, the change in blood vessels occurs long before actual changes in blood pressure can be detected. There's usually no known cause; only about 10 percent (or fewer) of cases of high blood pressure can be attributed to specific conditions, such as kidney or blood vessel abnormalities.

You don't want your blood pressure to be *too* low because that can result in dizziness or fatigue. But for most women, the lower the blood pressure, the healthier they'll be, says Marilyn M. Rymer, M.D., medical director of the Stroke Center at Saint Luke's Hospital in Kansas City, Missouri.

When you get your blood pressure taken, there are two numbers to consider. The first, higher number measures systolic pressure—the pressure that's generated when the heart is actually pumping blood. The second, lower number measures diastolic pressure—the pressure when your heart rests between beats.

Here's what the readings mean.

- Ideally, blood pressure should be below 120/80 milligrams per deciliter, although readings as high as 130/85 are considered normal.

- If your systolic pressure is 130 to 139, and the diastolic pressure is 85 to 89, you're heading into risky territory, especially if you have other risk factors for stroke or heart disease, such as obesity or a family history of high blood pressure, or if you're postmenopausal or African-American.

- A reading of 140/90 or higher means that it's time to take action. Even if only one of the numbers is high, you may need medical treatment.

BRINGING THE NUMBER DOWN

Many people require medications to control high blood pressure, but this isn't always necessary. "With a healthy lifestyle, many women can prevent hypertension from developing—or at least reduce its severity," says Samuel J. Mann, M.D., associate professor of clinical medicine at the Hypertension Center of New York Presbyterian Hospital–Cornell Medical Center in New York City and author of *Healing Hypertension: A Revolutionary New Approach*.

Here's what doctors advise.

Lifestyle Strategies

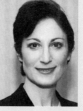 **Maintain a healthful weight.** "Excess weight is the biggest risk factor for high blood pressure," says Matthew Gillman,

---

WHAT WORKS FOR ME

DEBRA R. JUDELSON, M.D., is a cardiologist, medical director of the Women's Heart Institute at the Cardiovascular Medical Group of Southern California in Beverly Hills, and former president of the American Medical Women's Association. Here's what she does to make sure that her risks for high blood pressure and stroke are as low as they can possibly be.

I eat fewer processed foods these days, and I also go for a brisk walk every morning before I shower. This is my thinking time. By the time I'm dressed and ready to leave the house, my day is already planned.

I've also worked to reduce the stress in my life—and not just by using relaxation techniques. I've changed my entire life.

I used to be a type A personality. I was working incredibly hard—always in a hurry. Then, just before I turned 45, I began wondering why I was working so hard. I realized that I was trying to make a lot of money to pay for a fancy house and fancy vacations or other things I really didn't need. But I wasn't necessarily reaching my goal of happiness.

I stopped the 80-hour weeks. I now keep my office time limited. Sometimes I go in at 9 o'clock—it gives me time to spend time with the kids in the morning. I don't rush very much anymore. I have a degree of peace and comfort throughout the day that sustains me. ■

M.D., associate professor of ambulatory care and prevention at Harvard Medical School. Studies have shown, in fact, that men or women who lose as little as 10 pounds can send their blood pressure plummeting.

The only way to lose weight is to consume fewer calories than you burn. You can do this by eating smaller servings, consuming fewer high-fat foods (fat contains more calories than protein or carbohydrates), and avoiding snack foods. "Portion size is important, and be aware that manufacturers of processed low-fat foods tend to replace the fat in those foods with sugars, which also contribute to weight gain," he notes. At the same time, you'll need to exercise regularly to burn off the calories you consume. "Concentrate on increased physical activity," Dr. Gillman recommends. (For more information on healthy weight loss, see chapter 6.)

Keep your body moving. Even if you're at a healthful weight, regular exercise is among the best ways to prevent—or reverse—high blood pressure. Studies have shown, in fact, that men and women who are sedentary are 20 to 50 percent more likely to develop high blood pressure than those who are physically active.

How much exercise do you need? A total of at least 30 minutes a day of gardening, walking, jogging, bicycling, weight lifting, or other types of exercise is probably enough to keep blood pressure in check. (For more information on exercise, see chapter 5.)

If you smoke, try to quit. Every time you light up, your blood pressure climbs—and it stays elevated for an hour or more afterward. (For information on how to quit smoking, see chapter 8.)

Nutritional Treatments

Follow the DASH diet. It stands for "dietary approaches to stop hypertension," and it's considered one of the most effective ways to keep blood pressure in a healthful range. The diet calls for having:

- Eight to 10 daily servings of fruits and vegetables (each about $\frac{1}{2}$ cup)
- Seven to eight daily servings of whole grains (one slice of bread, or about $\frac{1}{2}$ cup)
- Two to three daily servings of low-fat or fat-free dairy foods (each 1 cup, or $1\frac{1}{2}$ ounces)
- Two or fewer servings of meat (each about 3 ounces)

The DASH diet is so effective that one study found that men and women who followed the eating plan were able to lower their blood pressure as much as they would have had they taken prescription drugs.

For more information on the DASH diet, visit the National Heart, Lung, and Blood Institute's Web site at www.nhlbi.nih.gov.

Cut way back on salt. The government's dietary guidelines call for limiting salt consumption to 2,400 milligrams daily (1 teaspoon). However, several recent studies suggest that this number may be too high. When men and women without high blood pressure lowered their salt intake by about a third of the recommended limit—to $\frac{2}{3}$ teaspoon, or 1,500 milligrams—their systolic pressure fell by 7 millimeters; in those with high blood pressure, the drop was 11.5 millimeters. People who lowered salt intake and followed the DASH diet had even better improvement.

"We eat huge amounts of salt in this country because of all the processed foods," says Dr. Judelson. When buying soups or other processed foods, look for the words "low sodium" or "sodium free" on the label. Avoid ultra-salty foods such as chips, pickles, and soy sauce, and use the salt shaker sparingly.

Eat fish two or three times a week. It's rich in omega-3 fatty acids, which have been shown to help lower blood pressure. Fatty fish has the largest amounts of omega-3s. This includes salmon, tuna, and sardines.

If you're not a fish eater, you can get the same beneficial fats by eating flaxseed or walnuts or using oils made with flaxseed, canola, or walnuts.

Imbibe moderately. Moderate drinking (one glass of wine or beer for women, no more than twice that for men) won't affect blood pressure and has been shown in several studies to be good for your heart and arteries. Drinking to excess, however, can cause long-term rises in blood pressure, and more than a drink a day increases the risk of breast cancer. So if you do drink, limit yourself to about $1\frac{1}{2}$ ounces of hard liquor, 5 ounces of wine, or a 12-ounce bottle of beer a day.

It's also a good idea to limit your coffee intake. Those who consume too much caffeine—in the form of coffee, tea, or caffeinated sodas—may experience rises in blood pressure of as much as 10 points. Limit yourself to about two servings of coffee, tea, or colas daily.

Keep cholesterol in check. It makes the arteries less elastic, and it also leads to accumulations of fatty material, called plaque, on the artery walls—the cause of heart attacks. As the arteries narrow, blood moves through them with greater force.

The best way to control cholesterol is to avoid saturated fats in the diet and increase your consumption of whole grains, legumes, and other fiber-rich foods. (For more information on controlling cholesterol, see chapter 13.)

Alternative Therapies

Drink hawthorn tea. It dilates blood vessels, which can result in modest drops in blood pressure, says Dr. Judelson.

To make a tea, steep 1 to 2 teaspoons of crushed herb in a cup of boiling water for 10 minutes. You can drink the tea several times daily.

Get in touch with "hidden" emotions. Folklore to the contrary, daily anxiety and stress don't play much of a sustained role in high blood pressure, even though they may affect blood pressure in the moment. However, emotions that are held deep inside may send blood pressure soaring, at least in some women.

"One-quarter to one-third of the hypertension cases I see are related to repressed or, so to speak, hidden emotions," says Dr. Mann. "These are people who have had childhood traumas or who cope with emotional stress by not dealing with it. They're the ones who are even-keeled—who never complain—and are actually less likely than most to feel depressed."

People whose hypertension is related to hidden emotions tend to achieve less success with blood pressure–lowering medication. "For some women, shifting attention to what has been hidden away

WHEN BAD THINGS HAPPEN TO HEALTHY WOMEN

Job Stress Raised Her Blood Pressure

In retrospect, Brita Hudson-Smith isn't surprised that her blood pressure rose to 140/90. When she was in her early thirties, she suffered the death of her mother. She also had gained weight, and she had a family history of hypertension. At the time, however, she was shocked to realize that her blood pressure had risen so high.

"You don't really pay attention to your risks until it happens to you," she says.

Her doctor immediately put her on hypertension medication, but she didn't work very hard at making basic lifestyle changes until she left her high-stress job at a suburban Philadelphia health organization a few years later.

"I started walking every day," she says. "I got involved in my community, and I read books about health and spirituality. I also meditated every day and became a vegetarian. It took time, but my blood pressure went down even further."

But the changes didn't last. When she started a new job the following year, her health routine fell apart. Her blood pressure rose higher than it had ever been. In fact, she wound up in the hospital after a test revealed that her blood pressure had risen to an alarming 170/100.

Hudson-Smith, now 51, admits that she struggles to find a balance between career demands and healthful living. "I keep saying a mantra to myself: 'I'm not going to let my job keep me from eating right and exercising.'"

She continues to take medication, but she also eases daily stress by visiting friends and doing things she enjoys, like flower arranging and going to the theater. "I know I don't have to do everything, that it's okay to let some things go," she says. "I write little notes to myself about the priorities in my life. I read them whenever I feel things getting crazy." ■

---

can rapidly lower blood pressure," says Dr. Mann. "Some can heal themselves, and others can benefit from consulting with a psychotherapist."

Medical Options

 Ask your doctor to check your blood pressure twice. Nearly one in four people, including women, suffers from "white-coat hypertension." In other words, their blood

pressure is usually normal, but it spikes when they visit the doctor, often because of simple anxiety. They could wind up being treated for hypertension that they don't have.

The opposite can also happen. It's normal for blood pressure to rise and fall periodically. It's possible for a woman to have normal blood pressure in the doctor's office, but soaring blood pressure at home.

"Always make sure that you really have hypertension before getting treated," advises Dr. Mann. The way to do this is to ask your doctor to take more than one blood pressure reading during your visit. Another option is to buy a blood pressure cuff and periodically check your own pressure at home.

Consider medications. If you aren't able to control your blood pressure with lifestyle changes, your doctor will probably advise you to take pressure-lowering medications. There are many classes of drugs to choose from. Some of the main ones are:

- Diuretics. Also called "water pills," they cause the body to eliminate water, which causes blood pressure to fall.

- Beta-blockers. They block the action of a body chemical called epinephrine, thereby slowing the heart rate and causing a drop in blood pressure.

- ACE inhibitors. They cause the blood vessels to stay dilated, allowing blood to flow with less force.

Blood pressure drugs are safe for most women, but they can cause a variety of side effects, including dizziness, dehydration, decreased levels of potassium, or sedation. They can even cause blood pressure to drop too low in some cases. Doctors usually resort to medications when lifestyle measures aren't effective, says Dr. Mann.

REDUCE YOUR RISK FOR STROKE

Heart disease and cancer get all the headlines, but stroke is the third leading cause of death in both men and women in the United States. Overall, one in six women will die of stroke, compared with one in 25 who will die from breast cancer.

About 25 percent of those who suffer from strokes are younger than 65, and more than half are women.

"We've done such a good job of educating women about breast cancer, but stroke is much more common," says Dr. Rymer.

There are two main types of stroke: ischemic strokes, which occur when a blood clot blocks the flow of blood through an artery in the brain, and

when to see a doctor

If you experience migraine headaches that are preceded by difficulty talking or partial paralysis on one side of your body, call your doctor right away. These types of migraines mean you may have a slightly higher risk of stroke, says Wayne M. Clark, M.D., director of the Oregon Stroke Center at Oregon Health Sciences University in Portland.

If you experience sudden numbness or weakness in the face, arms, or legs, or if you're having trouble speaking, walking, or maintaining your balance, get to an emergency room. You may have experienced a "mini-stroke" or stroke warning called a transient ischemic attack, which could potentially be followed by a full-fledged stroke.

If you're suddenly suffering from depression, and you haven't had depression in the past: This is sometimes caused by a "symptomless" stroke, especially in those 50 years and older.

If you notice that your pulse is irregular: This is sometimes caused by atrial fibrillation, an irregular heartbeat that increases the risk that blood clots will travel to the brain.

hemorrhagic strokes, which occur when brain blood vessels leak or burst.

The same strategies that lower blood pressure—such as cutting back on salt and eating a low-fat diet—also reduce the risk of stroke. It makes sense because high blood pressure damages arteries throughout the body, including those in the brain. Other stroke-preventing strategies include the following:

Home Remedies

 Quit smoking immediately. It's bad for blood pressure, and it's even worse for stroke. Studies have shown, in fact, that compared with nonsmokers, smokers have double the risk of having a stroke. If you quit, within 5 years your risk will be the same as that of a nonsmoker.

Take aspirin daily. It reduces the tendency of blood to form clots in the arteries, which can help prevent strokes. Aspirin is usually advised for those who have already had a stroke or who have a high risk for having one. Even if your risk for stroke is low, you may want to take a daily baby aspirin, which contains 81 milligrams, says Dr. Rymer. Of course, check with your doctor to make sure daily aspirin is right for you.

Nutritional Treatments

Take vitamin E. It is thought to be healthy for blood vessels and may reduce the risk of heart attack or stroke, says Dr.

Rymer. *Prevention* magazine recommends a dose of 100 to 400 IU daily separate from your multivitamin.

Get extra B vitamins. They lower levels of a chemical in the body called homocysteine. "High homocysteine levels may be as risky as high cholesterol," explains Wayne M. Clark, M.D., director of the Oregon Stroke Center at Oregon Health Sciences University in Portland.

Leafy green vegetables and beans are among the best dietary sources of folate and vitamins B_6 and B_{12}. You may want to take supplements as well. Look for a multivitamin that contains 1 milligram of folic acid, 25 milligrams of vitamin B_6, and 250 micrograms of vitamin B_{12}, Dr. Rymer advises.

Medical Options

Don't go in for a second round. In an international study that followed 6,105 stroke survivors for 4 years, those who took the blood pressure drug perindopril (Aceon) plus the diuretic indapamide had 43 percent fewer second strokes than those who took placebos.

Twenty percent of stroke survivors will have another one within 5 years—and second strokes are often more disabling, or deadly. "Now, we're finally seeing evidence that secondary strokes can be prevented," says Stanley Rockson, M.D., a cardiologist at Stanford University and a spokesman for the National Stroke Association. Discuss this with your doctor if you've had a stroke.

Diabetes

A few decades ago, a diagnosis of diabetes meant a lifelong sentence of dietary austerity—and a vastly increased risk of blindness, nerve damage, and other serious symptoms.

Things have improved dramatically since then. Diabetes is still a serious illness, but it can almost always be controlled—and one type may even be prevented and possibly reversed in some people through a combination of medications and important lifestyle changes.

"Diabetes is a very manageable disease—but it does take some work," says Karen E. Friday, M.D., an endocrinologist and associate professor of medicine at Tulane University Health Sciences Center in New Orleans.

Diabetes occurs either when the pancreas doesn't make enough insulin or when the insulin that is produced isn't efficiently used by the body's cells. Insulin is a hormone that transports energy-giving glucose, the sugar found in foods, into the cells. When insulin is in short supply, the cells don't get all the glucose they need. Instead, the glucose accumulates in the blood. Small amounts of glucose are essential for health, but at high levels it literally becomes toxic. Uncontrolled high blood sugar can lead to kidney failure, blindness, stroke, nerve damage, and heart disease.

There are two main forms of diabetes. Type 1—formerly called juvenile-onset or insulin-dependent diabetes—occurs when the immune system destroys beta cells, insulin-producing cells in the pancreas. Type 1 diabetes accounts for 5 to 10 percent of all diagnosed diabetes cases and is thought to be caused by genetic and environmental factors. People with type 1 diabetes need daily insulin shots or insulin delivered by a pump to manage their blood sugar.

The second form of diabetes, which accounts for 90 to 95 percent of all diabetes cases, is type 2, previously known as non-insulin-dependent or adult-onset diabetes. Those with type 2 have a condition called insulin resistance in which their bodies do not respond efficiently to insulin. Blame this one on lifestyle factors. People who are genetically susceptible and are overweight, eat a lot of processed foods, and don't get regular exercise have the highest risk of developing it. "It's mostly associated with obesity and sedentary lifestyles," says Mitchell A. Lazar, M.D., director of Penn Diabetes Center at the University of Pennsylvania School of Medicine in Philadelphia.

Other risk factors for type 2 diabetes include a

family history of the disease, age, and ethnicity: African-Americans, Hispanics, and Native Americans are more likely than Caucasians to get type 2 diabetes. Women with a history of gestational diabetes—a type of diabetes that occurs during pregnancy and then disappears—and those who have had a baby with a birth weight exceeding 9 pounds are also at an increased risk for later developing type 2 diabetes.

If you have diabetes, one of the most important things you can do, apart from controlling it, is to keep an eye on your heart health. People with diabetes have a very high risk of heart disease, as well as stroke.

Almost before anything else, doctors advise people with diabetes to get their other risk factors under control. These include:

- Elevated blood pressure. Be sure to keep it under 130/85.

- High cholesterol. The National Cholesterol Education Program of the National Institutes of Health recommends that people with diabetes keep low-density lipoprotein (LDL, the "bad" cholesterol) below 100. After this goal is reached, women should then try to get their high-density lipoprotein (HDL, the "good" cholesterol) over 50, and keep their triglycerides under 150.

- Pregnancy. About one in 20 pregnant women will develop gestational diabetes. Your doctor can screen for gestational diabetes around the sixth month of pregnancy. If you have it, you'll have to be especially vigilant about taking care of yourself later on.

Spice Up Your Metabolism

Cinnamon is more than a flavorful kitchen spice. There's good evidence that it can help prevent or at least delay the onset of type 2 diabetes.

In studies at the Nutrient Requirements and Functions Laboratory at the Agricultural Research Service in Beltsville, Maryland, lead scientist Richard A. Anderson, Ph.D., has tested more than 50 spices and herbs—including cinnamon, allspice, catnip, and turmeric—to see which ones make fat cells more responsive to insulin. The research is important because insulin-resistant cells can't take in enough energy-giving glucose from the blood, which can lead to diabetes.

"Cinnamon is the champ," says Dr. Anderson. It contains a substance called methylhydroxy chalcone polymer, or MHCP, which in laboratory studies increased glucose metabolism up to twentyfold.

In the future, the compound may be available in supplement form. For now, Dr. Anderson recommends eating ¼ to 1 teaspoon of cinnamon daily, particularly if you have high blood sugar, insulin resistance, or type 1 or type 2 diabetes. He suggests sprinkling cinnamon on your oatmeal and stirring it into foods, like yogurt, throughout the day, to reach the total amount.

"We've heard from people with diabetes who have begun adding cinnamon to their diets," he says. "They say it's the best thing they've tried since sliced bread." ∎

Catch It Early, Treat It Well

The goal of treating type 2 diabetes is straightforward: to keep blood sugar levels as normal as possible with a combination of lifestyle changes, or with lifestyle changes plus medications, possibly including insulin. Women with type 1 diabetes need to maintain a healthy lifestyle, too, and take insulin. If you have either type of diabetes, you will also be instructed by your doctor on how to monitor your blood sugar levels at home. Your physician also can check for kidney problems by measuring protein in the urine. This is important because diabetics have a higher risk of kidney disease. You should also go for yearly eye exams to check for early, treatable changes in the eyes.

The sooner diabetes is diagnosed, the better your chances of managing it effectively. With type 1 diabetes, people may be able to come off insulin early in the disease with the help of lifestyle changes and certain medications. And an early diagnosis for type 2 diabetes is important because if it continues uncontrolled for years, the high glucose and insulin levels eventually destroy the pancreas so it can't produce a sufficient amount of insulin. Once the pancreas is no longer producing insulin, there may be no going back—you might require medications for the rest of your life.

"But type 2 diabetes may possibly be reversed in some people, up to a point, if they lose weight and exercise," says Katherine D. Sherif, M.D., assistant professor of medicine at MCP Hahnemann University School of Medicine and director of the Center for Women's Health and Wellness, both in Philadelphia. In some cases, in fact, people are able to quit taking medications once they make fundamental changes in their diets and exercise habits, she adds.

It's important to recognize the early signs of type 2 diabetes because it's during the initial stages of the disease that reversing it may still be an option. Women need to be especially alert because they have a higher risk than men for developing heart disease if they have diabetes.

Your first clues, if you have type 2 diabetes, may be frequent trips to the bathroom and excessive thirst. Extremely high blood sugar may also be accompanied by fatigue and visual blurring. The main symptoms of type 1 diabetes are unexplained

Must-Have Monitoring

If you have diabetes, get these five checks regularly. If your doctor's office has a diabetes educator on staff, he or she can help teach you how to do these.

- Blood sugar self-monitoring (daily)
- Blood test for glycosylated hemoglobin (at least once a year)
- Foot check for sores or ulcers (performed by your physician at least once a year)
- Eye screening for retinopathy, a condition that can lead to blindness (once a year)
- Lipid panel (total cholesterol, HDL, LDL, and triglycerides) to check heart disease risk (once a year) ■

WHEN BAD THINGS HAPPEN TO HEALTHY WOMEN

She Traded In Her Candy Bars for a Treadmill

Sylvia Charity wasn't surprised when she first noticed the telltale signs: frequent bathroom trips, a raging thirst, and lightheadedness. Both type 1 and type 2 diabetes run in her family, and her mother recently died of complications from the disease.

Charity, a 52-year-old government supervisor in Hampton, Virginia, quickly had her blood sugar level tested. The test was positive. "My worst fear was confirmed—I had type 2 diabetes. I was heartbroken at first, then became very angry because I felt responsible for allowing my fear to become a reality," she says. "You really don't want to admit that this is happening to you."

Like many women her age, Charity had put on some weight over the years. She had slacked off on exercise, and she spent most of her days confined to a desk at work.

"After always being able to do whatever I wanted, like eating a piece of cake or having a banana split, I finally realized I was going to have to adjust my life," she says. "At first it felt like the end of the world, but now I know I can live with this."

Charity, who describes herself as a "chocoholic," stopped buying candy bars. She cut back on high-carbohydrate meals, and she always balanced the carbohydrates with small portions of meat and vegetables. She got her doctor's approval and started working out on a treadmill three or four times a week. She's now up to 25 minutes a session. "I've lost 23 pounds, and my blood sugar stays pretty much in control.

"This is not an overnight thing," she says. "Temptation is all around you. But I've got six grandkids that I want to be around to see. I know I need to get my priorities straight and to be in control of my life again." ■

weight loss and hunger, sometimes called "starvation in the midst of plenty." But if you are at risk for either form of diabetes, see your doctor regularly for checkups, even if you don't have any symptoms.

Preventing diabetes, of course, is a lot better than treating it later. Long before people actually develop the disease, the body's cells may be becoming increasingly resistant to insulin, mainly because of poor lifestyle habits.

"If we could get people to restrict calories, exercise, and eat right, in theory we could prevent type 2 diabetes," says Francine Ratner Kaufman, M.D., head of the division of endocrinology and metabolism at Children's Hospital of Los Angeles and vice president of the American Diabetes Association.

Lifestyle Strategies

If you don't have diabetes, the following lifestyle tips will help ensure that you never get it. Even if you've already been diagnosed with diabetes, you can use this guide to help control your glucose levels, reduce symptoms, and generally keep the disease at a manageable level.

Control your weight. It's easier to talk about losing weight than actually doing it. There's a good reason for this: Human beings have a genetic tendency to overindulge and hold on to every last calorie.

"Our genes aren't that different from those in our caveman ancestors," says Dr. Kaufman. "If a bison came along only once a week, those genes enabled us to survive by storing calories incredibly efficiently. Now, with a convenience store on every corner and fast food everywhere, we're still storing those calories efficiently, but it leads to obesity."

The problem with obesity is that it increases the risk of insulin resistance. This means that it's more difficult for glucose to enter the body's cells. The glucose sits in the blood and starts to poison the blood vessels, nerves, and pancreas. Insulin resistance is more likely to occur when body fat is stored in the abdomen rather than in the hips or buttocks—but any fat accumulation may be a factor. As little as 20 extra pounds of fat can make you insulin resistant.

The best way to lose weight is to follow *Prevention* magazine's weight-loss guidelines, which are discussed in detail in chapter 6. But one point is worth mentioning here: Diets that promise dramatic weight loss in a short period of time almost never succeed. Traditional diets, which involve a combination of physical activity and smart eating, may be slower, but they've been proven to work.

"I always try to be realistic when I advise a woman about weight loss. For example, I might

The Blues–Blood Sugar Connection

doctors have known for a long time that depression and diabetes seem to go hand in hand. But which comes first: the depression or the diabetes? A new study suggests that, in most cases, depression arrives earlier.

Scientists looked at dates from the medical records of 1,680 people with newly diagnosed type 2 diabetes and compared them with records for the same number of people without the disease. They found that those with diabetes had suffered significantly more bouts of depression prior to their diagnoses. In fact, in those who had been diagnosed with diabetes and depression, the depression came first three-quarters of the time.

"I'm not sure we can say that depression causes diabetes," says lead researcher Gregory A. Nichols, Ph.D., senior research associate at Kaiser Permanente Center for Health Research in Portland, Oregon. It's possible, he says, that both depression and diabetes are linked to a common factor—one that hasn't yet been identified.

If you have a family history of diabetes or if you have other risk factors for the disease, it's worth paying attention to your moods, Dr. Nichols says. "I'd consider depression a possible warning sign. If you notice you're depressed, get it treated—and get your blood sugar checked, too." ∎

say to aim for losing 10 percent of her weight over 6 months," says Dr. Sherif. "If you weigh 180, that means losing 18 pounds—which is just 3 pounds a month."

Do you have to keep losing weight to control diabetes? There are plenty of good reasons to reach and maintain your ideal weight, but there's a good chance that you'll notice significant improvements in blood sugar control in the meantime. If the diabetes is at an early stage, and your body's cells and insulin levels are close to normal, losing as little as 10 pounds may be enough to keep your blood sugar from getting into the diabetic range, says Dr. Lazar.

It's not always easy to tell at a glance if you're truly overweight or how much weight you might need to lose. Doctors recommend a tool called the body mass index, or BMI. We discuss this is more detail in chapter 6, but here's how it works. To find your BMI, multiply your weight in

WHAT WORKS FOR ME

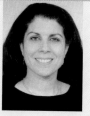

KATHERINE D. SHERIF, M.D., *is assistant professor of medicine at MCP Hahnemann University School of Medicine and director of the Center for Women's Health and Wellness, both in Philadelphia. She comes from a family of immigrants—and she saw firsthand what happens when people switch to the overabundant Western diet and lifestyle, which puts them at high risk for developing diabetes.*

My father is Egyptian, and our family members who eat the traditional diet of lots of fruits and vegetables and who get regular exercise are very healthy. But those who have sedentary lifestyles and eat a typical Western high-calorie, high-carbohydrate diet have developed diseases like heart disease, stroke, hypertension, diabetes, and high cholesterol. The transformation I've seen in just one or two generations is striking.

I've always tried to eat a healthful diet. For example, I have one of three breakfasts: Sometimes a couple of hard-boiled eggs and fruit, sometimes a cup of plain yogurt with soy protein powder and fresh fruit mixed in, and sometimes high-protein Egyptian beans with vegetables, which are a staple of the Egyptian diet in the countryside. Lunch might be a can of tuna fish and fruit, and my afternoon snack is typically roasted soybeans or string cheese with fruit. Dinner often consists of tofu and stir-fried vegetables, or a piece of fish or chicken, served with a salad or vegetables.

I also take multivitamins. I get 100 milligrams of B vitamins, 2,000 milligrams of vitamin C, 400 IU of vitamin E, and 2,000 milligrams of fish oil.

It's so hard sometimes to play sports or go to the gym, so I try to walk 10,000 steps daily. One mile is roughly 2,500 steps. I wear a pedometer throughout the day so I can show my patients how I incorporate exercise into my life.

If I park a little farther down the parking lot, I add 500 steps coming into the office and 500 steps going out. On weekends, I walk nine blocks from my house to the Philadelphia Art Museum. That's 2,500 steps there and 2,500 back. The exercise really adds up. ■

pounds by 703 and divide that number by your height in inches. Divide that number again by your height in inches, and you have your BMI. A BMI of 25 to 29.9 means that you're overweight. Anything above 30 is considered obese.

To make the calculations easier, check out the online BMI calculator of the National Heart, Lung, and Blood Institute. The Web address is www.nhlbisupport.com/bmi/bmicalc.htm.

Get regular exercise. It's among the best strategies for treating both types of diabetes, and evidence suggests it may also help prevent type 2 diabetes.

"Exercise has two beneficial effects. It alters muscle cells to improve their resistance to insulin, and it also allows sugar to get out of the blood into the skeletal muscle in the absence of insulin," says Dr. Lazar. If you exercise regularly, your cells will be less resistant to insulin and will take in more glucose, which in turn keeps blood sugar levels in a healthful range.

Getting regular exercise will also help you maintain a healthful weight, control your cholesterol, and keep your blood pressure numbers normal. It can dramatically reduce your risk of heart disease, which is important because women with diabetes are two to four times as likely to die from heart disease as those without diabetes.

For a complete guide to exercise, see chapter 5. Keep in mind, however, that even if aerobics classes or weight lifting isn't for you, simply walking for 40 minutes a day can reduce your risk of diabetes by an impressive 40 percent. If you walk for a full hour at a good clip, you can cut the risk in half.

Talk to your doctor before starting an exercise routine, particularly if you already have diabetes or if you haven't put on your walking shoes for a while. Your doctor might recommend that you have a stress test, just to make sure that your heart can handle the workouts.

"There's no reason to go from being sedentary to running a marathon," says Dr. Lazar. "Increase your pace gradually. Start by walking ¼ mile, then slowly increase the distance," he advises.

Nutritional Treatments

Eat natural foods. Humans didn't evolve to eat fast food and high-sugar, high-fat snacks. The ideal diet today is the same one that fueled our ancient ancestors: fiber-rich whole grains, fresh fruits and vegetables, and legumes—and the "good" fats, such as olive and flaxseed oils and the omega-3 fats, says Burt Berkson, M.D., Ph.D., adjunct professor of applied biology at New Mexico State University, founder of Integrative Medical Centers of New Mexico, and author of *Syndrome X* and *The Alpha Lipoic Acid Breakthrough*.

In the past, people with diabetes were advised to avoid desserts and other sugary foods. Nutritionists still worry about this, but research has shown that the key to controlling diabetes is to eat a balanced diet. Keep your overall diet healthy and have only small portions of cake, candy, cookies, and other sweets very occasionally.

According to the American Diabetes Association, the optimal diet includes 10 to 20 percent of daily calories from protein; 30 percent (or less) of total calories from fats with less than 10 percent coming from saturated fats; and the rest from complex carbohydrates, which are mainly found in fruits, vegetables, beans, and grains. If your LDL cholesterol is 100 or more, you need to take extra care to make sure your saturated fat intake is less than 7 percent.

Include more fiber in your diet. A study done at the University of Texas Southwestern Medical Center at Dallas Southwestern Medical School found that people who increased their fiber intake from 24 to 50 grams daily had dramatic improvements in blood sugar levels. In fact, the high-fiber diet was as effective as some diabetes medications.

Rather than try to figure out how much fiber is in different foods, you can simply try to get a total of 13 daily servings of a mixture of fruits, vegetables, beans, brown rice, and whole grain

More Vegetables, Less Meat

the mantra of diabetes experts is "low fat, high fiber." But what about meat? According to one study, people with diabetes might want to give up all meat, including fish and chicken, and fill their plates with hefty servings of vegetables instead.

Researchers from Georgetown University School of Medicine and the Physicians Committee for Responsible Medicine divided people with type 2 diabetes into two groups. Those in one group were given a low-fat vegan diet (consisting of whole grains, vegetables, legumes, and fruits, and no animal products), while those in the second group were given a low-fat diet that included fish and poultry. Both groups stayed on the diets for 12 weeks.

In the vegan group, fasting blood sugar levels dropped by 28 percent—more than twice the amount as those in the fish-and-poultry group. People in the vegan group also lost an average of nearly 16 pounds, compared with an 8-pound loss in the meat-eating group.

Even better, some of the people in the vegan group were able to discontinue or reduce their levels of blood sugar medications. None of the meat eaters, however, had similar benefits.

"Unlike the complex carbohydrates in a plant-based diet, refined foods, especially the sugars and fats, and calorie-dense foods, like meat and dairy products, are absorbed rapidly. This prompts blood sugar spikes that lead to increased insulin requirements and the accumulation of fat. Most people with type 2 diabetes are overweight, reflecting their intake of these refined foods, and have an increased risk for insulin resistance. The heavier you get, the more insulin resistant your cells become. The sugar that is in your blood because it can't get into the cells damages the nerves, pancreas, and arteries," explains Thomas J. Barnard, M.D., professor of human biology and nutritional sciences at the University of Guelph in Ontario. "Unrefined plant foods may interfere with carbohydrate and glucose absorption, resulting in lower blood sugar and lower insulin requirements. They are also sources of protective antioxidant nutrients, which are vital to the prevention and reversal of the arterial damage that is associated with diabetes. They are some of the most powerful tools we have against obesity and diabetes." ■

pastas, cereals, and breads. For optimal glucose control, try to get an equal mix of soluble fiber (found in oranges, grapefruit, prunes, cantaloupe, raisins, lima beans, oat bran, and granola) and insoluble fiber (found in some greens, vegetables, legumes, and whole grains).

Avoid sugary drinks. There's nothing wrong with having fruit juices or sodas on occasion, but they're brimming with sugar and little else. When you take in a lot of calories from sugar, you'll be less likely to get enough calories from wholesome, nutrient-packed foods, says Dr. Kaufman.

She advises people with diabetes to drink mainly water. When you do have a hankering for soda or a juice, look for products that are sugar-free—and drink them in moderation, no more than one a day, she advises.

Consider supplements. In the past few years, researchers have found that a number of essential nutrients can play a powerful role in controlling diabetes and related symptoms. You can't get enough of these nutrients from foods, however, so you'll need to get extra amounts in supplement form.

Protect Your Oral Health

gum disease may threaten more than your teeth and gums. Although not proven scientifically, it is thought that gum disease may be a trigger for the clinical onset of diabetes in individuals already predisposed to the disease. There is also evidence that gum disease can worsen the degree of control of diabetes.

Using data from the Third National Health and Nutrition Examination Survey (NHANES III), researchers found that among overweight adults with the highest insulin resistance levels, one in two also suffered from severe gum disease.

It's possible that gum disease, which is caused by chronic bacterial infections that affect the whole body, may somehow trigger insulin resistance. The process is believed to be due to inflammatory substances produced in response to the infection. Molecules of these substances prevent insulin from docking on its receptors on the cells' surface. This reduces the uptake of glucose by the cells and results in insulin resistance.

"Oral health is far more important than we previously thought," says Sara G. Grossi, D.D.S., assistant professor of oral biology at the School of Dental Medicine at State University of New York at Buffalo and director of the university's Periodontal Disease Research Center. "Gum disease may affect other conditions in the body, such as heart disease, stroke, respiratory diseases, and diabetes. Periodontal disease in people with diabetes constitutes a significant health risk since it could lead to difficulty in controlling blood sugar and therefore worsen diabetic status."

The best way to prevent gum disease is to brush and floss your teeth twice daily, eat a balanced diet rich in antioxidants—and visit your dentist regularly for checkups and teeth cleanings. Your dentist will advise you on the recommended frequency of your visits. ■

- Vitamin E. It strengthens immunity and plays a key role in preventing infections. This is important because people with diabetes are much more likely to get infections than those without the disease, says Dr. Berkson. Vitamin E also helps prevent heart disease, a common consequence of diabetes. People with risk factors for diabetes are advised to take 400 IU vitamin E daily. For those who already have the disease, the recommended dose is 400 to 600 IU daily.

- Vitamin C. It lowers blood glucose levels and helps insulin work more efficiently. Take 500 to 1,000 milligrams of vitamin C daily.

- Alpha lipoic acid. This is a cofactor for the enzyme that converts the broken-down glucose in the body's cells to a form that will be used to produce energy. It also helps prevent cells from becoming resistant to insulin. Dr. Berkson advises people with type 2 diabetes to take 400 to 600 milligrams of alpha lipoic acid daily. For prevention, take 100 milligrams daily. Important: If you're already taking medications for diabetes, talk to your doctor before supplementing your diet with alpha lipoic acid.

- B-complex vitamins. Take them if you're using alpha lipoic acid, which depletes B vitamins from the body. Look for a supplement that contains 100 percent of the Daily Value for all the B vitamins.

- Multimineral supplements. Look for a product that contains chromium, magnesium, zinc, and selenium. Chromium and magnesium improve insulin efficiency, zinc improves insulin produc-

tion in the body, and selenium helps protect the kidneys from damage. The recommended doses for people with diabetes are 400 micrograms of chromium, 30 to 40 milligrams of zinc, and 100 to 200 micrograms of selenium.

Alternative Therapies

Until recently, most physicians dismissed alternative healing techniques for serious conditions such as diabetes. But recent studies have shown that remedies outside of mainstream medicine, such as medicinal herbs and mind-body techniques, may play an important role in keeping diabetes under control.

Let go and relax. Simply taking a deep breath and relaxing your muscles may result in significant dips in blood sugar. A study of 18 people with diabetes found that relaxation exercises were able to reduce blood sugar levels by 9 to 12 percent.

"When you're under stress, the brain secretes hormones that make you more susceptible to all diseases, including diabetes," says Dr. Berkson.

There are many relaxation techniques to choose from. One of the easiest is called progressive relaxation. Begin by breathing deeply for a minute or two. Spend the next 10 to 15 minutes progressively relaxing all the muscles in your body, starting at your toes and working upward to your head. In your mind, imagine that the muscles are getting heavy, warm, and loose. By the time you're done, you'll notice that stress and tension have slipped away. If you do this every day, you may find that your blood sugar levels have dropped into a safer zone. (For more relaxation techniques, see chapter 7.)

Battle depression. Studies have shown that people with diabetes are twice as likely to suffer from depression than nondiabetics. Depression is a real problem because it makes people less likely to focus on the lifestyle changes that are needed to keep blood sugar under control.

If you've been feeling depressed or anxious, your doctor may recommend that you talk to a therapist or get a prescription for antidepressant medications. On the home front, really push yourself to get more exercise and to spend time with friends. They're among the best ways to ease depression.

Try milk thistle. It contains a compound called silymarin, which appears to improve insulin resistance and glucose control, says Dr. Berkson. He advises people with diabetes to get 140 to 210 milligrams of silymarin from standardized milk

thistle extract daily. The supplement label will tell you how much silymarin the milk thistle product contains.

Syndrome X: The Beginning of Diabetes

Long before people suffer from diabetes, their bodies have begun laying the groundwork for future problems. They may have what doctors refer to as insulin resistance or syndrome X, which leads to other problems, including high cholesterol and triglyceride levels, high blood pressure, and accumulations of fat. These conditions can increase the risk of diabetes as well as heart disease.

"People who are diabetic may have been insulin resistant for years," says Dr. Sherif. "One day, the pancreas just can't crank out enough insulin anymore. Blood sugar builds up, which leads to diabetes. And by that time, half of them also have developed coronary artery disease."

Does Television Cause Diabetes?

for years, doctors have known that an active lifestyle protects against diabetes and all of its life-threatening complications. But researchers at the Harvard School of Public Health wanted to find out if the reverse was true: Would long stretches of TV watching—the sedentary activity that consumes 40 percent of our leisure time—increase the odds?

They analyzed the viewing habits of nearly 38,000 men, ages 40 to 75, for more than 10 years. After adjusting for age, physical activity levels, alcohol use, and smoking, those who watched TV more than 4 hours a day doubled their odds of getting diabetes, compared with those who watched less than 2 hours weekly. Those who viewed 40 hours a week tripled their risk.

And if TV watching keeps you up late, you may face a second risk. Another study, from the University of Chicago, suggests that getting less than 6½ hours of shut-eye nightly raises the odds of insulin resistance, a diabetes precursor. ■

Researchers have found that insulin resistance and syndrome X have a common cause: the fat that accumulates through years of munching refined carbohydrates, which are generally found in snacks and other processed foods.

The problem with refined carbohydrates, and possibly with refined fats and excess protein, is that they're quickly turned into glucose in the body. The cells get overloaded with glucose, so the body stores it in the form of fat, explains Dr. Berkson.

That fat does more than cling to just the abdomen—or the hips, buttocks, thighs, and everywhere else. It promotes the production of a hormone called resistin, which essentially orders cells to ignore instructions from insulin to gobble up glucose that's circulating in the blood. In other words, it makes the cells resistant to insulin, one hallmark of type 2 diabetes. Although this mechanism is not proven, researchers think that resistin may be the link between obesity and type 2 diabetes.

"We're all at risk from syndrome X, which is caused by poor diets and lifestyles," says Dr. Berkson. "But you can reverse it, and sometimes type 2 diabetes as well, by eating a proper diet, taking nutritional supplements, getting regular exercise, and reducing stress," he explains. If you have a family history of diabetes, or if you have high cholesterol, high blood pressure, or abdominal obesity, it may be helpful to see your doctor for an oral glucose tolerance test. "It tells how your body handles sugars after eating," says Dr. Sherif. "If sugar levels don't drop after a couple of hours, it means that your body isn't handling glucose and you're probably insulin resistant."

The test may be helpful for women with a condition called polycystic ovary syndrome (PCOS), which causes symptoms such as irregular periods, unexpected weight gain, and acne outbreaks. Most women with PCOS are insulin resistant and have a very high risk of developing type 2 diabetes. If they're not treated, many do go on to develop the disease, says Dr. Sherif.

16

Cancer

Almost every week, another cancer myth makes the Internet rounds. You've probably seen e-mail cancer alerts about deodorant, shampoo, and even electrical appliances. It's enough to make women swear off consumer products forever. Your best bet is to delete those e-mail warnings—and empower yourself with facts. Doctors know what causes cancer, and those lists of "carcinogenic" goods looping through cyberspace usually have very little basis in truth.

What does count is how you live. If every woman ate well, exercised, didn't smoke, and safeguarded herself against infectious diseases, particularly the sexually transmitted kind, nearly three-quarters of cancer deaths among women would never happen.

"The majority of cancer risk can be attributed to lifestyle," says Therese Bevers, M.D., medical director of clinical cancer prevention at the University of Texas M. D. Anderson Cancer Center in Houston. Diet and smoking make up most of the risk pie, she explains, with inherited cancers accounting for between 5 and 10 percent of cases. "But even then, lifestyle or environmental factors may actually trigger it," she says.

Does that mean you'll stay cancer-free if you follow the rules of good health? Not necessarily,

says Mitchell L. Gaynor, M.D., director of medical oncology at the Center for Complementary and Integrative Medicine, affiliated with New York Presbyterian Hospital–Cornell Medical Center in New York City. But you greatly improve your odds.

Many Diseases, Similar Strategies

Cancer may sound like one disease, but it's actually dozens of diseases that attack different organs and spring from different causes.

What all cancers share, though, is the uncontrolled growth and spread of abnormal cells—cells that eventually destroy the body if they aren't stopped.

Your immune system is uniquely equipped to recognize and destroy deviant cells before they become cancerous. Your detoxification system, which is controlled by the liver, rids your body of cancer-causing toxins. But sometimes this arsenal of defenses fails, due to poor diet, illness, lack of exercise, or stress. That's when cancerous cells may slowly begin accumulating. "A tumor is the manifestation of a process that may have taken decades to happen," says Dr. Gaynor.

That's why keeping your body, mind, and spirit in potent fighting shape is the key to preventing cancer and to living with cancer once you have it.

"If you get cancer, the healthier you are, the less likely you'll be to have other medical conditions that might interfere with treatment, and the better you'll be able to get through it," says Marilyn Leitch, M.D., a surgical oncologist, professor of surgery at the University of Texas Southwestern Medical Center, and medical director of the University of Texas Southwestern Center for Breast

Care in Dallas. "You don't have to die from cancer."

Here's how to lower your general cancer risk, plus ward off the most common women's cancers.

YOUR CANCER PREVENTION PLAN

Someday, you may be able to get a shot that would protect you against cancer the same way you get a shot against tetanus. Scientists are working on it. In fact, it's one of the hottest areas of medical re-

Turning Out the Lights May Help Turn Off Cancer

the hormone melatonin—which is secreted by the pineal gland at night when it's dark, and is curtailed by light—has been lauded as everything from a promising sleep aid to the fountain of youth. But its greatest potential may lie in its potency against breast cancer.

In a recent laboratory study, Steven M. Hill, Ph.D., professor in the department of structural and cellular biology at Tulane University Health Sciences Center in New Orleans, and the Edmond and Lily Safra Endowed Chair for Breast Cancer Research, gave female rats a preparation to induce breast cancer. Then he treated them with a combination of melatonin and 9-cis-retinoic acid, a derivative of vitamin A. The animals given the treatment developed significantly fewer tumors than those that didn't get the treatment. In addition, the onset of tumors was delayed from 5 to 7 weeks.

The vitamin A derivative is a known cancer fighter, and adding melatonin to the mix ap-

peared to make it even more effective, Dr. Hill explains.

Besides its ability to prevent or delay breast cancer, melatonin may aid in the treatment of existing breast tumors by altering estrogen receptors and by starving tumor cells of the hormone they need for growth. Dr. Hill isn't suggesting that women take melatonin supplements to prevent or treat breast cancer. But it might make sense to encourage the pineal gland to produce as much of this healing hormone as possible by turning out the lights when the sun goes down and going to sleep early. No easy task in today's busy world.

"By getting up at 5:00 every morning and staying up until 11:00 or 12:00 every night, with artificial lights on, you're giving your pineal gland only a short period in which to make melatonin," says Dr. Hill. He suspects, in fact, that melatonin deprivation may explain why some reproductive cancers are on the rise. ■

search today. Until a breakthrough occurs, however, your best bet is to do everything you can to lower your risk—starting with dietary changes.

Nutritional Treatments

Eat wholesome foods. Like so many lifestyle diseases, cancer risk can be reduced by good eating. The American Cancer Society recommends having five or more servings of fruits and vegetables daily, plus plenty of other plant-based foods, such as whole grain breads, rice, pasta, and beans. Prepare low-fat meals, and limit your consumption of meat, particularly high-fat red meats.

Women who try to overhaul their diets all at once often get frustrated and fail. Dr. Leitch advises making the changes slowly. For example, substitute fruit or vegetables for french fries one day; on another, replace red meat with fish, whole grains, or legumes. "You can't go on a grapefruit diet for the rest of your life, nor would you want to," she says. "But if you have a more comprehensive plan that lets you eat enough to feel satisfied, then you're more likely to stick with it over time."

Stack your odds with superfoods. "I think the most exciting advance in the next decade will be predicting who's at risk for cancer, and preventing it largely through nutrition," says Dr. Gaynor. Scientists have found that many foods contain protective antioxidants and phytonutrients, which boost your body's natural defenses against carcinogens. Some of the best include:

- Tomatoes and tomato sauce. They contain lycopene, a plant pigment that blocks the harmful effects of naturally occurring molecules called free radicals. Lycopene has been linked to reductions in lung, breast, colon, cervical, and other cancers.

- Fish and flaxseed. They contain omega-3 fatty acids, which fight cancer by inhibiting the body's production of prostaglandins, chemicals that promote tumor growth and inhibit the ability of the immune system to detect cancers. Oily fish such as tuna, salmon, mackerel, cod, and halibut contain the most omega-3s. Or you can eat 2 tablespoons of flaxseed oil daily.

- Cruciferous vegetables. Cabbage, broccoli, cauliflower, Brussels sprouts, and kale contain formidable cancer fighters, including sulforaphane and indole-3-carbinol. Dr. Gaynor recommends having six servings of cruciferous vegetables weekly.

- Mushrooms. They're packed with compounds called polysaccharides, large, chainlike molecules that have both antitumor and immune-stimulating properties. Enoki and maitake mushrooms contain the largest numbers of these molecules.

- Olive oil. It contains anthocyanins, flavonoids, and phenols, which are known cancer combatants. They're not bad for your heart, either.

- Green tea. Studies have shown that people who drink about 4 cups of green tea daily have a lower risk of cancer than those who don't drink tea.

■ Garlic. Along with scallions, leeks, and onions, it contains sulfur compounds, which have anticancer properties.

Use vitamins as needed. If you're eating at least six to eight servings of fruits and vegetables daily, you're probably getting enough immune-boosting, cancer-fighting nutrients. But if your diet needs a little help, you may want to consider taking a multivitamin that contains 100 percent of the Daily Value for most nutrients (including the recommended daily allowance of B vitamins), as well as separate daily supplements of the following: 5,000 IU of vitamin A; 400 IU of vitamin D; 500 milligrams of vitamin C; 100 to 400 IU of vitamin E; plus calcium (500 milligrams a day for women under 50; 1,000 milligrams for women over 50) if you don't get three servings of milk, cheese, or yogurt every day.

Lifestyle Strategies

Get physical. Regular exercise can reduce your risk of a variety of cancers, including colon, breast, endometrial, and ovarian cancers.

"You should get at least 30 minutes of moderate-to-heavy physical activity a day," says Dr. Leitch. (For a complete guide to fitness, see chapter 5.)

Do Low-Calorie Diets Prevent Cancer?

before you sit down to your next big meal or hit the refrigerator for a midnight snack, consider this: Eating much less than you usually do could potentially add years to your life and prevent or delay the development of cancer or other diseases.

For more than 10 years, scientists at the National Institute on Aging in Baltimore have been studying two groups of 60 male and 60 female rhesus monkeys. Animals in one group are allowed to eat as much as they want, while those in the second group consume about a third fewer calories.

Preliminary results suggest a dramatic difference between the groups. Of the 60 well-fed monkeys, six have developed cancer. In the restricted-calorie group, only two have developed cancer. Other animal studies have shown similar effects.

It's possible that calorie restriction significantly slows cell division in the body, which reduces the likelihood of diseases that rely on cell proliferation, such as cancer and endometriosis, says Mark Lane, Ph.D., head of the Nutritional and Molecular Physiology Unit of the Laboratory of Neurosciences at the National Institute on Aging and principal investigator of the NIA's primate calorie restriction and aging project.

Animals who eat less also have lower incidences of heart disease, cataracts, and ulcers. They live longer, too. "In human terms, you'd see an average increase in life span from age 80 to 100, and the maximum age limit would rise from 120 years to 140 years," Dr. Lane says.

Should you reduce your calorie intake by one-third? Probably not. "That would mean skipping a meal a day every day for the rest of your life," says Dr. Lane. "It's just not realistic." ■

Live lean. "Excess weight gain has been associated with increased breast cancer risk," Dr. Bevers says.

Every woman knows just from looking in the mirror if her weight is close to what it should be. In scientific terms, a body mass index (BMI) of 25 to 29.9 is considered overweight, and anything over 30 is obese. To calculate your BMI, multiply your weight in pounds by 703. Divide that number by your height in inches. Divide that number again by your height in inches, and you'll have your BMI. A woman who's 5 foot 5 is overweight if she weighs between 150 and 179 pounds. (For more information on weight control, see chapter 6.)

Take a stress break. When you experience stress in your life, the body produces higher amounts of stress hormones, which suppress immunity and increase the likelihood of cancer. Soothing stress with relaxation strategies, such as yoga or meditation, not only appears to prevent some cancers but also helps prevent relapses in those who have already had cancer.

"Get in touch with your essence," says Dr. Gaynor. "Make a list of things in your life that

Views That Heal

mother Nature's beauty calms frayed nerves and soothes tired eyes. But can its magic have an effect on cancer and other diseases?

Absolutely, says Richard Enoch Kaufman, M.D., assistant clinical professor of internal medicine at Yale University School of Medicine. "Even having a hospital window with a view of nature, or having flowers in a room, is healing," he says.

Research suggests that people who are able to experience nature have an increase in immune activity. Nature also activates hormones that promote healing and neuropeptides that ease pain. One study showed that hospital patients who had a view of nature had shorter stays, less need for pain relievers, and fewer complaints during recovery.

Many of the nation's cancer wards have gone beyond providing pleasant views—they actually bring nature inside. At Marin General Hospital in Greenbrae, California, for example, patients about to undergo radiation treatments can look through a wall-length window from the waiting room into a sea of multihued foliage. They can hear the soothing sounds of a stone fountain. Paths and benches are arranged throughout the Healing Garden for those who wish to enter.

"The patients are vulnerable. They're usually wearing their gowns and are right in the throes of the most intense part of their treatment," says Leslie D. Davenport, manager of the hospital's Institute for Health and Healing Humanities Program. "The garden gives the feeling of being in a private inner sanctum."

To heighten the connection between nature and healing, the plants and trees in the garden are selected for their cancer-curing properties. One example is yew, a tree that yields a medication (taxol) that's used to treat ovarian and breast cancers.

"One cancer patient took home a cup of water from the fountain and put it in a bowl on her home altar," Davenport recalls. "It somehow represented her path to wellness—out of the artificial, harsh, technological world to a more natural place of healing." ■

serve you and things that don't—and try to get rid of those things not serving you. Play music that you find relaxing. Try yoga, deep breathing, guided imagery—anything that relaxes you." (For a stress-reduction action plan, see chapter 7.)

Medical Options

 Get a complete checkup. If you've never had a formal cancer risk assessment, now's the time to do it, says Dr. Bevers. "Knowing your risk for certain cancers allows you to pay attention to specific risk reduction strategies and screening techniques that are right for you," she says.

Your doctor can perform the assessment, but you can also do it on your own on the Internet. Visit the Web site of M. D. Anderson Cancer Center at www2.mdanderson.org/app/risk. Or check www.yourcancerrisk.harvard.edu/index.htm, the Web site for Harvard's Center for Cancer Prevention. To learn more about your risk for specific cancers such as breast, ovarian, uterine, and cervical cancers, visit the Web site of the

WHAT WORKS FOR ME

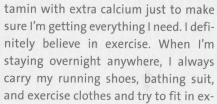

JULIE R. GRALOW, M.D., *is assistant professor of medical oncology at the University of Washington School of Medicine in Seattle and coauthor of* Breast Fitness: An Optimal Exercise and Health Plan for Reducing Your Risk of Breast Cancer. *Here's what she does to reduce her own risk of cancer.*

I try to practice what I preach on cancer prevention, but I'm the first to admit I'm not perfect. I don't smoke, but I do drink a glass or two of wine a week. A little bit is enjoyable, and it relaxes me.

I travel around the world a lot for work, and I try to be reasonable about my diet. I don't eat much meat, but I do eat fish. But I'm always struggling to get enough fruits and vegetables. In hotels, if I'm ordering room service, I have some control. During business meetings, I often order the vegetarian plate. Airport lounges now offer baskets of fruit, so I take some along. It's a little more work to get what you need, but it can be done.

Of course, there are days I look back and am mortified by what I've eaten, so I take a multivitamin with extra calcium just to make sure I'm getting everything I need. I definitely believe in exercise. When I'm staying overnight anywhere, I always carry my running shoes, bathing suit, and exercise clothes and try to fit in exercise, even if it's only at the hotel gym or around the neighborhood. I've actually jogged around the Kremlin and through Shanghai.

At home, I run a couple of times a week, and my husband and I try to plan an event every weekend, such as a bike ride or hiking. We've climbed nearby Mount Rainier and Mount Hood, and occasionally we've biked 50 miles a day. Every August I participate in a sprint triathlon (swimming, biking, running) as part of Team Survivor, a group of female cancer survivors I work with.

To reduce stress, I make sure to schedule quiet time. I love novels, and I read a couple nights a week and on weekends. I'm also a big fan of massages, and I try to get them whenever I can, especially when I'm traveling in Asia. ■

Women's Cancer Network at www.wcn.org, which also provides an online assessment of cancer risk.

BREAST CANCER

It's true that breast cancer strikes more women than any other kind of cancer. But your overall risk is probably much lower than you think, and there are ways to make it lower still.

About one in eight women will develop breast cancer during her lifetime. Hereditary factors, such as carrying the BRCA1 or BRCA2 breast cancer gene, account for 5 to 10 percent of all breast cancers. The rest are mainly due to what you eat and how you live.

Here's an anti-breast-cancer plan that will tilt the odds in your favor.

Nutritional Treatments

Have 10 daily servings of fruits and vegetables. In one recent study, women at high risk for breast cancer increased their daily intake of fruits and vegetables from 5.8 servings to 10 or more servings. After 2 weeks, re-

Women Blame Stress for Breast Cancer

Science has found strong links between cancer and diet, genes, and lifestyle. But cancer survivors tend to finger something else: stress. Do patients' beliefs—even when not scientifically proven—help them survive?

To find out, Donna Stewart, M.D., professor at the University of Toronto and chairperson of women's health for the University Health Network, surveyed nearly 400 breast cancer survivors who had been disease-free for at least 2 years. They were asked what they felt was the cause of their cancers, and why the cancers hadn't recurred.

Stress was overwhelmingly named as the leading culprit, cited by 42 percent of the respondents. Known scientific risk factors—such as genetics (26.7 percent), environment (25.5 percent), hormones (23.9 percent), and diet (15 percent)—trailed considerably.

"We know that stress alters immune function, and these women may in fact be partly right that stress contributed to their cancers," says Dr. Stewart. "But the evidence isn't very clear."

When the women were asked why their cancers hadn't returned, 60 percent credited their positive attitude. This was followed by diet (50 percent), healthy lifestyle (40.3 percent), exercise (39.4 percent), stress reduction (27.9 percent), and tamoxifen (3.9 percent).

Dr. Stewart and her colleagues concluded that patients' personal beliefs about the cause of their cancers—even when their opinions were at odds with scientific evidence—were important in helping them cope with and manage the disease and that these beliefs should be worked with and not be discounted by doctors. ∎

searchers found that free radical damage to the DNA in the women's white blood cells had dropped by 21.5 percent.

When choosing fruits and vegetables, look for those that contain a variety of phytochemicals, says Caroline L. Apovian, M.D., director of nutrition and weight management at Boston Medical Center, and associate professor of medicine at Boston University School of Medicine. Some of the best include citrus fruits and berries, cruciferous vegetables (such as broccoli and cabbage), leafy green vegetables, tomatoes, and yellow and orange vegetables.

Get more fiber in your diet. Dietary fiber helps reduce the amount of estrogen that circulates in the blood, and it reduces estrogen's impact at the cellular level, says Dr. Apovian. Over a woman's lifetime, this can reduce the risk of breast cancer. Fiber also makes the stools bulkier, which can allow the body to excrete estrogen more efficiently.

All plant foods contain fiber. When you plan your menus, be sure to include plenty of fruits, vegetables, whole grains, legumes, and nuts. *Prevention* magazine recommends 25 to 35 grams of fiber per day for general good nutrition.

Get "good" fats in your diet. Diets that are high in animal fats and high in foods, such as margarine, that contain trans fatty acids have been linked to higher breast cancer rates. Replace these with monounsaturated fats, such as those in olive and canola oils, or with omega-3 fatty acids, such as those in fish and flaxseed.

Drink moderately or not at all. Research suggests that woman who have two drinks a day may increase their risk of breast cancer by 25 percent. If your overall breast cancer risk is average, it's probably safe to have a drink or two on occasion. "One drink a day may be too much for women who already have breast cancer or for those at high risk," says Dr. Apovian.

Lifestyle Strategies

Get up and go. Don't underestimate the power of physical activity to safeguard you against breast cancer. Even a little bit of exercise can help—but the harder you exercise, the greater your protection. Brisk walking or jogging for 3 or more hours a week can lower your breast cancer risk by 30 percent.

"I recommend exercising for at least a half an hour, 3 or 4 days a week," says Julie R. Gralow, M.D., assistant professor of medical oncology at the University of Washington School of Medicine in Seattle and coauthor of *Breast Fitness: An Optimal Exercise and Health Plan for Reducing Your Risk of Breast Cancer.* "Then augment that with a bike ride or something else on weekends or other days."

Stay slim. One reason exercise is so crucial is that it controls fat, a tissue that produces large amounts of estrogen—and estrogen, as we've seen, increases the risk of breast cancer. Fat is even riskier after a woman reaches menopause, when the incidence of breast cancer rises.

"If you're 150 pounds, and then you gain 15 pounds at menopause, your risk increases," says Dr. Gralow.

Medical Options

℞ Use hormone replacement therapy (HRT) for a limited time. Women who have reached menopause may be advised to undergo HRT in order to reduce the risk of osteoporosis; supplemental estrogen also reduces hot flashes and other types of menopausal discomfort. However, there's some evidence that women who use hormone replacement therapy for an extended time may have a higher risk of breast cancer.

Studies indicate that limiting HRT to less than 5 years—just long enough to get through the period of hot flashes and menopausal mood swings—won't elevate the odds of getting breast cancer and will still probably protect against osteoporosis to some extent.

See your doctor regularly. You'll want to have an annual breast exam and mammogram, starting at age 40. If you have a high risk for breast cancer, your doctor may recommend starting mammograms earlier. You'll also want to practice monthly self-exams on your breasts throughout your life.

Some women, including those with dense breast tissue, may benefit from having a yearly MRI. Women who have a very high risk for breast cancer may be advised to undergo a procedure called ductal lavage, which can detect malignant cells years before a tumor shows up on a mammogram.

Consider chemoprevention. If you have a strong family history of breast cancer or you've had it yourself, talk to your doctor about taking tamoxifen, a selective estrogen receptor modulator that can reduce a woman's risk of developing the disease by almost 50 percent. Preliminary studies suggest that another drug, raloxifene, may be similarly beneficial.

LUNG CANCER

Preventing lung cancer can be summed up in two words: Don't smoke. If we all heeded this advice, lung cancer cases among men and women alike would drop by 80 percent.

Your chances of getting breast cancer are greater, but lung cancer is more likely to kill you if you get it. In fact, it's now the number-one cancer killer of women, mainly because more women are starting to smoke at an earlier age, when their lungs are most vulnerable.

"Mutational changes in the lungs start to develop right off the bat, so it's worth quitting earlier rather than later," says Anne L. Davis, M.D., a pulmonologist and associate professor of medicine at New York University School of Medicine and an attending physician at Bellevue Hospital, both in New York City. "Quitting smoking is the most important thing a woman can do."

If you've smoked for years, and you've smoked a lot, your risk of lung cancer is naturally greater than if you never smoked. But the risk drops dramatically once you quit and your lungs start repairing the smoke damage. In just 10 years, your risk may be up to half that of a smoker. Even if you wait until middle age to quit smoking, you can reduce your risk considerably.

For tips on giving up the habit, see chapter 8. Or point your browser to the American Lung Association's free online smoking cessation program at www.lungusa.org/ffs.

Nutritional Treatments

Eat your way to lung health. The chemical compounds in fruits and vegetables can protect the lungs from cancerous changes. In one study, women who ate more than six daily servings of fruits and vegetables were able to reduce their lung cancer risk by 21 to 32 percent.

Some of the best choices include cruciferous vegetables (such as cabbage and broccoli), citrus fruits, and vegetables high in carotenoids (such as tomatoes, winter squash, and carrots). Apples and onions are also good choices because they contain a compound called quercetin, which has been shown to reduce lung cancer rates.

Cook with curry. It contains curcumin, a compound that appears to detoxify smoking-related carcinogens in lung tissue.

Lifestyle Strategies

Exercise early or late. "Exercise is good for your lungs, but my only warning is to avoid exercise outside in highly polluted areas," says Dr. Davis. If you can't avoid the fumes from urban traffic or industry, at least get your exercise in the early morning or later in the evening, when traffic is lighter.

Check for radon. After smoking, radon is the main cause of lung cancer. It's formed during the

The Power of Acceptance

am putting myself in God's hands."

For years, when doctors heard cancer patients say these words, they felt that they were surrendering to almost certain death. Better to display a fighting spirit, it was assumed, than to accept the disease. But what sounds like resignation may actually be an effective coping style.

"We used to think that fatalism meant that someone believed that they were going to die and that there was nothing they could do," explains Ellen G. Levine, Ph.D., director of psychosocial oncology research at California Pacific Medical Center in San Francisco and affiliate member of the Cancer Center at the University of California, San Francisco. "But

for a certain group of women, that may not be so."

Dr. Levine and former graduate student Cory Fitzpatrick, Ph.D., assessed the coping styles of 120 women with breast cancer. Contrary to the prevailing notion that fatalism means giving up, the researchers found that adopting a fatalist attitude was linked to feelings of control, acceptance, spirituality, and engagement in religious practices. The women also reported a higher quality of life and less depression and anxiety.

"A better way to think of fatalism may be as spiritual acceptance," says Dr. Levine. "The attitude seems to be 'I'm doing everything I can; now it's up to God. I trust there will be spiritual help along the way.'" ■

natural breakdown of radium in rocks and soil, and it gets trapped in basements and other airtight spaces. If you live in a high-radon area, or if you just want to make sure that your house doesn't have elevated levels of this odorless, radioactive gas, look in your phone book for a testing service.

Medical Options

Rx Get tested right away. One reason lung cancer is so deadly is that the most common diagnostic test, a chest x-ray, isn't sensitive enough to detect tumors when they're small enough to be cured. If you're 60 years or older and you're a smoker or former smoker, talk to your doctor about getting an annual CAT (computerized axial tomography) scan, where a doughnut-shaped machine takes pictures of cross-sections of your body, called "slices." However, these screenings are not generally covered by health insurance.

A study of 1,000 heavy smokers found that low-radiation CAT scans detected suspicious nod-

ules in the lungs more reliably and earlier than standard chest x-rays.

COLORECTAL CANCER

For some reason, people often think that cancers of the colon or rectum (colorectal cancers) are more likely to strike men than women. The opposite is true: slightly more women now die from colorectal cancer each year than do men.

However, this is one type of cancer that can almost always be prevented. "If you get tested and have a reasonable diet, you shouldn't get colorectal cancer," says Ernestine Hambrick, M.D., founder of the Stop Colon-Rectal Cancer Foundation in Chicago.

Most colorectal cancers begin as a polyp, a tissue growth inside the colon or rectum. Over many years, they may gradually change to cancer.

"Usually there's adequate time to prevent cancer by removing polyps before they turn cancerous," says Mary Elizabeth Roth, M.D., a clinical professor at Wayne State University School of Medicine in Detroit and vice president of medical

Rye Protects against Colon Cancer

the next time you eat a deli sandwich on rye, you might be enjoying powerful protection. A recent study in Finland looked at 17 people who ate either about four slices of whole grain rye or the same amount of refined bread, every day for 4 weeks. Researchers found that the whole grain rye re-

duced levels of bile acids—digestive fluids that are thought to promote colon cancer—by an average of 26 percent.

Unfortunately, most of the rye bread in the United States is made from refined flour. To get the benefits from rye, check the labels and look for the term "whole rye flour" or "whole rye meal." ∎

affairs at Sacred Heart Hospital in Allentown, Pennsylvania. Even a malignant polyp, if caught before the cancer spreads, can be removed almost all the time for full recovery.

"That's why it's so important to assess your risk and get tested regularly," says Dr. Roth.

Medical Options

Have regular tests. Doctors advise people with average risk for colorectal cancer to get a digital rectal exam as part of their annual physical exam along with a fecal occult blood test, starting at age 50. For a more thorough screening starting at age 50, *Prevention* magazine recommends that you undergo, every 10 years, the testing procedure called colonoscopy. Recent research has found that colonoscopy is the most effective method of screening for colon cancer. During a colonoscopy, a slender, flexible lighted tube is inserted through the rectum. It allows the doctor to see any abnormalities throughout the large intestine. It's important to also have a flexible sigmoidoscopy every 3 to 5 years. During this test, the doctor gently inserts a soft, bendable tube about the thickness of the index finger into the anus (rectal opening) to examine the rectum and lower colon.

If you have a high risk of colorectal cancer—because you have a family history of colon cancer, for example, or if you have inflammatory bowel disease—you may be advised to start having the tests at an earlier age, and having them more often.

Talk to your doctor about hormone replacement. "Women who have been on estrogen replacement therapy—even those who have been on it for just 1 year, starting at age 60 or 70—have a lower incidence of colon cancer," says Dr. Roth. "The lowest rate is among those who've been on it since menopause."

Nutritional Treatments

Eat plenty of fiber. Cereals and breads contain fiber, but most of it is too refined to protect your colon from carcinogens. "The best sources of fiber are raw fruits and vegetables," says Dr. Roth. "Fiber literally cleans away potential carcinogens from your intestine."

One study found that people who ate more than six daily servings of fiber-rich fruits and vegetables had a 40 percent lower risk of colorectal cancer than those who only ate two daily servings.

Cut way back on fat. The saturated fat in meats, butter, and other animal foods may cause cellular changes in the intestine that can lead to cancer.

Eat grilled foods sparingly. Meat that's charred on the grill (or in the broiler) produces cancer-causing compounds that can increase the risk of colon cancer, says Dr. Roth. She recommends grilling only on occasion. When you do grill, don't let the flames touch the meat, which increases the production of cancer-causing compounds.

Take folic acid. Studies have shown that taking 400 micrograms of folic acid (the synthetic form of folate) daily may reduce the risk for colon cancer.

Get extra calcium. This essential nutrient is believed to bind to toxic bile acids released from the liver. This is important because bile acids may trigger cancer when they come into contact with the colon wall.

The best dietary sources of calcium include low-fat milk and cheese, fortified cereals or soy milk, and vegetables such as broccoli and turnips. You also may want to take a calcium supplement. Dr. Gaynor recommends taking 1,500 milligrams daily if you're postmenopausal and you aren't undergoing hormone replacement therapy. Younger women can take 1,000 milligrams daily.

Home Remedies

Keep regular bowel habits. If you exercise regularly, drink plenty of fluids, and get enough fiber in your diet, your bowel movements will naturally stay regular. This is important because constipation may increase the risk for colon cancer by allowing harmful substances to linger in the intestine, says Dr. Roth.

UTERINE OR ENDOMETRIAL CANCER

A woman's body produces estrogen, which offers significant protection to your heart and bones. But too much estrogen can boost the risk of uterine and other reproductive cancers, which usually strike after menopause. In fact, high exposure to estrogen over many years may be your single biggest risk factor for uterine cancer.

If you started menstruating before age 12, entered menopause after age 50, never gave birth, and have a history of infertility, you've been exposed to relatively large amounts of estrogen over time—and your chances of getting uterine cancer are elevated.

You can't change your menstrual or reproductive history, but there are other ways to reduce your lifelong exposure to estrogen. Here's what doctors recommend.

Lifestyle Strategies

Maintain a healthful weight. Fat tissue does more than hug your thighs and hips. It converts certain hormones into estrogen. Women who are obese are two to five times more likely to develop endometrial cancer than are slimmer women. (For more information on achieving—and maintaining—a healthful weight, see chapter 6.)

Nutritional Treatments

Follow a low-fat diet. Foods that are high in fats, particularly animal fats, can raise your risk of uterine cancer in two ways. Fatty foods lead to weight gain—and fat tissue itself, as we've seen, increases the risk of cancer. High-fat foods also appear to boost the body's production of estrogen.

Research has shown that women who consume diets low in fat and high in complex carbohydrates have a reduced risk for developing endometrial cancer, says Linda R. Duska, M.D., a gynecological oncologist at the Gillette Center for Women's Cancers at Massachusetts General Hospital in Boston.

Medical Options

Consider birth control pills. Taking oral contraceptives for up to 5 years defends against endometrial cancer—not only while you're using them but for years afterward. Most birth control pills contain progesterone, which helps reduce the body's exposure to estrogen. It's the same reason that pregnancy—which shifts the hormonal balance toward greater levels of progesterone—also safeguards the uterus.

Add progesterone to hormone replacement therapy. There's no question that the use of supplemental estrogen after menopause has given new meaning to the term "golden years." But taking estrogen without balancing it with progesterone may increase the risk for endometrial cancer.

"It's pretty clear that a lot of uterine cancer is preventable with the use of progesterone during estrogen replacement," says Joanna M. Cain, M.D., chairperson of the department of obstetrics and gynecology at Pennsylvania State University in Hershey.

Be wary of tamoxifen. Used to prevent breast cancer, it acts like estrogen in the uterus, sometimes encouraging growth of the uterine lining and slightly raising the risk of endometrial cancer. If you're taking tamoxifen, have a yearly

Speak Up to Relieve Cancer Pain

about 90 percent of people with cancer have at least moderate pain at some point in their illness, but half don't find relief.

New research shows that a frank talk with your doctor could make all the difference. Researchers at the University of California, Davis, studied 67 people with cancer pain. Counselors met with half of the group to set pain relief goals and rehearse what to say at future doctor visits. The other half received standard pain control advice. Two weeks later, after all the patients had seen their doctors, those who had received coaching felt 20 percent less pain. Those who'd reported severe pain now described it as moderate.

"Cancer patients should know that their physi-

cians are just as concerned about symptoms such as pain as they are about treating their cancer directly," says lead study author Richard L. Kravitz, M.D., director of the university's Center for Health Services Research in Primary Care. "Don't be afraid to tell your doctor."

To help ease cancer pain, take these steps.

Ditch these myths. Cancer patients worry that treating pain may keep their doctors from treating their cancer aggressively or that they'll become addicted to pain medicines. Neither is true.

Set goals. For example, you may hope to sleep through the night without pain. Rehearse. Have a run-through with a friend or relative before your doctor visit. ■

gynecologic exam—and be sure to report any abnormal bleeding to your doctor.

Report unusual bleeding to your doctor. A number of conditions, many of them harmless, can cause abnormal menstrual bleeding. With endometrial cancer, however, abnormal bleeding is almost a given. "If you're bleeding abnormally, especially after menopause, contact your doctor," says Dr. Duska.

See your gynecologist. Starting at age 18, visit a gynecologist every year for a pelvic exam and Pap test. If you are under age 18 but are sexually active, you should go earlier.

The Pap test is most effective at detecting cervical cancer (in the lower uterus), but it may detect endometrial cancers as well. If you have the hereditary form of colon cancer or are at risk for it, your chance of developing uterine cancer is also higher. Get an annual endometrial biopsy—a test that looks for cancerous changes in the tissue lining the uterus—beginning at age 35.

OVARIAN CANCER

"The most significant factor related to ovarian cancer is the number of ovulations that you have

The Benefits of Healing Retreats

I n 1995, Nancy J. Raymon and Donna Farris founded Healing Odyssey, a retreat and follow-up support program for female cancer survivors. Since then, they have witnessed again and again how group support can powerfully transform and extend the lives of women with cancer.

Raymon, an oncology clinical nurse specialist and director of program development at the Hoag Cancer Center in Newport Beach, California, decided to demonstrate the effectiveness and long-term benefits of weekend retreats. She surveyed 41 women, mostly breast cancer survivors, who were to participate in a retreat held in a remote location. The retreat included a coping with fear and sexuality workshop, a spirituality session, yoga, meditation, and guided imagery sessions, nature walks, a Saturday-night celebration, and an Empowerment Walk.

The survey looked at physical, psychological, social, and spiritual well-being. Raymon and a colleague evaluated participants before the retreat, directly afterward, 6 weeks later, and again at 6 months.

"We found a statistically significant increase in all four quality-of-life domains following the retreat," says Raymon. What's more, the effects remained strong after 6 months.

Raymon believes that healing retreats are effective because more and more patients are now living long lives with cancer. Many are looking to sharpen their survival skills and maintain long-term physical, psychological, and spiritual health by connecting with others.

"Cancer has become more of a chronic disease, unlike in the past, when most people either died or were cured," says Raymon. "These retreats are designed to help people deal with the challenging emotional and psychological issues of survivorship. It's also building a community of support and learning practical tools for moving forward with life." ■

WHEN BAD THINGS HAPPEN TO HEALTHY WOMEN

She Survived Both Breast and Ovarian Cancers

Corinne Beacham-Greene considers herself blessed. Not just because she's still alive and active after a devastating diagnosis of breast cancer in 1988 and a more recent diagnosis of ovarian cancer. Rather, she says, she treasures what she's learned on her path to wellness.

"I value every day, and I try to stay cognizant of the miracles that happen all the time," she says. "Most days everything works right in our bodies. That's a miracle."

Beacham-Greene was 35 years old when she first noticed a lump in her breast 14 years ago, while she was rocking her 3-year-old son to sleep. She had a lumpectomy, chemotherapy, and radiation, and the tumor disappeared.

Then, in 1998, she noticed pain and severe bloating in her abdomen. After seeing her primary care physician for 4 months with these symptoms, her primary care physician ordered a sonogram. At that point, she was quickly diagnosed with advanced ovarian cancer, and she underwent a total hysterectomy. She still receives chemotherapy. "I'm trying to keep the cancer under control until a treatment comes along that works; my doctor calls it 'coexisting' with the disease," she says. "I put myself in God's hands, and I focus on my children and husband. My goal is to be the best person I can, and not give the cancer any more than I've already given it."

In addition to healthful living, including not eating red meat, Beacham-Greene incorporates a few complementary approaches into her healing strategy, such as yoga and visualization. "When I have chemotherapy, for instance, I visualize it as white light going through my body, instead of poison," she says.

More important, she says, are the profound relationships that have been made richer and stronger through adversity—relationships with other cancer survivors, as well as with her children and husband.

"We're a very close, tight-knit family, and we don't take each other for granted," she says. "My kids have a developed a different level of awareness about what's important. My husband and I are still very passionate about each other. I think that's what's kept me going." ■

over a lifetime," says Dr. Cain. "Things that suppress ovulation—such as birth control pills, having children, breastfeeding, later menstruation, or early menopause—will all decrease your risk."

About 10 percent of ovarian cancers are genetic. If your mother, sister, or daughter has had ovarian cancer or breast cancer, particularly at a young age, or if you've had breast cancer yourself, your chances of getting ovarian cancer are greater.

Whatever your initial risk, following the general anticancer plan that we discussed at the beginning of this chapter will go a long way toward providing lifetime protection. In addition, here are some other strategies that you'll want to follow.

Medical Options

Rx **Get tested regularly.** Have an annual pelvic exam and Pap test starting at age 18. The exams are particularly important after age 65, when half of all ovarian cancers show up. Pap tests, which are best at finding cervical cancer, sometimes detect advanced ovarian cancers as well.

If you have a family history of cancer, you may want to visit a genetic counselor to find out if you carry the BRCA1 or BRCA2 gene. These genes raise the risk for both ovarian and breast cancers.

"You'll want to discuss what you're going to do if you have the gene," says Dr. Cain. "Doctors recommend removing the ovaries after a woman is done having children. If someone's not at that point yet, we can test with transvaginal ultrasound (with a small instrument inserted into the vagina) and a CA-125 screen every 6 months." CA-125 is a blood protein that's sometimes elevated in women with ovarian cancer. These tests are recommended only for women with a higher-than-average risk of ovarian cancer, Dr. Cain adds.

Enroll in a clinical trial. "If you carry the BRCA genes, my recommendation is to be involved in a study," says Vicki Seltzer, M.D., chairman of obstetrics and gynecology at Long Island Jewish Medical Center and North Shore University Hospital in New Hyde Park, New York, and past president of the American College of Obstetricians and Gynecologists.

Your doctor can tell you how to enroll in a clinical study. Or contact the American Cancer Society at www.cancer.org or (800) ACS-2345.

Report symptoms immediately. "Many women have subtle symptoms, such as mild nausea, a little diarrhea that doesn't get better, or a slight pain in the pelvic region, about 6 months to a year before they're diagnosed with ovarian cancer," says Dr. Cain.

Other symptoms of ovarian cancer include long-term swelling of the abdomen, unusual vaginal bleeding, pelvic pain or pressure, back pain, leg pain, or digestive disorders, such as gas, indigestion, or stomach pain.

Chances are, the symptoms will turn out to be nothing to worry about, but having prompt checkups can ease your mind and also aid your chances of recovery if it turns out to be ovarian cancer.

Review reproductive options with your doctor. Having one or more pregnancies is one way to reduce the risk for ovarian cancer, especially if your first baby arrives before you're 30. If you breast-feed for a year or more, you'll improve your odds further.

This doesn't mean that women should rush into having children before they're ready. The goal is to reduce your body's long-term exposure to ovulation, and this can be achieved with the use of birth control pills. Women who take birth control pills for more than 5 years are 60 percent less likely to get ovarian cancer than women who have never used them.

CERVICAL CANCER

Your mother and grandmother probably worried more about cervical cancer than you do. Thanks to the development of Pap tests, which allow for early detection, deaths from cervical cancer plummeted by nearly three-quarters between 1955 and 1992.

But don't let vigilance blip off your radar screen. Your risk may be higher than you think, particularly if you or your partner has been sexually active outside the relationship, or at other times in your lives.

The leading cause of cervical cancer is infection with HPV—the sexually transmitted, and often symptomless, human papillomavirus. The more sexual partners you and your partner have had, the greater your likelihood of HPV infection.

"All women may be at higher risk for HPV than they believe," says Dr. Seltzer. Even if you've had few sexual partners in your life, your significant other may unwittingly harbor the infection.

So far, there isn't a sure way to prevent HPV. The use of condoms can help, but it's possible for HPV to be transmitted during skin-to-skin contact with an infected area, such as skin of the gen-

Pap Test Update

If you went for your annual Pap test recently, you may have found your gynecologist using a new type of test called the ThinPrep. Unlike the conventional method for Pap testing, the ThinPrep test "rinses" the instrument used to collect cells into a container of liquid. When the sample reaches the lab, a special process separates the cervical cells from any accompanying debris and then applies a thin layer of cells to a slide.

The result is a slide that is clearer and easy to read. ThinPrep has been around for a few years, so why are doctors only switching now? Because when ThinPrep first became available, it was more costly, and though it was picking up more abnormalities, these were mostly low-grade lesions, which often resolve without treatment.

But several things have changed since then. Nearly 300 insurers now reimburse for all or part of liquid-based tests. Here are more positives: Yale University School of Medicine is now encouraging its physicians to use a liquid-based Pap test because research suggests that ThinPrep does indeed result in higher-quality slides and fewer unsatisfactory or limited slides that require a repeat Pap. The majority of studies published in the past 2 years have confirmed that ThinPrep does detect a higher percentage of low- and high-grade precancerous lesions than conventional Pap tests.

Today, 41 percent of all Pap tests administered are ThinPrep tests, according to a company spokesperson. The big, still unanswered question is whether ThinPrep detects the most common cancerous or invasive lesions (called squamous cell) better than the usual Pap test.

"While in theory it should be better at picking up invasive cancer, I think it's still open to question," says Kenneth Noller, M.D., professor and chairman of the department of obstetrics and gynecology at Tufts University/New England Medical Center in Boston. There simply aren't enough data yet, explains Dr. Noller, a consultant on Pap tests for the American College of Obstetricians and Gynecologists. "Even in studies of 100,000 women, the number of invasive cancers is so small that comparisons between the two tests are difficult," he says. "There are, however, some preliminary data that ThinPrep picks up more glandular lesions (adenocarcinoma) than the traditional Pap test," he says. This type of cancer is rarer and may occur higher up in the cervix than squamous cell cancer. ■

ital area not covered by the condom, even if symptoms aren't apparent. Doctors are currently working on an experimental vaccine, and within a few years it could be available. "If successful, it will pretty much wipe out cervical cancer," predicts Dr. Duska.

Here are some other important strategies.

Medical Options

 Have an annual Pap test. One of the most important things you can do is have a Pap test every year, beginning at age 18

or when you first start having intercourse, whichever comes first. Pap tests can detect the signs of cervical cancer long before it becomes a real threat.

"Cervical cancer is almost completely preventable with regular Pap tests," says Dr. Seltzer. It can also be successfully treated when abnormalities are detected early.

It's not uncommon for mild dysplasias (precancerous cell abnormalities) to show up during Pap tests. These abnormalities don't always become cancerous. They may even disappear by themselves. If you have a positive test, don't be

Drumming Up Cancer Immunity

group drumming is used as a part of healing rituals around the world. It sounds more like a quaint relic of medicine's unenlightened past than a modern cancer fighter. But drumming circles could soon find their way into oncology's arsenal of potent new weapons.

Barry Bittman, M.D., is medical director of the Mind-Body Wellness Center in Meadville, Pennsylvania. He and his colleagues have looked at group drumming and its effects on stress levels and immune function.

To enhance camaraderie and lightheartedness, participants in the studies were first asked to pass around, faster and faster, plastic "shaker eggs" filled with sand or gravel until the eggs invariably fell to the floor—and the group erupted into laughter. Participants were then asked to drum together in rhythm to their own names,

varying the tempo and pace. This was followed by a guided imagery session in which members played their drums as the facilitator told stories.

The researchers found that people who drummed had a reduction in stress levels and an increase in their immune response, including a rise in natural killer cell activity. Natural killer cells are the body's main cancer-fighting cells.

Apart from the physical effects of drumming, it's also a powerful community-building tool, says Dr. Bittman. It allows participants to reveal feelings that may be hard to air verbally.

Dr. Bittman now uses drumming circles with his cancer patients, both to help them destress and to give voice to their pain and fears.

"Chemotherapy, radiation, and surgery are certainly valid therapies, but there's also a fourth tool—a whole-person component that provides coping strategies, community, and stress reduction," he says. ∎

surprised if your doctor doesn't seem too concerned. He or she might schedule a follow-up Pap test to keep track of changes.

If the dysplasia is more advanced, your doctor will probably remove the abnormal cells. It's a simple procedure that can be done right in the office, either with the use of liquid nitrogen (cryosurgery) or with a cone biopsy.

Lifestyle Strategies

 Don't light up. If you smoke, do everything possible to quit right away. Doctors believe that tobacco smoke creates chemicals that damage DNA in cervical cells. If you smoke, you're twice as likely to get cervical cancer as a nonsmoker.

Nutritional Treatments

Consume retinoids. Found in a wide variety of fruits and vegetables, retinoids such as vitamin A and beta-carotene ap-

pear to slow the growth of epithelial cells in the cervix, which is where most cancerous and precancerous abnormalities occur.

SKIN CANCER

We all like that sun-kissed look, but our love affair with the sun is a prime health hazard. Skin cancer is the most common of all cancers.

"Heredity plays a role, and the more irregular moles you have, the more likely it is that you may develop melanoma," says Diane Berson, M.D., assistant clinical professor of dermatology at New York University School of Medicine in New York City. "But protecting yourself from the sun is the most important thing you can do."

Fortunately, most skin cancers are highly curable, especially nonmelanomas, such as basal cell and squamous cell carcinomas, which account for the majority of cases.

Malignant melanomas are less common, but they're also less curable. Catching them early is your best shot at making a complete recovery.

Vaccine Boosts Skin Cancer Survival

a recent study looked at 62 men and women with high-risk melanoma who had been given a new anticancer vaccine. Five years later, 55 percent were still alive. Without the vaccine, researchers estimate, only 20 percent of the patients would have been expected to survive.

The injectable vaccine, which was made from the patients' own chemically altered cancer cells,

seems to stop the spread of the disease by activating the immune system to attack active cancer cells, explains lead study author David Berd, M.D., professor of medicine at Thomas Jefferson University in Philadelphia.

More studies are planned, and the vaccine may be ready for marketing within the next few years. ■

Wearing sunscreen is essential, of course. It's especially important to start using it early because 80 percent of sun exposure occurs before you're 18. *Prevention* magazine recommends wearing, at all times, a waterproof, sweat-proof sunscreen with at least 15 SPF and full ultraviolet A (UVA) and ultraviolet B (UVB) protection. Apply it 20 minutes before exposure and reapply every 2 hours. You should also avoid the sun as much as possible between 10:00 A.M. and 4:00 P.M. (For a complete guide to skin care, see chapter 9.) Practicing healthy habits, such as refraining from smoking and eating a low-fat diet, will contribute to the overall health of your skin, including reducing cancer risk and having fewer wrinkles.

Dr. Berson recommends having an annual skin exam by a dermatologist, starting in adulthood. *Prevention* recommends seeing a dermatologist for a head-to-toe skin cancer check at least every 3 years between ages 20 and 40. If you've had skin cancer or are at high risk because of family history, start exams earlier and get them more often.

It's also important to check your skin monthly. When looking at moles, remember the letters A (asymmetry), B (border irregularity), C (changes in color), and D (changes in diameter). If you notice any one of these changes, you could have a higher risk for developing melanoma.

Nonmelanomas often start as pale or pink, waxlike, pearly nodules, or as red, scaly patches. Report to your doctor any skin changes, including scaling, oozing, or bleeding from bumps or moles. "Skin cancer is the one cancer that shouldn't be missed, because it's visible," says Dr. Berson.

It's also worth drinking a few cups of green tea daily or using skin-care products that contain green tea extract. Green tea is rich in antioxidants, which have been shown to prevent skin cancer in laboratory mice. Some researchers believe green tea is probably just as effective in humans.

17

Osteoporosis

One of the scary things about osteoporosis, a bone-thinning condition that primarily affects women after menopause, is that it develops over decades without causing overt symptoms. It doesn't hurt. You won't see any visible signs. But year after year, the bones get progressively weaker. You won't suspect there's a problem until you actually fracture a wrist, hip, or spinal bone or notice a substantial decrease in your height.

Osteoporosis is incredibly common. Your risk of developing it rises with age, especially in the first 5 to 7 years after menopause, when drops in estrogen may result in a 20 percent loss of bone mass. For women 50 years and older, the risk of suffering an osteoporosis-related bone fracture at some point is about 50 percent.

The good news? Even if you have risk factors for osteoporosis—such as a family history of the disease, a thin or small-framed body, a history of irregular or skipped periods, smoking or drinking excessive amounts of alcohol, not getting enough calcium, being inactive, or having taken steroids or other bone-thinning medications—the odds for preventing it can be very much in your favor.

"Osteoporosis is a disease of heredity and lifestyle," says Bess Dawson-Hughes, M.D., di-

rector of the calcium and bone metabolism laboratory at the USDA Human Nutrition Research Center on Aging at Tufts University in Boston. "You can't do much about heredity, but you can prevent much of it with lifestyle modifications."

Nutritional Treatments

Throughout your life, bone cells called osteoblasts are continually adding new bone to your skeleton while cells called osteoclasts demolish old bone in order to supply the rest of your body with much-needed calcium.

The prime bone-building years are between childhood and early adulthood. In other words, at that time new bone is added to your skeleton faster than old bone is destroyed. By age 30, your bones are as dense and strong as they'll get. After that, bone loss gradually begins to outpace bone construction. Everyone—male or female—needs an adequate level of estrogen to build bone during their youth. Estrogen deficiency in premenopausal women is a significant risk factor for bone loss, and once a woman reaches menopause, declines in the body's estrogen cause the bones to lose calcium and break down at an accelerated rate.

"Whether you get enough calcium and build adequate bone mass early in life or not, your body will start reabsorbing bone from your skeleton during your perimenopausal and postmenopausal years, which can lead to osteoporosis," says Ethel Siris, M.D., director of the Toni Stabile Center for Osteoporosis at Columbia Presbyterian Medical Center in New York City. "If you enter menopause with a lower bone mass, obviously you'll be at a disadvantage," Dr. Siris notes. The body uses the reabsorbed bone to keep your blood calcium at a healthy level to sustain life.

Get enough calcium. Calcium is important throughout your life, but your needs for this important mineral change over time.

If you're 50 years or younger, you should be getting 1,000 milligrams of calcium daily through your food, plus a supplement if needed. If you're older than 50, you need 1,500 milligrams daily. That's a lot of calcium, but Mother Nature is generous—many delicious, wholesome foods are brimming with it, says Robert R. Recker, M.D., director of the Osteoporosis Research Center at Creighton University School of Medicine in Omaha, Nebraska. Dairy products are your best bet, followed by calcium-fortified juices, breads, and cereals.

How much calcium can you get in your diet? Consider this: Just three daily servings of low-fat or fat-free milk, cheese, or calcium-fortified soy milk or orange juice will provide more than 1,000 milligrams of calcium. When you add the calcium that you get from other foods, such as legumes or salad greens, you'll get the calcium that your bones need to stay healthy—provided you eat all those foods day in and day out.

Consider supplements. Even women who eat healthful diets most of the time don't always get enough calcium. This is especially true of women who don't eat dairy foods—either because they don't care for the taste or because they find them hard to digest. If you aren't getting enough calcium in your diet, it's fine to make up the difference with supplements, says Dr. Siris.

She sometimes advises women to take chewable supplements, such as Tums (an antacid that's calcium-based) or Viactiv soft chews, as a portion of their daily calcium intake. You can also choose to take traditional calcium supplements. Supplements in any form are often overkill, Dr. Siris notes, because your body is able to absorb only a certain amount of calcium at one time and then excretes the excess. Genetics play a role in determining how much calcium your body can actually use for optimal bone density, Dr. Siris explains. Your body never fully absorbs all of the calcium you ingest, but taking calcium in several servings or doses throughout the day will optimize absorption.

"You might think you're getting 900 milligrams of calcium at breakfast if you drink a glass of milk—which has about 300 milligrams—and take a 600-milligram supplement, but in reality you're only absorbing somewhat less," she says.

One more point about supplements: Those that contain calcium carbonate should be taken only with meals in order to prevent stomach upset. Supplements that contain calcium citrate, on the other hand, can be taken anytime.

Be aware of the calcium robbers. Salt, caffeine, and protein play a role in removing calcium from your body. To safeguard your calcium stores, cut back on processed, canned, and fast foods, plus chips, pickles, and other items that are high in salt, says Dr. Dawson-Hughes. The upper daily limit for salt is about 2,400 milligrams, assuming you consume 2,000 calories daily.

Dr. Dawson-Hughes also advises drinking no more than two cups of coffee a day—although adding milk to coffee will replenish the calcium that's lost due to the caffeine. It's also helpful to eat moderate amounts of protein. Women between the ages of 30 and 50 are advised to get about 10 to 15 percent of their total caloric intake from protein each day.

Lifestyle Strategies

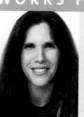

Get a little sun each day. Every time sunshine strikes your skin, the body produces vitamin D, which aids in the absorption of calcium. You get some vitamin D in fish oil, egg yolks, and fortified milk, but few other foods contain this vital nutrient—so getting a little bit of sun makes good sense.

If you don't get much sun, you may want to take a multivitamin that contains vitamin D—or take a calcium supplement with vitamin D added. The recommended daily dose of vitamin D is 400 IU. Women over 70 should take 600 IU.

Get plenty of exercise. Aerobic exercise is good for everyone, but for protecting the bones, you can't beat weight-bearing or resistance exercises, which are essential for increasing or maintaining bone mass.

What's the best exercise? You have plenty to choose from. Felicia Cosman, M.D., clinical director of the National Osteoporosis Foundation and asso-

---

WHAT WORKS FOR ME

FELICIA COSMAN, M.D., *clinical director of the National Osteoporosis Foundation and associate professor of medicine at Columbia University in New York City, shares her secrets for keeping her bones strong.*

My mother was diagnosed with osteoporosis in her early sixties. She suffered compression fractures of the spine, which resulted in height loss and back discomfort. That puts me at greater risk, so I've developed a personal strategy to prevent osteoporosis.

First, I make sure to get enough calcium each day. I don't drink milk, so I have 4 to 6 ounces of calcium-fortified juice at breakfast—it provides about 200 milligrams of calcium. Reduced-fat dairy products offer as much calcium as regular dairy products, so at other meals I eat about 1 to 1.5 ounces of reduced-fat cheese, which adds another 300 milligrams. I take one 500-milligram Viactiv chew, and I probably get another 200 milligrams from other foods in my diet, which includes about five servings of fruits and vegetables a day.

I don't take vitamin D supplements, but I get outside in the sunshine most days during the week, and I wear sunscreen.

Exercise is a big part of my routine. I go to the gym at work three times a week—either during lunchtime or right after work. I jog on the treadmill for 25 to 30 minutes, and I do weight training for my back, upper body, and legs.

I also plan to have a bone-density test as I approach menopause in the next decade. ■

ciate professor of medicine at Columbia University in New York City, advises women to run, walk, ski, or dance. In fact, any activity that gets you on your feet and moving against gravity for 30 minutes five times a week will keep or modestly increase your bone mass. (For details on starting an exercise program and sticking with it, see chapter 5.) For additional benefits, add 15 minutes of muscle-strengthening exercises, such as lifting weights. (For a complete guide to bone-building exercises, see the photos and instructions on page 216.)

If you smoke, make every effort to quit. Cigarettes damage the bones in several ways. Smoking lowers levels of estrogen, which hastens bone loss. In addition, women who smoke may absorb less of the calcium in their diets. (For details on how to quit, see chapter 8.)

Drink alcohol in moderation, if at all. Having more than a drink or two a day will interfere with the bones' ability to absorb calcium. Heavy drinking is even more detrimental because it often results in poor nutritional intake overall, which can increase the risk of osteoporosis and fractures.

Medical Options

 As we've seen, the body's levels of estrogen decline at menopause. Combined with the natural bone loss that occurs with age, this can vastly increase your risk for osteoporosis and related bone fractures. Women who have reached menopause need to follow all of the bone-protection strategies that they depended on when they were younger—plus some that are unique to this stage of life.

"It's good to have an ongoing dialogue with your physician about your bone status throughout your life," says Dr. Siris. "Simply taking calcium and exercising won't stop osteoporosis. You need to discuss your risk factors and what you can do for protection."

Get a bone test. Around the time you've reached menopause and have one or more risk factor for osteoporosis, you'll probably want to undergo a test called central DEXA (dual energy x-ray absorptiometry), which measures bone density of the hip and spine. If you don't have any risk factors for osteoporosis, you can probably put off the test until you're between the ages of 60 and 65, says Dr. Cosman. *Prevention* magazine recommends that women have a baseline bone-density test at the first signs of menopause—or earlier if they have one or more of the risk factors for osteoporosis. If you're 50 or older, the test may be covered by your health insurance.

If you're still in your thirties and forties, there's no reason to have a bone-density test as long as you eat a nutritious diet, get regular exercise, have a healthy lifestyle, and don't have any risk factors for osteoporosis.

Ask your doctor about taking estrogen replacement. You may already be on estrogen replacement therapy if you have been experiencing menopausal symptoms, such as hot flashes. If not, ask your doctor if you should be taking supplemental estrogen for maintaining and increasing your bone mass. Estrogen replacement therapy may be particularly important for those postmenopausal women who have low bone density. "If you are uncomfortable

WHEN BAD THINGS HAPPEN TO HEALTHY WOMEN

She Made Up for Lost Time—And Bone

About 12 years ago, Linda Harrigan, now a 51-year-old Washington lobbyist, felt a pain in her hip during aerobics class. The pain was bad enough to send her to her doctor. Even more shocking was the diagnosis: osteoporosis.

"My reaction was total surprise," she recalls. "I thought, 'This is an old woman's disease.'"

While the reasons for her condition weren't surprising (she had undergone a hysterectomy, which had halted her body's production of bone-building estrogen), she didn't understand why her doctor hadn't recommended supplemental estrogen or extra calcium to offset the bone loss.

"I was angry," Harrigan says. "But I'm also a fighter. I never gave up, and I never stopped to be emotional."

As soon as she got the news, Harrigan went on a bone-strengthening regimen. She began getting 1,800 milligrams of calcium daily, from high-calcium foods and supplements, and she launched into an exercise plan that included walking, cycling, lifting weights, and running on a treadmill. Because she has brittle bones, she stays away from pounding activities, such as horseback riding or running on hard surfaces.

Harrigan also decided to begin low-dose estrogen replacement therapy, and she gets a bone-density test every 2 years. Because she has a family history of breast cancer, however, she may discontinue the use of estrogen and begin taking an osteoporosis-stopping drug.

"I've been told that my spine is what you'd find in a 90-year-old, so I worry sometimes that my body will start to crumble and fall apart. But I'm very upbeat about it. I just went for my yearly checkup, and I'm still 5 foot 10, and my posture is excellent. I've been blessed." ∎

with choosing estrogen, there are alternatives you can discuss with your physician," Dr. Cosman notes.

Take medications to prevent bone loss. Most women can prevent osteoporosis by maintaining a healthful lifestyle—but if you already have it, your doctor may recommend medications that will prevent further bone loss.

In addition to estrogen, the FDA has approved a number of drugs for the prevention and treatment of osteoporosis. These include the selective estrogen receptor modulator raloxifene (Evista), alendronate (Fosamax), calcitonin (Miacalcin nasal spray), and risedronate (Actonel). Each of these drugs reduces bone loss and also increases bone density.

"If you're 65 or older and have osteoporosis, you'll probably want to take one of these drugs after you go off estrogen replacement," says Dr. Cosman. "If you don't have osteoporosis, you might not need drugs. Just continue your prevention program."

Strengthen Your Bones with Exercise

There are two main types of exercises for building and strengthening bones: weight-bearing exercises, in which you move your body against gravity, and strength-training and resistance exercises, which are considerably more strenuous. Here are some of your choices. If you do have osteoporosis, check with your doctor before starting an exercise plan. Physical activity is good for you, but you'll probably be advised to limit certain activities—such as those that require bending your back forward, or high-impact exercises such as tennis or running.

Walking

This is among the best weight-bearing activities. When you walk, your legs are required to bear most of your weight, increasing stress on bones in the legs and hips. Researchers aren't sure why, but the stress felt by bones during exercise stimulates the bone-building cells, osteoblasts, to make new bone.

Walking is easier to do than many types of exercise, and it's an excellent way to retard bone loss as you age. Women who regularly walk throughout their lives have higher bone density than women who are sedentary. They also have a fracture rate that's 30 percent lower.

Doctors advise taking a 30-minute walk 5 days a week. You don't have to do it all at once: Two 15-minute walks will give the same benefits. To increase the intensity of your workout—and increase the bone benefits—walk faster, or choose an uphill route.

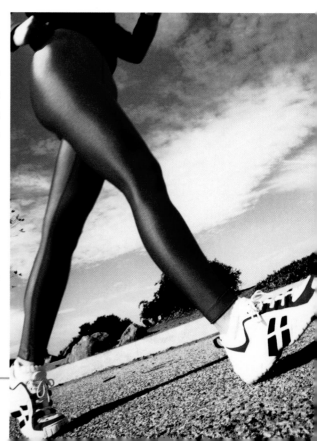

Running

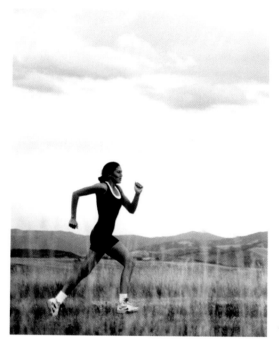

This is a high-impact exercise. It stimulates more bone growth than walking—about three times more, according to recent studies. If your bones are already strong, high-impact activities (which include aerobics, dancing, and tennis) are a good choice. If, however, you've already been diagnosed with osteoporosis, ask your doctor if your bones are strong enough for high-impact activities.

Many women incorporate high-impact activities into their regular walks—for example, by breaking into a run for a minute or two, then slowing back to walking speed. To give your body time to adjust to the vigorous exercise, start out by running for just 10 seconds. If it feels comfortable, gradually increase the time. Even a small amount of high-impact activity will prompt significant bone growth.

Gardening

You don't have to belong to a gym to get the bone-boosting benefits of resistance exercises. Activities such as lawn care and gardening require a lot of digging, pulling, and pushing. They're two of the best bone-preserving activities you can do.

Remember, though, to take it easy. If you haven't done yard work for a while, rest frequently to prevent overexertion—and drink plenty of water to prevent dehydration.

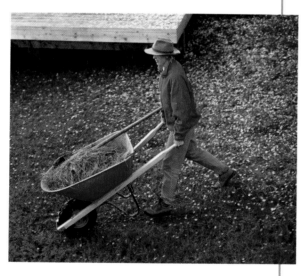

continued

Strengthen Your Bones
with Exercise *continued*

Jumping Jack

If your bones are already strong and healthy, jumping is a good way to increase hip density. In fact, doing this type of exercise for 2 minutes daily can increase bone density in a matter of months.

Jumping jacks are good for beginning jumpers. Find a flat surface, either indoors or out. Avoid slippery spots or extremely hard surfaces, like concrete or tile.

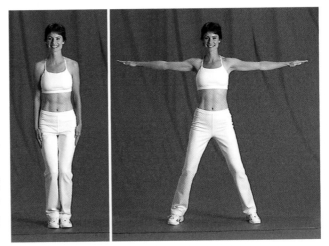

Stand with your feet together and arms at your sides (left). Bend your knees slightly, and jump while simultaneously moving your arms and feet out to the sides. Your feet should be approximately 3 feet apart. Your arms should be parallel to the floor (right). Land on the balls of your feet with your knees slightly bent.

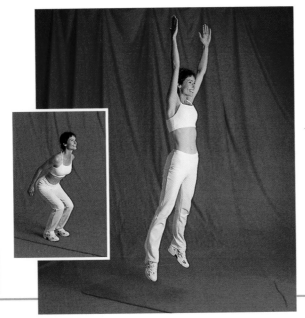

Power Jump

If you've been doing jumping jacks for at least 4 weeks, and you're sure you can jump and land safely, the "power jump" is worth a try.

Stand with your feet hip-width apart and your elbows bent slightly at your sides (far left). Bend your knees 4 to 6 inches, then jump straight up. As you jump, extend your arms up over your head, as if you were reaching toward the ceiling (near left). Land on the balls of your feet, keeping your knees slightly bent.

Seated Reverse Fly

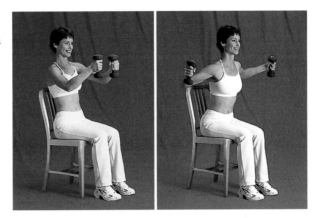

This simple exercise will strengthen your shoulders and back.

Sit in a chair with your feet flat on the floor, hip-width apart. Hold a dumbbell in each hand, with the weights at chest level. Hold them about 12 inches from your body, with your palms facing each other as though you were holding a beach ball. Your elbows should be slightly bent (near right). Bend forward from your hips about 3 to 5 inches.

Keeping your back flat and your spine straight, slowly squeeze your shoulder blades together and pull your elbows as far back as possible (far right). Pause, then slowly return to the starting position. Repeat the exercise 8 to 12 times. Rest a moment, then do 8 more.

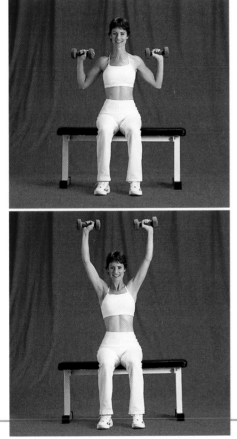

Overhead Press

This offers plenty of lifting and lowering—and lowering weights is what really counts when it comes to stimulating bone growth, according to researchers at California State University in Los Angeles.

While sitting, hold a weight in each hand (top). Start with the weights at shoulder height; your palms should be facing forward. Raise the weights above your head without bringing them together or locking your elbows (bottom), then bring them back down to your shoulders.

Important: Don't try to lift weights that are too heavy. The weight should be challenging, but not overwhelming. If you find you can easily repeat the exercise more than 12 times, move to a heavier weight. If you can't do eight repetitions, the weight is too heavy. This advice on weight selection pertains to the military press exercise here, as well as the exercises requiring dumbbells, above and on pages 220 and 221.

continued

Strengthen Your Bones with Exercise *continued*

Squat

A type of resistance exercise, squats are an excellent way to strengthen the thighs—and new research suggests that the more muscle you have, and the less fat, the higher your bone density will be. Here's how to do them.

Stand with your feet shoulder-width apart (near right). Bend your knees and squat, as though you're sitting; hold your arms in front for balance. Slowly lower your buttocks until your thighs are almost parallel to the ground (far right). Don't let your knees extend beyond your toes. Hold the position for a second, then rise.

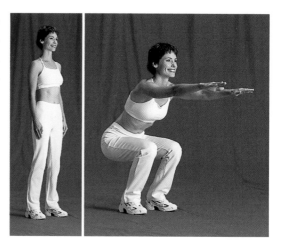

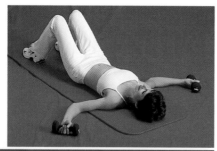

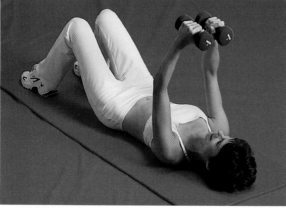

Chest Fly

This exercise improves chest and shoulder strength, as well as your posture.

Lie face-up on an exercise mat, with your knees bent, feet hip-width apart, and toes straight ahead.

Holding a dumbbell in each hand, extend your arms out to the sides, with your palms facing up and your hands at chest level (top). Bend your elbows at about a 45-degree angle.

Keeping your wrists straight and your lower back pressed into the floor, slowly lift both arms up and toward the center of your body in a sweeping arc (bottom). Make sure not to lift the dumbbells directly over your head, and don't straighten your arms.

Stop just before the weights touch in midair over your chest. Pause, then slowly lower the weights. Repeat the exercise 8 to 12 times. Rest a moment, then do them again.

Wrist Flexion

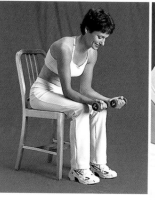

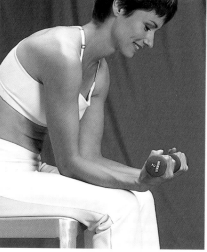

Osteoporosis is responsible for 250,000 wrist fractures each year. This easy exercise will strengthen the wrists and protect against carpal tunnel pain, sprains, and other injuries.

Sit in a chair, your feet hip-width apart. Holding a dumbbell in each hand, place your forearms on top of your thighs so your palms are facing up (left). Your hands will hang over your knees.

   Slowly bend your wrists, curling the dumbbells up toward your arms (right). Your wrists and hands should be the only things moving. Bring your hands up as high as is comfortable. Hold, then slowly lower. Repeat the exercise 8 to 12 times. Rest, then repeat the exercise.

Wrist Extension

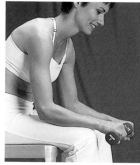

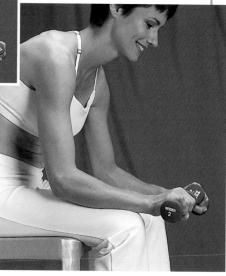

Like wrist flexions, this exercise will both strengthen and protect your wrists.

Sit in a chair with your feet hip-width apart. Holding a dumbbell in each hand, place your forearms on top of your thighs so that your palms are facing down (near right). Your hands will hang over your knees.

   Slowly lift the dumbbells, bringing your knuckles up toward your arms (far right). Your wrists and hands should be the only things moving. Go as far as is comfortable. Hold, then slowly lower. Repeat the exercise 8 to 12 times. Rest, then repeat the exercise.

18

Alzheimer's Disease

Occasional forgetfulness is one of the disconcerting signs of middle age. Maybe you occasionally misplace the car keys or find yourself racking your brain for a word that's just beyond reach. Deep down, you may worry that these flashes of forgetfulness are the beginnings of Alzheimer's disease.

The worry is understandable. About one in 10 Americans over age 65, and almost half of those over 85, suffer from this debilitating brain condition. Sixty-five percent are women. Medications can ease some of the symptoms for a time, but there isn't a cure, and scientists still aren't sure of what the underlying causes are. While researchers have found that people with Alzheimer's have abnormal tangles in and around nerve cells in the brain, which interrupt their normal connections and result in mental and physical deterioration, it isn't clear what triggers these changes in the first place.

Most memory problems, of course, are entirely normal—although research has shown that you can minimize the lapses with a little help. (For more information on memory problems, see page 432.) Even if you have a greater risk for developing Alzheimer's disease—because it runs in your family, for example, or you've had a serious head injury in the past—you may be able to reduce that risk.

"There's no proven way yet to prevent Alzheimer's disease, but there are positive signs of progress," says Linda A. Hershey, M.D., professor of neurology and pharmacology at the School of Medicine at State University of New York at Buffalo and chief of neurology at Veterans Affairs Medical Center in Western New York Healthcare System.

Most neurological problems take decades to develop. The earlier you start strengthening and protecting your brain, the better your chances of staying healthy throughout your life, says Dharma Singh Khalsa, M.D., president and medical director of the Alzheimer's Prevention Foundation in Tucson.

"The brain is not a computer," says Dr. Khalsa. "It's flesh and blood like any other organ—and it depends on the same things to keep it healthy."

Nutritional Treatments

Eat smart. The same foods that are healthy for the heart and arteries are also good for the brain, Dr. Khalsa says. He advises people to eat an abundance of fresh fruits, green leafy vegetables, whole grains, and soy foods. They're rich in protective phytochemicals, plant-based nutrients that may protect brain cells from future damage.

Reduce the fat in your diet. Ideally, fewer than 20 percent of your total calories should come from fat, especially if you have a family history of Alzheimer's disease. "Fat plugs up arteries in the brain and reduces bloodflow," says Dr. Khalsa. A high-fat diet also increases damage from free radicals, harmful oxygen molecules that damage tissues in the brain and other parts of the body.

Take a vitamin E supplement. High doses of vitamin E daily may delay mental declines in Alzheimer's patients. It's also possible that vitamin E may play a role in preventing the disease, says Gary W. Small, M.D., director of the Center on Aging at UCLA.

For prevention, doctors advise taking 400 to 800 IU of vitamin E daily. For those who have started developing symptoms of Alzheimer's, doctors recommend a higher dose—usually 2,000 IU daily.

Vitamin E is safe for most people, but it may increase the effects of blood-thinning medications, such as warfarin (Coumadin). If you're taking these medications, check with your doctor before supplementing your diet with vitamin E.

Get extra vitamin C. Like vitamin E, it's an antioxidant that blocks some of the effects of cell-damaging free radicals. It's fine to take 1,000 to 2,000 milligrams of vitamin C daily, says Dr. Khalsa.

Consider an over-the-counter supplement. A product available in pharmacies and health food stores, phosphatidylserine (PS), is thought by some researchers to reverse certain types of age-re-

Focusing on Fish May Help to Focus the Brain

Our ability to bond with animals may be hardwired into our brains. Now researchers at Purdue University in West Lafayette, Indiana, believe that they've found a way to harness the healing power of this inner circuitry to benefit those with Alzheimer's disease.

In one study, scientists placed glass tanks of brightly colored fish in three nursing homes, then studied the effects on 60 men and women with Alzheimer's disease.

"Two problems with Alzheimer's disease are that people often wander aimlessly or get lethargic—and it's hard to get them to eat," says Nancy E. Edwards, Ph.D., assistant professor in Purdue's School of Nursing. "The fish tanks had a sedating, calming effect on wandering patients, so they'd sit down longer and eat." The tanks had the opposite effect on the lethargic patients— they were more likely to stay awake, which also made it easier for them to eat.

In fact, patients who watched the fish ate up to 21 percent more than the non–fish watchers. Some patients who had previously been unresponsive were even prompted to talk.

It's not clear why watching fish had the effects it did. The researchers speculate that human beings may have an intrinsic need to bond with animals and that watching the fish fulfilled some deep-seated spiritual, emotional, or even physical need. ■

lated memory loss. One study has shown, in fact, that people who took PS had an improvement in their ability to remember names. Dr. Khalsa advises taking 100 to 300 milligrams of PS daily.

Home Remedies

Take ibuprofen. Because brain inflammation appears to play a role in the development of Alzheimer's disease, taking ibuprofen (such as Motrin or Advil) may delay its onset—or even prevent it entirely. Because ibuprofen may cause side effects, be sure to talk to your doctor before using it as part of an Alzheimer's prevention plan, Dr. Hershey says.

Stay physically active. In a 5-year study of people ages 65 and older, Canadian researchers found that those who exercised vigorously at least 3 days a week were up to 50 percent less likely to develop Alzheimer's disease and 40 percent less likely to suffer other symptoms of mental decline than their sedentary counterparts.

Even those who did only light activity such as easy walking had a much lower risk, says lead re-

Why Early Diagnosis Is Vital

families often wait 3 to 4 years—dutifully fishing car keys out of sugar bowls and nodding at the same tale repeated over and over in a single conversation—before they seek professional help for a loved one exhibiting the early signs of dementia. Those 3 to 4 years could cost dearly. Here's why.

There are three stages of dementia. Stage 1, in which the patient begins to exhibit confusion, depression, irritability, anxiety, difficulty with everyday tasks, and social withdrawal, but is still able to live on her own, lasts 2 to 4 years. Most families mistakenly attribute this stage to normal aging. A doctor's opinion is frequently not sought until stage 2, which is often marked by troublesome behaviors such as agitation, paranoia, or aggression and by more serious cognitive and physical slippage and a need for more care. By the time someone reaches stage 3, they often require around-the-clock care.

Families who receive an early diagnosis of Alzheimer's while their loved one is still in stage 1 may be able to slow down the progression of the symptoms by as much as a year or more with medications such as Cognex, Aricept, Exelon, and Reminyl, says Steven Potkin, M.D., director of neuropsychiatric research at the University of California, Irvine, Medical Center. "Their loved one consequently gets to stay home longer and functions better than she otherwise would."

New evidence suggests that if you miss that window of opportunity, the new drugs may not work as well. In a recent study, patients with mild to moderately severe Alzheimer's who received Exelon improved after 6 months; expectedly, those given a placebo didn't.

"But then the researchers gave the placebo group Exelon, and checked in with both groups over the next year and a half," says Dr. Potkin. "Much to their surprise, while the original placebo group improved with Exelon, they never did as well as the people who had been given the drug from the beginning." ■

WHEN BAD THINGS HAPPEN TO HEALTHY WOMEN

To Care for Her Dad, She Had to Care for Herself First

When Debby Gunsolley attended her parents' 50th wedding anniversary, she noticed that her father seemed confused. In the months that followed, he acted unusually nervous. He often sat alone without speaking, and he kept misplacing his keys.

Soon afterward, a visit to a neurologist revealed that her father was in the initial stage of Alzheimer's disease.

The next 3 years were emotionally and physically draining. Gunsolley, a 53-year-old school librarian's aide in South Sioux City, Nebraska, found herself working two shifts: one at her job, and the other helping her mother care for her dad. Things got even worse when her father suffered a small stroke that left him debilitated. Finally, the family realized that it was time for him to go to a nursing home.

"There's a lot of burden on caretakers," Gunsolley says. "Every day you think you've got it under control, and then, all of a sudden, you're in tears."

She got alarmed when she noticed that her own health was suffering. She had gained 15 pounds and was developing high blood pressure.

To combat stress and bolster her physical well-being, Gunsolley started exercising regularly—mainly running, swimming, and walking. She tried to eat better and began taking vitamin C, vitamin E, and B-complex supplements upon the recommendation of her doctor.

She also realized that it was time for her to start appreciating the small, everyday joys.

Her father has since passed away, but Gunsolley continues to do her best to take care of herself and maintain a positive perspective. "I had to learn to laugh," she says. "I have bad days, but little things don't bother me now. I've learned to enjoy life more." ■

searcher Danielle Laurin of Laval University in Quebec. "We need more research, but exercise may work by improving bloodflow to the brain (hence providing more nutrients), which keeps brain cells healthy and alive."

Exercise your brain. "Reading the paper and discussing it, doing crossword puzzles, or taking up a hobby—such as art, music, or learning a foreign language—increases the connections between brain cells and decreases your chance of getting Alzheimer's," says Dr. Khalsa.

Alternative Therapies

Take a break from stress. "Chronic stress raises levels of the hormone cortisol, which is toxic to the memory center of the brain," says Dr. Khalsa. Cortisol decreases the brain's ability to use glucose, blocks the effects of neurotransmitters, and actually injures and kills brain cells. He advises people to manage stress by meditating, doing stretches, or simply sitting quietly for a few minutes before they begin their day.

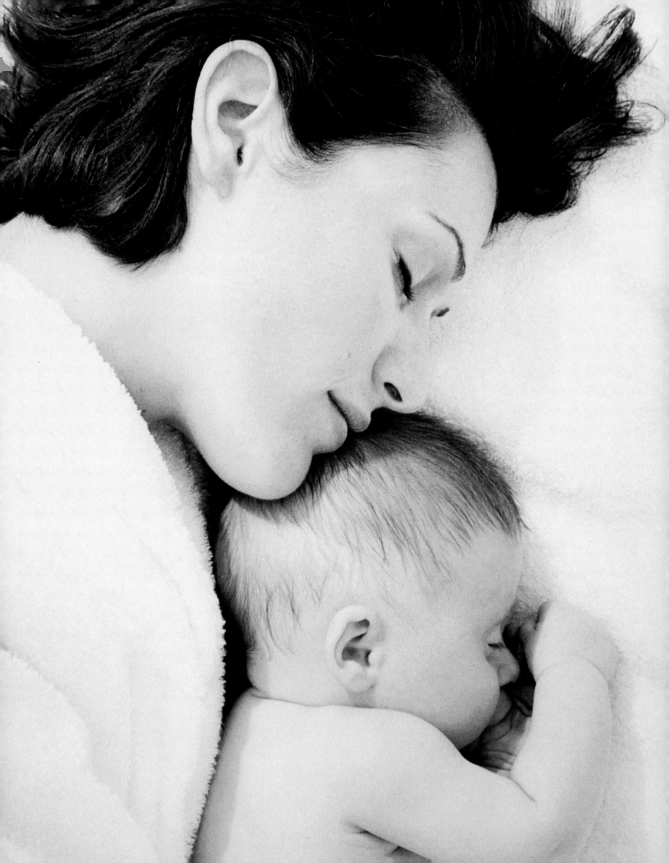

HORMONAL

WELLNESS:

THE BEST-EVER

LIFE-STAGE

STRATEGIES

PMS and Menstrual Discomforts

Each month during your reproductive years, a flurry of activity takes place within and around your reproductive organs. A single egg passes from an ovary to a fallopian tube, where it lies in wait for sperm. While the egg waits, the ovary releases estrogen and, a bit later, progesterone, in order to create a nourishing and protective nest in the lining of the uterus.

Some say a woman peaks at this premenstrual time of the month—that is, she is not only physically "ripe" but also emotionally and intellectually at her best.

Should the egg remain unfertilized, the uterine lining begins its monthly regenerative ritual by trickling out blood vessel–constricting substances called prostaglandins. The chemicals stimulate contractions that release the uterine lining—and trigger cramps that may start as early as a week before the period begins and continue until menstruation is done.

Because prostaglandins have inflammatory and pain-causing effects, many women also experience a touch of nausea, bloating, headaches, diarrhea, or breast tenderness.

What's Normal and What's Not

The cramps, fluid retention, and occasional moodiness that many women experience before and during their periods are nothing more than signs that their reproductive systems are following their normal, healthy patterns, says Ronald Young, M.D., director of the division of gynecology at Baylor College of Medicine in Houston.

But there may be other changes that aren't so healthy. Severe menstrual pain, called dysmenorrhea, for example, warrants a checkup with your gynecologist or family doctor because it could be a sign of endometriosis, uterine fibroids, or pelvic inflammatory disease.

Emotional changes can be just as telling. A little moodiness is one thing, but the onset of menstruation shouldn't leave you feeling morose or out of control. Severe emotional swings are often signs of physical problems, including diabetes and thyroid disorders.

More than 150 physical and emotional changes have been linked to the menstrual cycle. When women are otherwise healthy, menstrual-related changes in their physical or emotional health are often caused by lifestyle factors, such as stress, nutritional deficiencies, or a lack of sleep, says George J. Kallins, M.D., assistant clinical professor in the department of obstetrics and gynecology at the Keck School of Medicine of the University of Southern California in Los Angeles and coauthor of *Five Steps to a PMS-Free Life.*

Because the menstrual cycle can trigger such a wide range of signs and symptoms, there is no cure-all. However, doctors have identified more than 300 treatment options for menstrual or premenstrual discomfort. It's worth being optimistic because you're sure to find some simple remedies that will work for you.

Home Remedies

Sometimes even small changes can have profound effects on the way you feel. Women have always treated PMS and menstrual discomfort with home remedies—simple, time-tested strategies that can make a difference. Here are some things you may want to try.

Take ibuprofen right away. Ibuprofen blocks the body's production of pain-causing prostaglandins—and it's much less likely than other pain medications to cause side effects.

If you start taking ibuprofen at the first sign of symptoms, you'll have protective levels of the medication in the bloodstream, which will prevent the discomfort from getting worse later on, says Melvin V. Gerbie, M.D., professor of clinical gynecology at Northwestern University Medical

School and professor of medicine at Prentice Hospital, both in Chicago.

He advises taking 400 milligrams of ibuprofen four times daily. Start taking it 2 days before your period, and keep taking it until the time in your cycle when the cramps usually stop—usually about the second day after menstruation begins.

Water down bloating. Fluid retention caused by high hormone levels can cause uncomfortable swelling in the abdomen, breasts, and ankles. It sounds paradoxical to drink a lot of water when you

when to see a doctor

If you're experiencing so much discomfort before or during your period that you can't function normally, make an appointment to see your doctor. Mild menstrual discomfort may be normal, but if it's interfering with your life, there's probably an underlying problem that needs to be addressed, says Melvin V. Gerbie, M.D., professor of clinical gynecology at Northwestern University Medical School and professor of medicine at Prentice Hospital, both in Chicago.

If you've been having depression, anxiety, or irritability for more than 3 months, or if the feelings aren't limited to the 7 to 10 days before your period: You could be confusing clinical depression with PMS. Make an appointment to see a psychologist or psychiatrist, or discuss it with your current health care provider.

If you're having cramps as well as irregular or heavy bleeding, or if the blood is coming out in clots: You could have physical problems that need looking into.

feel like a sponge, but water acts as a diuretic and removes excess fluid from the body, says Dr. Kallins. He advises drinking at least eight full glasses of water daily before and during your period.

Avoid cigarette smoke. Research has shown that even secondhand smoke can make premenstrual discomfort worse. In one study, Chinese researchers looked at 165 female nonsmokers, all newlyweds. None of the women had a history of menstrual discomfort. In the months after marriage (and their exposure to secondhand smoke by household members), there was a significant increase in premenstrual lower-back pain and abdominal discomfort.

Nutritional Treatments

Estrogen regulates the body's metabolism of a variety of nutrients, and it also affects the body's ability to absorb them. New evidence suggests that levels of calcium, vitamin D, iron, and other key nutrients may rise and fall in synchrony with estrogen fluctuations. Some researchers believe that short-term nutritional deficiencies are responsible for some of the premenstrual symptoms that have perplexed doctors for decades.

More than 10 major studies, for example, have shown that supplementing the diet with calcium or vitamin B_6 can relieve menstrual or premenstrual symptoms in women who usually don't get adequate amounts of these nutrients.

Supplements can only do so much, of course. Every woman should eat a healthful diet and maintain adequate levels of vitamins and minerals

throughout the month, not just before and during the menstrual period.

"Don't think about getting enough fresh fruits and vegetables—and avoiding processed foods—only when your symptoms hit," says James G. Penland, Ph.D., a research psychologist and PMS researcher at the USDA Human Nutrition Research Center at Grand Forks, North Dakota. As extra insurance against PMS discomfort, however, it's fine to use supplements containing no more than the daily recommended intakes.

Get enough magnesium and vitamin B_6. "One of the reasons that these two nutrients are so highly recommended for PMS is that they help assure a healthy supply of the mood-regulating brain chemicals serotonin and dopamine," says Dr. Kallins. Research suggests that these chemicals, called neurotransmitters, also play a role in easing or preventing physical symptoms, including bloating, headaches, acne, and cramps.

You can get a lot of magnesium and vitamin B_6 from figs, raisins, corn, and bananas. To be on the safe side, Dr. Kallins advises women to supplement their diets with 350 milligrams of magnesium and 100 milligrams of vitamin B_6.

The B vitamins work together, which means that supplemental B_6 won't be helpful unless you also have adequate amounts of the other B vitamins. So it's a good idea to take a multivitamin or a B-complex supplement, he says.

Ease breast pain with a nutritional combo. If your breasts get tender as your period approaches, you might want to try a remedy suggested by Mary Jane Minkin, M.D., clinical professor of obstetrics and gynecology at Yale

WHEN BAD THINGS HAPPEN TO HEALTHY WOMEN

Her Monthly Discomfort Led to a New Life

When Charis Lindrooth was a schoolteacher in Kutztown, Pennsylvania, she found that any stress and disappointments that she felt during the month would climax in the days before her menstrual period.

"I'd feel fine the rest of the month, and then, a few days before my period, I'd habitually dwell on everything so much that I'd make myself physically sick," says Lindrooth. "When depression set in really hard, it sent me off on a crazy sugar binge."

She finally mustered the discipline to quit eating sweets—and it made a remarkable difference in how she felt. She also consulted an herbalist, who gave her black cohosh and black haw for her moodiness, and ginger and cardamom for her digestive problems.

"I also started on chamomile and lemon balm tea, which really helped resolve my anxiety," she says. "After taking these herbs for a month, it felt like suddenly something was really healed inside me."

Lindrooth was so inspired by the changes that she decided to study nutrition and body work. Eventually she left her job as a teacher and went on to become a chiropractor—and she's getting ready to complete a degree in herbal medicine.

"I sometimes tell people that the call to my vocation came through my uterus," she laughs. ■

University School of Medicine and coauthor of *What Every Women Needs to Know about Menopause.*

Take 1,000 milligrams of evening primrose oil, 400 to 800 IU of vitamin E, and 100 milligrams of vitamin B_6 daily. This supplement combination reduces the pain and inflammation that are triggered by surges in prostaglandins during the menstrual cycle, she explains.

Focus on the "top four" proteins. Many of the foods that Americans depend on for protein— mainly meat and dairy foods—are also high in fat, which has been linked to menstrual cramps. Better sources of protein include fish, soy foods, egg whites, and legumes, says Dr. Kallins.

These foods provide more than just protein, he adds. Soy foods and legumes are rich in phytoestrogens, plant-based chemicals similar to the estrogen that women produce naturally. Fish is rich in omega-3 fatty acids, which help regulate mood, and egg whites provide an abundance of protein with virtually no fat.

Don't give in to cravings for sugary food. Many women crave candy, baked goods, and other sweet foods before and during their periods. Indulging in these foods causes a rapid rise in blood sugar, which in turn can cause your energy and mood to crash. Highly processed carbohydrates, such as bagels, potato chips, and sodas, aren't much better because they supply a lot of calories and not a lot in the way of important nutrients. If you fill up on "empty" calories, you may find that you're not getting enough important nutrients to prevent menstrual discomfort.

It's fine to give in to cravings on occasion, but only if your diet consists mainly of fresh fruits and vegetables, whole grains, and other nutritious foods. The fiber in a plant-based diet is especially helpful because it helps remove excess estrogen from the body, which will go a long way toward reducing menstrual and premenstrual discomfort, says Dr. Kallins.

Take advantage of healing oils. We mentioned earlier that chemicals called prostaglandins are responsible for some of the pain and discomfort that occur before and during your period. But there are actually several types of prostaglandins, including some that inhibit pain and inflammation. Flaxseed, hemp, and borage oils, available in health food stores, stimulate the body's production of "good" prostaglandins. Adding these oils to your diet may inhibit cramps, bloating, and breast tenderness. These oils aren't used for cooking, but you can add them to salads, shakes, or other foods. Try to get a total of 3 teaspoons of one or more of these oils daily all month.

Alternative Therapies

Most women experience some degree of premenstrual stress. As it turns out, stress is not only a symptom of PMS but also a cause of it.

THREE THINGS I TELL EVERY FEMALE PATIENT

GEORGE J. KALLINS, M.D., assistant clinical professor in the department of obstetrics and gynecology at the Keck School of Medicine of the University of Southern California in Los Angeles and coauthor of *Five Steps to a PMS-Free Life*, offers the following tips for controlling PMS and menstrual discomfort.

1 DON'T TAKE ANTIDEPRESSANTS UNLESS YOU'VE TRIED CALCIUM FIRST. Scientific studies have shown that calcium supplements—about 1,200 milligrams daily—can reverse menstrual-related mood swings, depression, and anger. The mineral also reduces the discomfort of cramps and headaches.

EXERCISE OFTEN. "I see in my patients that those who exercise regularly experience less menstrual symptoms than those who don't,"
says Dr. Kallins. Natural chemicals called endorphins are released during exercise. Known as "feel good" chemicals, endorphins can help ease cramps, breast tenderness, and other types of menstrual discomfort.

2 For the best endorphin "rush," Dr. Kallins advises women to focus on aerobic exercises, such as fast walking, bicycling, or swimming. Try to exercise for 20 to 30 minutes at least four times a week.

LIMIT INDULGENCES. Women who eat a lot of sweets or fast food, or who consume caffeine or alcohol regularly, tend to have more menstrual and premenstrual discomfort than those who eat a healthier diet. "Don't think of it as depriving yourself," Dr. Kallins advises. "Think of it as a gift you're giving yourself to feel more balanced on every level." ∎ **3**

When we experience stress, the adrenal glands take progesterone and make cortisol, a stress hormone, out of it. This results in low levels of progesterone—and low progesterone is thought to be a primary cause of menstrual cramps and PMS symptoms.

To reduce your risk of suffering from stress-related PMS, try to develop and practice stress reduction strategies every day.

Each woman has a different approach to reducing stress. Some of the most helpful are meditation, taking hot lavender-scented baths, and getting at least 8 hours of sleep every night. Other helpful strategies include the following:

Press away symptoms. For centuries, Asian healers have practiced reflexology, a technique in which one "adjusts" the body's internal organs by pressing certain points on the feet, hands, and ears. In one study, women with PMS underwent foot, hand, and ear reflexology sessions in which practitioners manipulated the trigger points that correspond to the uterus and ovaries; other women in the study were given "sham" treatments at inappropriate trigger points. The women who received the real treatment had a significant reduction in symptoms, says Terry Oleson, Ph.D., director of the department of behavioral medicine at the California Graduate Institute in Los Angeles.

To find a professional reflexologist in your area, go to the Reflexology Association of America's Web site at www.reflexology-usa.org.

Practice progressive relaxation. An easy way to relax and let go of tension is to tense and then relax each muscle in your body. The technique, known as progressive relaxation, is simple.

While you're lying down, contract the muscles in your feet. Hold the tension for a moment, then relax. Then move up to the calves . . . the knees . . . the thighs . . . and onward up to your head. It takes about 15 to 20 minutes to work through the whole body. At the end of each session, you'll find that your levels of physical and emotional tension will be substantially reduced.

Imagine a beautiful light. Another way to practice progressive relaxation is to lie down and visualize a golden-white light running down like a waterfall, says Dr. Oleson. Imagine that the light is pouring through your head, then through your face, the back of your head, and your neck. Gradually let it pass down through each region of the body until finally it runs out from your feet.

"Give yourself a good 15 minutes to settle your body down," says Dr. Oleson. "Remind yourself that you deserve this gentle self-care every day."

Combine exercise with meditation. Women who exercise tend to have less PMS or menstrual discomfort than those who are sedentary. To get even more benefits from exercise, Dr. Kallins recommends making it "mindful." In other words, focus all your thoughts on your body—the stretching of your muscles, the slap of your feet on the mat or pavement, the breath going in and out of your lungs—and not on the things that are troubling you.

The idea, he explains, is to use your movements to put yourself into a kind of mild trance. When your mind is relaxed, you'll be more in touch with your body and feelings—and that's the first step to managing them more effectively.

Prevent cramps with dang gui. An herb traditionally used by Asian healers, dang gui appears to improve circulation, which helps remove pain-causing chemicals from the body. It also boosts levels of magnesium, iron, and B vitamins. This herb, also known as Chinese angelica, works slowly and can be used safely long term. Use it for a month before judging its effects. Take three doses a day, with meals, in any of these forms: dried root, 1 gram boiled in water; tincture 1:5, 1 teaspoon or 5 milliliters; tincture 1:1, 20 drops; tableted root, one 500-milligram tablet. You can find angelica tincture and tablets at most health food stores. Avoid products made of the leaves or seeds—buy only products made from the root. And don't buy a product containing other herbs.

Use vitex supplements. The fruit of the chaste tree, vitex is a popular folk remedy for PMS—and one study suggests that it may work. In a German study, women suffering from PMS were given 20 milligrams of dried vitex extract daily. After taking the supplements for three menstrual cycles, more than half of the women reported a dramatic reduction in headaches, irritability, and other symptoms of PMS.

Vitex is available in health food stores and some pharmacies. Try taking two 500-milligram tablets twice daily for a few months to see if it helps. (The seeds—also called the berries—are the most effective part.) If it does, you'll have to keep taking it: In the study, women who took vitex and then gave it up had a return of symptoms within 3 months.

Try black cohosh. If you're approaching menopause and your menstrual and premenstrual symptoms are getting worse, black cohosh, an herb, may help. It helps modulate the effects of a woman's hormones and may prevent the extreme "swings" that cause discomfort. It seems to be especially helpful for women who are approaching menopause, says Dr. Kallins. If you're post-menopausal, check with your doctor before taking this herb, as it may cause bleeding, he adds. And don't use black cohosh if you're taking estrogen in any form.

Take two 500-milligram dried root tablets three times a day. And don't take this herb if you're already on hormone replacement therapy.

Reduce anxiety with kava kava. "This herb isn't for everyone because it has powerful tranquilizing effects," says Dr. Kallins. But it's an excellent remedy for women who suffer from intense anxiety or insomnia during their menstrual cycles.

"I recommend taking 500 to 1,000 milligrams of kava kava tablets on an as-needed basis, three times a day," advises Dr. Kallins. Just be sure not to combine it with alcohol or sedating medications or to drive while you're using it, he adds.

Medical Options

Rx Most women can control menstrual or premenstrual discomfort with changes in lifestyle or diet—but some can't. Since there are other causes of severe pain, consultation with a knowledgeable physician is imperative before you start a medication for pain. If your symptoms aren't getting better, here are some medical options that might make the difference.

WHEN BAD THINGS HAPPEN TO HEALTHY WOMEN

A Meat-Free Diet Banished Menstrual Pain

Barbara Swanson is an energetic and healthy woman, but for a long time she had such unbearable menstrual cramps that she routinely missed 2 days of work a month.

"When my period hit, I couldn't do anything but lie uncomfortably on the couch in front of the television," says Swanson, an administrative assistant in Washington, D.C. "I had to take a lot of over-the-counter pain pills, which only seemed to make me sleepy."

In 1997, Swanson received a postcard calling for women to participate in a Georgetown University study that was looking at the link between vegan (meat- and dairy-free) diets and pain-free periods. She volunteered—and several cooking classes, a restocked pantry, and two menstrual cycles later, her cramps were markedly reduced, she could function at work, and she was up off the couch and jogging.

Swanson has stuck with the vegan diet ever since. "I have some great cookbooks that I use for making simple dinners," she says. For desserts, she enjoys soy ice cream and soy yogurt, and she has even found vegan versions of fast foods, like faux burgers and hot dogs.

She was also pleased to get an additional bonus from the vegan diet: Soon after giving up meat and dairy, she lost 5 pounds—and the weight never came back. ∎

Take high-dose ibuprofen. Available by prescription, ibuprofen tablets that contain 800 milligrams appear to be more effective than taking four over-the-counter pills containing 200 milligrams each.

"It's a mystery why, but it seems to make a difference," says Dr. Gerbie.

Try birth control pills for 6 to 12 months. "For some women, the Pill ends all the discomfort because it stops the hormone fluctuations that occur with ovulation—and it stops the lining of the uterus from building up so much," says Dr. Gerbie.

In many cases, taking the Pill for 6 months to a year will balance the hormones and relieve symptoms for good.

Be sure to let your doctor know if you're using the Pill only for menstrual or premenstrual discomfort, and not for birth control, because you'll need a different dosage, Dr. Gerbie explains.

Consider antidepressants. Some women have a severe form of PMS known as premenstrual dysphoric disorder, which has the same force as major depression. A number of prescription antidepressants have been shown to reduce symptoms of this serious condition by more than 50 percent.

A medication that seems to be especially helpful is fluoxetine (like Sarafem). You'll probably be advised to take it during the time between ovulation and the onset of your period, or you will take it the entire month.

Contraception

Contraceptives are incredibly effective. When used correctly and consistently, all of the leading contraceptives have been shown to prevent pregnancy more than 99 percent of the time.

So why is it that 50 percent of unwanted pregnancies occur in those who use contraceptives?

In most cases, it's because people are using products that really aren't right for them, says Mitchell Creinin, M.D., associate professor in the department of obstetrics, gynecology, and reproductive sciences at the University of Pittsburgh School of Medicine. When birth control seems inconvenient, for example, or when it causes worrisome side effects, people simply won't use it.

There are many different types of contraception. By knowing what's out there and choosing products or practices that suit your personality and lifestyle, you'll be able to get maximal protection without sacrificing comfort.

Every woman knows what's best for her, so don't let doctors or other health care advisors limit your options in advance, says Dr. Creinin. "Your doctor doesn't pay your bills, take care of your kids, deal with your in-laws, or have a relationship with your husband or partner," he adds.

Don't put too much weight on hearsay, either. Just because your sister or mother or most of the women in your book club prefer a certain method does not mean that it's the right one for you. With so many options to choose from, don't accept anything less.

The Right Match for Every Woman

Start by asking yourself if you need protection from just unwanted pregnancy or if you also need protection from sexually transmitted diseases (STDs), says Erica Gollub, D.P.H., an epidemiologist and contraceptives educator at the University of Pennsylvania in Philadelphia.

Some STDs cause infertility, some increase the risk of uterine cancer, and still others can threaten your life. "You have to recognize that they're out there, and if you have any doubt in your mind that your partner has undisclosed relationships, your safest bet is clearly the male or female condom," says Dr. Gollub.

If condoms aren't for you, other "barrier" methods of birth control, such as a diaphragm combined with spermicide, work much better than nothing, Dr. Gollub says. On the other hand, birth control pills or other methods of hormonal contraception, along with intrauterine contraceptives, may increase your risk for STDs because they alter the cervical mucus.

If you are in a mutually monogamous relationship and can use hormonal methods of birth control, you'll have to educate yourself about the pros and cons of using these products. We'll discuss this more in just a bit.

Another concern to keep in mind is whether you're planning to get pregnant in the future—and how soon you'll want it to happen. Fertility will usually return immediately upon stopping use of the Pill or a barrier method; even an intrauterine contraceptive or implant can be removed and assure a relatively quick return of fertility. However, the injection method of contraception known as Depo-Provera, which is given every 3 months, may delay pregnancy for 10 months after it's discontinued. Those using a newer product, Lunelle, which is injected once a month, may regain fertility in about 3 months.

Your Guide to Contraceptive Options

As you review your options, here are some other questions to ask yourself.

- Do I have the discipline and personality for this method?

- Does this method take away from or add to the pleasure of sex?

- What are the short-term and long-term costs?

BARRIER METHODS

Barrier methods are among the oldest and safest form of birth control. A barrier contraceptive's mission is to prevent a sperm from ever meeting up with an egg. Barrier forms of contraception include the diaphragm, cervical cap, sponge, and condom. The chemicals in spermicidal foams, jellies, and films also act as barriers.

Perhaps the most exciting evolution in barrier contraception was the female condom, which was approved in 1993 by the FDA for preventing pregnancy and also preventing disease.

"Women like the female condom because it makes them feel in control," says Dr. Gollub. You place the closed end—an inner ring—up in the vagina as far as it will go, then guide your partner's penis into the outer ring. When used correctly, it can prevent pregnancy as effectively as the male condom, and it may be even more effective in preventing disease since it covers more of the female genitalia.

Another promising development is an improved version of the cervical cap, a thimble-shaped cone that is placed in the vagina and held in place with suction against the cervix. Softer and smoother silicone caps are replacing the original rubber ones, and you will also soon see caps with a one-way valve that lets out a woman's natural secretions but doesn't allow other secretions to get in. Older caps can be worn for 2 days, but the newer models can stay in place for 5 to 7 days. The increase in convenience makes them a very attractive option.

Barrier contraceptives haven't proved in studies to be quite as effective as the Pill or other hormonal methods, but as long as they're used in combination with spermicides or other barrier chemicals, they're nearly as good.

Here's some expert advice on using barrier contraception.

Get the proper fit. Diaphragms and cervical caps come in different sizes. If yours feels uncomfortable or loose, ask your doctor for a refit, says Dr. Gollub. Always assume you will need a different size after childbirth, abortion, or gaining or losing 10 pounds, which changes the size of your cervix.

Select safe lubricants. Many barrier methods are designed to be used with spermicides or lubricants. Lubricants can increase pleasure. They also provide additional protection against pregnancy and may decrease the odds that a condom will break.

Be sure to use commercial lubricants, such as K-Y Jelly and Astroglide. Nonoxynol-9 is a fairly effective ingredient in spermicides that also has a lubricant effect.

Don't use household products, such as Vaseline, Crisco, or whipped cream. They can cause condoms to break down, and they provide no spermicidal effects.

Get ready ahead of time. If you find that fussing with a contraceptive disrupts the moment, remember that a diaphragm can be inserted 6 hours ahead of time. The female condom can be inserted up to 8 hours in advance, and the cervical cap can be inserted 2 to 3 days before a romantic encounter.

Remember to remove them. More than a few women have left diaphragms or caps in place long past their allotted time, which can result in

bladder or even blood infections. It may be worth writing a note to yourself and putting it on the bathroom mirror or somewhere else where you'll see it, suggests Dr. Gollub.

ORAL CONTRACEPTIVES

The Pill has been in use for more than 40 years, and it's getting safer all the time. That's because the dose of hormones in the Pill has been falling as clinicians have become wiser about deciding who can and cannot use it. In fact, doctors have found that birth control pills even offer some health benefits that are unrelated to contraception.

There are two basic forms of oral contraceptives: the combination pill and the mini-pill. Combination pills contain synthetic estrogen and progestin, which are hormones similar to those already produced in a woman's ovaries. These pills prevent ovulation from taking place. Combination pills are available as monophasic pills, which provide estrogen and progestin at the same doses throughout the pill pack, and as biphasic and triphasic pills, which vary the amount of hormones over the course of the month.

Mini-pills contain progestin only. They do not consistently stop ovulation. They do, however, thicken the mucus over the cervix to prevent sperm from entering the uterus. They also stop the uterine lining from growing, which makes it more difficult for the egg to get implanted. These pills are usually used by women who are concerned about the possible health risks—such as heart disease, stroke, or breast cancer—of estrogen-based pills.

It's important for women to weigh some of the risks of using birth control pills with some actual health benefits. For example, women who use birth control pills may have a reduced risk of colon, endometrial, and uterine cancers. The estrogen in the Pill also protects against the bone-thinning disease called osteoporosis, says Joseph Goldzieher, M.D., distinguished professor of obstetrics and gynecology at Texas Tech University Health Sciences Center in Amarillo.

Because combination pills prevent ovulation, they can relieve or prevent menstrual pain, ovarian cysts, or fibroids. They can also prevent the hot flashes, headaches, irregular bleeding, vaginal dryness, and other symptoms that may occur in the years preceding menopause.

Birth control pills are very effective—but only if you remember to use them. Here are few ways to keep with the program.

Pack your pills. Carry extras in a pill pack just in case you forget your morning dose. You can keep the pills in your purse, wallet, or backpack, where you'll always have easy access to them.

Take them on a strict schedule. Progestin-only pills prevent pregnancy by thickening the cervical mucus. This effect lasts only for 24 hours, so it's important to take the pills at the same time every day. If you doubt your ability to stick to a regular schedule, you may want to choose another type of contraception.

Use an automated system. If you have trouble remembering to take the Pill, ask your doctor about the brand Mircette. The pills come with a computerized card, which beeps when it's time for the next dose.

A new hormonal form of birth control. The FDA recently approved a new type of contraceptive called NuvaRing. The 2-inch flexible plastic ring is inserted in the vagina and provides a continuous low-dose combination of estrogen and progestin. As with oral contraceptives, there is an increased risk of heart attack, stroke, and blood clots. Women who smoke or have a history of

when to see a doctor

 If you're taking the Pill or other hormone-based contraceptives and you experience chest pain, blurred vision, or leg pain, call your doctor immediately. The symptoms could be caused by inflammation, a blood clot, or even a stroke, says Mitchell Creinin, M.D., associate professor in the department of obstetrics, gynecology, and reproductive sciences at the University of Pittsburgh School of Medicine. Women who take the Pill have a slightly increased risk of developing these conditions, compared with women who don't use hormonal contraception, although the actual risk is still very small.

If you're developing acne or have unpredictable bleeding: These are common side effects of contraceptive hormones, and changing the dosage (or the medication) will probably resolve the problem.

If an intrauterine device becomes visible: The device has fallen out of position, and you'll want to get it repositioned immediately to prevent damage to the uterus or intestine. Avoid sexual intercourse or use an alternative method (like condoms) until you can talk to your health care provider about other contraceptive options.

blood clots or cardiovascular problems should not choose these products.

A woman inserts the ring herself and removes it after 3 weeks so that menstruation can occur. Each month, a new ring is inserted for continuous protection. You need a prescription to get Nuva-Ring, so check with your doctor if this form of birth control appeals to you.

LONG-ACTING HORMONAL METHODS

For many women, the nicest thing about long-acting hormonal methods of birth control is privacy. Nobody will find your pills, your partner won't feel an IUD string or the rim of a diaphragm, and there's no messy spermicide, says Robert Hatcher, M.D., professor of gynecology and obstetrics at Emory University School of Medicine in Atlanta and senior author of *Contraception Technology*.

The latest in long-acting contraceptives is Lunelle, an injection that combines estrogen and progestin. It's been available to American women since 2000.

"My patients have loved this contraceptive," says Dr. Creinin. "It's basically the same formulation as classic birth control pills, but you only need a monthly shot instead of having to take pills every day."

Depo-Provera has been available since 1992. The amount of hormones is higher than in other hormonal contraceptives, and it contains only progestin, rather than a combination of estrogen and progestin. It may cause unpredictable menstrual spotting, and it's also been linked to weight gain and bone loss in some women.

However, if you're one of the women who can use Depo-Provera without side effects, consider yourself lucky: It's the most fuss-free contraceptive available in the United States, offering 3 months of protection with one shot.

If you're thinking of using a long-term hormonal contraceptive, here are a few points to keep in mind.

Consider self-injections. If you have trouble fitting a monthly doctor's visit into your schedule, bear in mind that some doctors will provide a 6- to 12-month supply of injections, which you can administer to yourself at home, says Dr. Creinin.

Ask about needle-free options. Long-acting hormonal contraceptives are available in patch or implant forms (such as Norplant). If you want the protection of hormonal contraceptives but could do without the shots, ask your doctor if one of these products would be right for you.

INTRAUTERINE DEVICES

There's a good reason that many women appreciate an intrauterine contraceptive. Once it's inserted, it can be left alone for 5 years or more. It virtually stops monthly bleeding and cramps, and it's more effective than getting your tubes tied—and it's totally reversible, besides.

A recently approved product called Mirena contains a slow-release hormone called levonorgestrel, which mimics the effects of progesterone. This intrauterine contraceptive is more than 99 percent effective.

"The hormone is released locally in the uterus," says Dr. Creinin. "The amount of hormone that gets into the rest of your body is only about 10 percent of the amount that comes from taking birth control pills. This means that there's less potential for side effects."

Another intrauterine contraceptive is the Progestasert. It releases a form of progesterone identical to the hormone released by a woman's ovaries. It's slightly less effective than Mirena, however, and needs to be replaced once a year, compared with Mirena's 5-year span.

You can also use an intrauterine contraceptive that contains no hormones. Instead, it contains a lot of copper, which sterilizes any sperm it encounters. In fact, it has the unique ability to prevent pregnancy even if it's inserted 5 to 7 days after unprotected sex. If you're in a bind, ask your gynecologist to install one immediately. If you like it, you can leave it in for 12 years. The copper intrauterine contraceptive is more than 99 percent effective. The one drawback is that it may increase menstrual bleeding or cramping.

OTHER CONTRACEPTION OPTIONS

Tubal sterilization, a permanent procedure, is reserved only for those women who know that they don't want to have any (or any more) children. A small incision is made in the abdomen. The surgeon then seals the fallopian tubes, thereby creating a permanent roadblock on the egg–uterus highway.

Women who are most likely to regret getting their "tubes tied" are those under the age of 25, those who have divorced and then remarried, and those who rushed into the procedure after pregnancy or an abortion.

Even if you already have children, don't dis-

count the possibility that you may want to have more later on, especially if you happen to divorce and then remarry. Long-term, reversible methods, such as an intrauterine contraceptive, or a vasectomy for the spouse of a woman in a mutually monogamous relationship, might be better for you, says Dr. Creinin.

Some women depend on the "withdrawal method" for birth control, which can be a very unreliable method. However, family-planning clinics sometimes teach women the symptothermal method. It's a system of observing menstrual cycle patterns and abstaining from sex before and during ovulation. The more data you take using this method (such as body temperature, the appearance of vaginal mucus, self-cervical examinations, and urine tests), the more effective it becomes, says Dr. Gollub.

"It's a valuable educational tool for every woman to learn," she says. "It can also be quite moving to be so aware of your body's changes throughout the month."

EMERGENCY CONTRACEPTION

Emergency contraception is based on the reality that a woman, no matter how careful she tries to be, might find herself getting pregnant against her will. She might be forced to have sex; condoms can break; and a diaphragm can slip. And sometimes passion dissolves a firm "no" into "oh, yes."

The first thing to know about emergency contraception pills (ECPs) is what they are not. They are not meant to be a regular contraceptive method. Nor are they used to terminate pregnancies. As with some other contraceptives, ECPs either prevent ovulation or alter the uterine lining to prevent the implantation of an egg. You can think of them as very strong, fast-acting birth control pills.

To be effective, the pills have to be taken according to strict guidelines. For example, you might be told to take the first dose within 72 hours (or sooner) after unprotected sex, followed by another dose 12 hours later. The pills are unlikely to cause serious side effects, but some women may experience nausea, vomiting, abdominal cramps, headache, breast tenderness, or dizziness.

The American Medical Association and the American Fertility Society are pushing to make ECPs available over the counter. Until then, you need a prescription from your doctor, family-planning clinic, or hospital emergency room.

Here are some additional emergency strategies to keep in mind.

Get checked for infection. If you had unplanned sex outside of a mutually monogamous relationship, you might be at risk for an STD. The symptoms don't always show up right away (or at all). The only way you'll know you're infected is to have your doctor give you an exam.

Go to the source. If you want immediate information about emergency contraception, call the toll-free hot line (888) NOT-2-LATE. Or visit www.not-2-late.com, a Web site provided by the Office of Population Research, Princeton University. You'll find a lot of information about emergency contraceptives, along with lists of health care providers who prescribe them.

Get emergency pills in advance. "The effectiveness of ECPs drops off every minute after unprotected sex, and then drops off very rapidly after 72 hours," says Dr. Goldzieher. Since your physician may not be able to see you immediately or the pharmacy may be closed, you may want to get the pills in advance and keep them in a safe place. "I wish every woman carried emergency contraception, just like she might carry around a tube of lipstick," says Dr. Goldzieher.

Pregnancy

Every single day of your entire pregnancy, you are contributing to your child's well-being. You do so by what you eat, how you stay fit and relaxed, and how you practice prenatal care.

You're doing more than supporting a developing baby over 9 or 10 months. You're also growing as a woman and a mother-to-be, says Deborah Issokson, Psy.D., a psychologist specializing in reproductive mental health at the Boston University Nurse-Midwifery Education Program. Dr. Issokson is also the author of the postpartum chapter in the book *Our Bodies, Ourselves for the New Century*.

"The most important advice I can give is not to rush through 40 weeks trying to get everything ready for the baby," she says. "Focus instead on your personal development. Pregnancy is an incredibly reflective time when your sense of being a woman, a wife or partner, and even an employee is evolving to a new level. Make the time and space for that natural shift, and you'll feel emotionally your best before, during, and after pregnancy. Emotional well-being can also translate into physical well-being."

Get the Best Support

Whether you are having a first child or your fourth, getting good prenatal education is one of the smartest parenting decisions you'll make. Birth classes allow you to gain vital new information. Plus, you'll have the chance to talk about the experience with other pregnant women. The more you learn about the physical and emotional changes that other women undergo during pregnancy, the better prepared you'll be to cope with your own.

Birthing educators offer private instruction, classes in hospitals (usually six 1-hour sessions or a 1-day class), and weekend-long retreats, says Sally Reilly, codirector of the Academy of Certified Birth Educators, based in Olathe, Kansas.

Start with a broad-based class that will prepare you, physically and emotionally, for anything that might come up. The class should offer instruction on a variety of relaxation and comfort measures and breathing techniques, as well as discussions and role playing to help you and your partner focus on various scenarios.

Look for the same spirit of flexibility and objectivity in choosing your primary pregnancy caregiver—the person who conducts prenatal exams and attends your birth. Whether you choose an obstetrician, a family practitioner, or a nurse-midwife, try to sense whether her aim is to mold you into a good patient—or a smart mother.

Many women prefer to work with nurse-midwives because they tend to put a strong focus on empowerment and education. Women who work with nurse-midwives generally need significantly less medical intervention, including C-sections and labor induction, says Marion McCartney, R.N., a practicing nurse-midwife and director of professional services at the American College of Nurse-Midwives in Washington, D.C.

Nurse-midwives have access to the same general technology for prenatal evaluation and labor as doctors, but the Centers for Disease Control and Prevention reports that there is a lower rate of infant mortality when nurse-midwives attend labors, compared with those attended by obstetricians.

To get the best possible care, visit your prenatal caretaker every month up until your 32nd week. After 32 weeks, see her twice a month, then once a week after your 36th week.

Concerns for Older Moms and Higher-Risk Pregnancies

Many women today are getting pregnant when they're in their thirties and forties, and for the most part the pregnancies are uneventful. "Even women in their early fifties today are expected to have routine and normal pregnancies," says Ronald J. Wapner, M.D., a high-risk obstetrician and medical geneticist and director of Maternal Fetal Medicine at MCP Hahnemann University in Philadelphia.

However, women who are over age 35 do have a slightly increased risk for fetal chromosome abnormalities. There's also a higher risk if they've had children with a birth defect or a chromosome abnormality such as Down syndrome, says Dr. Wapner.

If you fit this profile, see a specialist in genetics to assess specific risks before you conceive. You'll also want to consider additional screenings once you get pregnant, such as the chorionic villus sampling (CVS) test in your 11th to 13th weeks, or an amniocentesis procedure in your fourth month.

Here are some additional issues older women may face.

- Diabetes. The body produces anti-insulin hormones during pregnancy, which can result in a temporary condition called gestational diabetes. It can also aggravate preexisting diabetes. Women who are 40 years or older have a 7 percent chance of developing gestational diabetes, compared with 1.7 percent for a woman in her twenties. To avoid complications that can be caused by uncontrolled blood sugar—such as an oversize baby—be sure to get dietary advice from a nutritionist or a perinatal specialist.

- High blood pressure. If you have hypertension, it's important to get it under control before you conceive, says Dr. Wapner. Since your heart will be pumping more blood when you're pregnant, you may develop high blood pressure for the first time. You'll need extra rest to avoid a serious complication called preeclampsia, which can rob a fetus of bloodflow.

■ Premature or low-birth-weight babies. Both are common among older moms because they're more likely to be carrying twins or triplets. There are also preterm births because of maternal illness, like high blood pressure. Uncontrolled blood pressure or unhealthy lifestyle factors can also increase the risk of premature or low-birth-weight babies.

■ Repeated miscarriage. Losing a baby may be your body's way of coping with genetic abnormalities. As a woman gets older, miscarriages occur more frequently because there are more genetic abnormalities of pregnancy. It may also be a sign of irregularly shaped reproductive organs, a hormone imbalance, or an immune system disorder.

A Healthy Pregnancy

Regardless of your age when you conceive, the following advice will help ensure a safe and healthy pregnancy.

Take folic acid supplements. All women who are thinking about getting pregnant should take a minimum of 400 micrograms of folic acid daily. Folic acid helps prevent spinal cord defects.

Stay fit before and during pregnancy. Regular exercise can keep blood sugar under control, and women who are fit generally have lower blood pressure. In addition, getting in shape will

improve your stamina to push out a baby. Check with your doctor first, but if you aren't currently exercising, you might want to start out by walking. Start at an easy pace—so you don't break a sweat—for 10 to 15 minutes at a time the first week. Add a few minutes each week as you feel comfortable, gradually working up to an hour most days, if possible. Stop walking and contact your caregiver immediately if you become short of breath or have uterine cramping. And make sure to drink plenty of water before, during, and after exercise to prevent dehydration and overheating.

Gain a healthy amount of weight. You want to gain 5 to 7 pounds in the first 13 weeks of pregnancy; 10 to 14 pounds in the second 13 weeks; and 10 to 14 pounds in the last trimester. Being too thin or overweight can complicate pregnancy, especially if you have gestational diabetes or high blood pressure.

Don't smoke, and avoid alcohol. Smoking and drinking can raise the risk of miscarriage, birth defects, and low-birth-weight babies. Ideally, women should avoid alcohol and tobacco even before they conceive, says Dr. Wapner.

Eat wholesome foods. Every pregnant woman needs to do her best to get a nutritional diet. It should include lots of fruits and vegetables, whole grains, and other healthful foods. You'll certainly want to avoid excessive amounts of sweets or highly refined (and nutritionally "empty") foods.

Get enough rest. Women who are at risk for preeclampsia or other health problems will usually be advised by their doctors to curtail their

WHEN BAD THINGS HAPPEN TO HEALTHY WOMEN

Difficult Pregnancy Led to Lifestyle Improvements

Marla Hardee Milling knew that her pregnancies—one when she was 35, the other at 37—wouldn't be easy. She had received 52 radiation treatments for Hodgkin's disease when she was in her early twenties, and she knew that women in their mid- to late thirties were well past their childbearing prime.

In addition, Milling, a director of communications at Mars Hill College near Asheville, North Carolina, discovered during her first pregnancy that she was a carrier of the group B strep bacterium, which could potentially infect her unborn children.

During her second pregnancy, gestational diabetes proved to be yet another challenge. Milling accepted the fact that she would require extensive prenatal testing. And she also knew that she would have to make some sweeping lifestyle changes—such as giving up her favorite sweets. "I became more aware of my body," she says. She walked more, ate a lot more fresh vegetables, and reflected on her physical and emotional changes in the journal she kept.

"All of the little things that were different— even things like fatigue and nausea—made me aware of the miracle that there was a child inside of me," she says. "Besides, a few uncomfortable symptoms were nothing compared to the challenge of a life-threatening illness."

She used her age as an asset as well. "Being an older mother, I was emotionally prepared. I was so mentally and spiritually ready to have children, it was actually the best I ever felt in my life, despite the so-called problems." ∎

working hours. But regardless of risks, listen to your body—and be prepared to slow down when you're feeling fatigued.

Feeling Well on Every Level

Between the time your future child is conceived and the time you deliver, your uterus will expand to 1,000 times its prepregnancy size. Your body will be producing 25 percent more progesterone and 100 percent more estrogen. These tremendous physical changes can result in nausea, backache, headaches, digestive difficulties, and fatigue—not to mention potentially overwhelming emotional ups and downs.

Women who mentally prepare themselves for motherhood generally feel better physically as well as emotionally, Dr. Issokson says.

"Women need to stay connected with their bodies and natural rhythms, with their partners, and with other women who want to talk about the birth and mothering experience," says Dr. Issokson. "Things like journal writing, yoga, swimming, gardening, good self-care, connecting with other women, and talking about what they envision for themselves as mothers are all activities that reflect where women are spiritually and physically when they are pregnant. If they ignore the reflective and spiritual aspects of pregnancy, then women often end up feeling disconnected from themselves—and they feel disconnected from their bodies as birth approaches."

To get in harmony with your mind and body during this important time, here are a few worthwhile strategies.

Allow yourself to feel ambivalence. "I don't think there's any way to go through a life-altering event such as childbearing without some internal conflict, even in the most planned and wanted pregnancy," Dr. Issokson says. It's normal and healthy for women to acknowledge their anticipated losses—like how much they're going to miss sleeping late on Sundays, or giving up a degree of sexual intimacy or the loss of freedom and spontaneity that comes with a child-free life. Admitting and coming to terms with these and other losses and changes will help a woman accept the entire experience of having a baby—the difficulties along with the joy.

Give yourself time to bond. When you're pregnant, set aside time to bond—not only with your spouse but also with your baby-to-be. Try a "story time and music box" ritual every night. Here's how it works.

You and your husband take turns reading. It can be anything from children's books to baseball scores, as long as you are addressing your future child. Afterward, play a music box on your stomach. As the fetus matures, it will respond with a flurry of activity when it recognizes these sounds. Later, as soon as your baby emerges from the womb, playing the music box will orient and comfort your just-born child.

Reduce nausea naturally. One study found that 90 percent of pregnant women had less nausea when they took ginger. Fresh ginger tastes great when it's added to stir-fries, soups, and spicy baked goods, and it's entirely safe during pregnancy.

Because nausea usually increases when the stomach is empty, it's important for women to eat frequent, small meals during pregnancy, says Mary Lake Polan, M.D., Ph.D., professor and chairperson of the department of gynecology and obstetrics at Stanford University School of Medicine.

Don't lose sleep because of back pain. "During pregnancy, the tissues that support the spine and pelvis naturally get soft in order to allow the pelvis to open for delivery. This, along with the extra strain from her changing center of gravity, strains a pregnant woman's back," says James Cable, M.D., a back injury specialist with the Texas Back Institute in Plano.

He advises pregnant women to sleep on their side with the knees slightly bent. Put one pillow between your legs and another beneath your abdomen for extra support.

Know when to consider therapy. "Mental health services should be a routine part of everyone's prenatal care," says Dr. Issokson. "Pregnancy and birth trigger a lot of issues for women. Some issues are old ones that have never been resolved or that have crept back up, and some issues are new. While not everyone needs therapy, a few sessions with a counselor or therapist can create a wonderful opportunity for women to sort through these issues. For a woman who has a history of depression or anxiety, trauma, violence, or eating disorders, a prenatal session with a therapist can help her evaluate her risk factors for postpartum difficulties, like postpartum depression," she says.

Therapists can help with many different issues: the previous loss of a child, anxiety about birth, or the sense of vulnerability that so many women experience. If you suffer depression after giving birth (postpartum depression), working with a therapist is among the smartest things you can do.

Increase communication with your partner. "Discuss what you both think parenthood will ultimately be like, and what your fan-tasies are. Along with these ideal expectations, understand what you both perceive as your roles and responsibilities," suggests Dr. Issokson.

You might, for example, discuss who will be responsible for getting up in the middle of the night when the child cries. Or you might discuss the types of discipline you believe in or who will take days off from work when it's time to visit the pediatrician.

If your relationship has problems, this is the time to seek couples therapy and commit to getting your relationship as a couple in good working order, adds Dr. Issokson. "Don't fall for any fantasies that a baby will make your marriage better. Babies add stress to every relationship. The stronger, healthier, and more communicative a relationship is, the better it is able to handle the stress of new parenthood."

22

Childbirth

The personal touches that were planned for bringing Maureen Angelino's child into the world created the confidence, comfort, and sense of sacredness that she hoped for.

In Allentown, Pennsylvania, her husband and the midwives collaborated like old friends—to offer loving massages, assistance into the whirlpool, or just standing by to change the CD. And when the baby was ready, the warmth of her husband's hands was the first sensation that his son experienced outside the womb. The honor of snipping the umbilical cord went to his 4-year-old brother.

Marla Hardee Milling, who lives in Asheville, North Carolina, needed an entirely different birth plan. Potentially lifesaving procedures were arranged to protect both mother and baby from complications. Medical interventions abounded.

Two different women, two different birth plans. Obviously, no two births are exactly alike. Every woman creates in her mind the ideal situation and circumstances for giving birth. Things can always change, of course, sometimes at the last minute. Planning for childbirth is important, but so is maintaining a spirit of flexibility.

Conceiving a Birth Plan

Women use words like "peaceful," "powerful," or "beautiful" to describe their birthing experiences, but there are also practical considerations: the kinds of support you get, which procedures you do or don't want, and the type of setting that you feel comfortable in, says Marion McCartney, R.N., a practicing nurse-midwife and director of professional services at the American College of Nurse-Midwives in Washington, D.C.

Creating a birth plan will help you think through the decisions that will one day come together to create the optimal scenario. It's a way of clarifying your expectations and ensuring that everyone is working together to fulfill your needs.

To create a birth plan that will help make your childbirth dreams come true, here are some points to keep in mind.

Get information from a variety of sources. Read about the kinds of births that are offered in hospitals, at birthing centers, or at home. Learn about the pros and cons of different medical interventions, from "natural" vaginal births to cesarean sections. Ask the mothers in your life to tell you their birth stories. Or check out some real-life birth plans, which are posted online at www.childbirth.org. Always discuss your birth plan with your midwife or physician during your pregnancy, and be realistic about their response. If your caregiver is reluctant to accommodate your plan, you need to find out why and either revise the plan or look for a person who is comfortable with your wishes.

Look into C-section rates. There are many situations when surgical delivery, known as cesarean birth, or C-section, is essential. But if a hospital or clinic has a C-section rate that approaches one in four births, as opposed to the more reasonable rate of one in 18, it may be a sign of overuse of medical interventions, says Mindy

when to see a doctor

When contractions settle into some sort of a pattern, it's time to call your doctor or midwife. Labor is about to begin, says Mary Lake Polan, M.D., Ph.D., professor and chairperson of the department of gynecology and obstetrics at Stanford University School of Medicine.

When contractions noticeably increase in strength and occur about every 4 to 5 minutes for 60 seconds at time, and this pattern has continued for 30 to 60 minutes: You may be entering the final phase of labor, and you'll need professional assistance.

When your water breaks: It's time to get to the hospital or birthing center—or, if you're giving birth at home, to have the assistance of your doctor or midwife.

Smith, M.D., professor in the department of family practice at Michigan State University in Lansing and author of *20 Common Problems in Women's Healthcare.*

Understand the pros and cons of medications. Epidural anesthesia is highly effective at relieving discomfort in your pelvic area, but it reduces the amount of control a woman has during delivery—and it increases the odds that you'll need a C-section or a delivery with forceps. Drugs that induce labor can decrease the anxiety of waiting, but they may increase your need for pain medication, which carries some risk to the unborn child.

Many women want to avoid the use of drugs during childbirth, and that's fine. Just be sure to plan ahead. If you want to utilize acupressure to manage pain, or nipple stimulation to increase uterine contractions, consider making it part of your birth plan.

Decide about episiotomy. A surgical incision in the area between the vagina and anus, episiotomy is often performed to make more room for the baby to pass. Some doctors perform episiotomies routinely. They feel that even though the incision may take several months to heal, it's a safer option than risking tissue tears, which sometimes occur during childbirth.

Other doctors, however, maintain that natural tears heal as easily as surgical incisions and are less likely to extend into the rectum. They also cite statistics that indicate that about 20 percent of first-time moms can make it through childbirth without tearing. This soars to 80 percent for subsequent births.

WHEN BAD THINGS HAPPEN TO HEALTHY WOMEN

Hiring a Birth Coach Avoided Repeat Delivery Stress

During her first pregnancy, Nancy Battis was immediately hooked up to machines. An electronic monitor was threaded into the uterus and attached to the baby's scalp. She was tethered to an IV and told to stay on her back—where she remained for hours.

It wasn't the kind of childbirth she imagined.

A public relations consultant based in Kansas City, Battis had wanted a more comfortable, intimate birth. She felt that she needed someone there to talk her through the experience, and she had hoped for an environment that made her feel as though she was having a healthy, natural delivery. Instead, it felt as though she was having a serious medical procedure.

The next time she got pregnant, Battis hired a professional labor coach and birth advocate known as a doula. She also crafted a detailed birth plan. There was to be no IV or internal birth monitor to restrict her movements. She arranged to have a whirlpool ready, and the doula made sure there was in the room a birthing ball, which Battis practiced using before the birth. "It was almost like she predicted my every need," Battis says.

"It's not that the labor wasn't hard," she adds. "But all of us—my doula and my husband and the medical staff—got through the hard times together. My doula kept us beautifully focused."

To locate a doula in your area, visit the Doulas of North America (DONA) Web site at www.dona.org, e-mail the organization at Referrals@dona.org, or call (888) 788-DONA. ∎

If you're adamant about not having an episiotomy, there are a number of nonsurgical options, such as using a warm compress to soften the tissue prior to delivery or receiving a daily perineal (the area between the vagina and the anus) massage during the last 6 weeks of pregnancy. Perineal massage works best for first-time mothers, who are more likely to tear. Nurse-midwives are trained in the technique and can show you (or your spouse) how to do it at home.

To cover all bases, women sometimes indicate in their birth plans that they want to try nonsurgical measures first—but they'll opt for the incision if there's too much distress to them or their babies.

Discuss the birth plan with your doctor or midwife. Plan on doing this around the sixth or seventh month of pregnancy.

Create an easy-to-read outline. It's not uncommon for women to create birth plans that fill an entire journal. But when it's time for the birth, the doctor or midwife isn't going to have time to read all of your thoughts. To make things easy, condense the birth plan into a one- or two-page outline that can be read at a glance. Make duplicates so that everyone who will be present will have a copy.

Advice from a Birth Coach

The early part of your labor, called the latent stage, typically lasts between 6 and 18 hours. You might experience painful, irregular contractions or regular, nonpainful ones. The latent phase doesn't result in cervical dilatation, but it can hurt, keep you awake, and seemingly go on forever. At this time, you want your labor coach to be nearby, and you may feel better if you stay busy around the house, says Mary Lake Polan, M.D., Ph.D., professor and chairperson of the department of gynecology and obstetrics at Stanford University School of Medicine.

Following the latent stage, you'll have approximately 4 to 8 hours of active labor. That's when the contractions increase in intensity and the baby makes its way down into the birth canal. Once you are fully dilated, expect to deliver in less than 6 hours—or in as little as 30 minutes, Dr. Polan says.

"Labor takes a lot of support physically and emotionally," says Sally Reilly, codirector of the Academy of Certified Birth Educators, based in Olathe, Kansas. Here's what birth coaches advise.

Fill your mind with positive images. Try to clear your mind of worry and all the clutter that you normally carry around. Try to visualize the baby coming through—and imagine how healthy the baby is, Dr. Smith advises.

Ask about birth balls. These air-filled physical therapy balls are often used to help women feel more comfortable and to gain control, from the earliest stage of labor to the actual delivery. Getting on your hands and knees and leaning over the ball helps reduce back pressure, while sitting on the ball opens the pelvis for babies who are having a more difficult time getting through, says Reilly.

Water down discomfort. Laboring in a tub of water can significantly reduce your pain. Immersion supports the mother's weight, reduces the opposition to gravity, and reduces pressure on the abdomen. It also relaxes the pelvic floor muscles. In addition, laboring in water can increase the rate of dilation. If a tub isn't available, you can use the shower while sitting on a birth ball, says Reilly.

Create a soothing environment. Take full advantage of relaxation aids, such as aromatherapy mists in a scent you find relaxing, your favorite music, soothing "hot pads" made from rice-filled socks gently warmed in a microwave, or simply your comfiest nightgown.

23

Infertility

Women naturally have a drop in fertility starting around age 30, when there's a reduction in the quantity and quality of eggs. Research has shown that one out of seven women between ages 30 and 34 will have trouble conceiving. Between ages 35 and 39, the odds change to one in five, and by the time a woman reaches 40 to 45, they're one in four.

While "infertile" has come to mean a delay or difficulty getting pregnant, it rarely means a woman is unable to conceive, says Ken Gelman, M.D., a reproductive endocrinologist and clinical assistant professor of medicine at the University of Miami.

Lifestyle factors play a surprisingly large role in a woman's ability to conceive. Losing or gaining weight, quitting smoking, or giving up alcohol, for example, can increase the chances of conception. When self-care isn't enough, medication or surgery can often make the difference.

For more difficult cases, assisted reproduction wonders such as in vitro fertilization and artificial insemination can make parents out of people who at one time would have been considered sterile. Since 1981, assisted reproductive technologies have made possible the births of more than 70,000 babies.

How aggressively a woman chooses to treat infertility depends largely on how much cost—in terms of time, money, risk, and emotion—she is willing to invest. Regardless of the medical options, every woman who is trying to get pregnant needs to maintain a diet and lifestyle that will push the odds in her favor.

Lifestyle Strategies

Hit a hormone-safe weight. Fat cells in the body stimulate an overabundance of estrogen, which inhibits ovulation. Not enough fat, on the other hand, also inhibits estrogen. "Fertility is not supported by extremes at either end of the weight spectrum," says Dr. Gelman. "A body mass index (BMI) between 20 and 27 seems to be the best range to foster fertility." To calculate your BMI—and to take steps to achieve the appropriate weight—see chapter 6.

Exercise moderately. Women who exercise especially vigorously—by running marathons, for example—may experience delays or disruptions in ovulation. "Limit yourself to 45 minutes of daily workouts, such as strength training, walking, biking, or aerobics," says Dr. Gelman.

Keep your environment pure. Limit your exposure as much as possible to photography chemicals, pesticides, solvents, dust from treated wood, or heavy metals, such as mercury or lead. Environmental toxins have been linked to infertility in women and sperm abnormalities in men. If you or your spouse has to work with these or other toxins, wear a respirator or breathing mask and protective gloves and clothing, and always ensure that there's adequate ventilation.

Don't smoke—and avoid secondhand smoke. It reduces the production of eggs as well as sperm.

Drink lightly. One study has shown that among women who consumed alcohol while trying to conceive, the probability of conception dropped more than 50 percent when compared with women who abstained from alcohol.

Giving up alcohol is a good way to promote fertility. If you continue to drink, limit yourself to three drinks a week, says Dr. Gelman. On specific days when you're trying to conceive, avoid alcohol altogether, he adds.

Switch to decaffeinated coffee or tea. Studies have shown that beverages with caffeine can cause delays in conceiving, and they may increase the risk of early miscarriage.

Nutritional Treatments

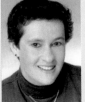 **Take prenatal supplements.** They contain a number of conception-supporting nutrients, including magnesium, B vitamins, and vitamins C and E. In fact, the chemical name for vitamin E, tocopherol, means "to bring forth offspring."

THREE THINGS I TELL EVERY FEMALE PATIENT

ALICE DOMAR, Ph.D., director of the Mind/Body Medical Institute for Women's Health at Beth Israel Deaconess Medical Center in Boston and assistant professor of medicine at Harvard Medical School, gives this special advice to women who are trying to get pregnant.

1 **TRY TO RELAX DEEPLY FOR AT LEAST 20 MINUTES A DAY.** Some of the most restorative techniques are prayer, guided-meditation tapes, and deep abdominal breathing.

SET PARAMETERS BEFORE YOU START TREATMENT. Infertility treatments are expensive and time-consuming, and sometimes risky to the health of the woman and the baby. Couples should set specific time (and cost) limits based on how far they want to go to achieve pregnancy. Knowing these limits in advance will help reduce long-term stress. **2**

3 **RALLY SUPPORT.** Infertile couples often feel isolated and alone. Ask your doctor at the fertility center to recommend a local support group. Or contact the National Fertility Association, 1310 Broadway, Somerville, MA 02144-1774 for information about group meetings in your area. ■

Supplement manufacturers don't make specific prenatal formulations for men, but there are a few key nutrients that can help boost a man's fertility. They include zinc (30 milligrams daily), copper (3 milligrams daily), L-carnitine (2 to 3 grams daily), and vitamin C (1,000 milligrams daily).

Men who want to be parents shouldn't take more than the recommended daily amount of 30 IU of vitamin E, Dr. Gelman adds. It may lower sperm counts when it's combined with vitamin C. It's always best to check with your doctor before taking any new supplements.

Eat natural foods. To support overall health and fertility, not only do you need the full spectrum of required daily nutrients, but you also need good digestion to absorb them, says Mercedes Cameron, M.D., a family practitioner at the Women's Place at St. Mary's Hospital in Grand Junction, Colorado.

She advises women who are trying to conceive to eat three to six daily servings of digestion-friendly whole grains, such as brown rice, oats, and barley, and nine daily servings of fresh fruits and vegetables. Make sure that you get 70 grams of protein daily. The protein can come from beans, nuts, eggs, lean meats, or cheeses. Buy organic foods whenever possible; it will reduce your exposure to hormone-disrupting chemicals that may be used by industrial farms, she says.

Mind-Body Techniques

Women who are facing infertility often feel anxious, depressed, and discouraged. Apart from disrupting their peace of mind, these and other negative emotions can also disrupt the way the body functions.

"Emotional distress can impair ovulation or cause the fallopian tubes and uterus to contract to the point where an egg is prevented from implanting," says Alice Domar, Ph.D., director of the Mind/Body Medical Institute for Women's Health at Beth Israel Deaconess Medical Center in Boston and assistant professor of medicine at Harvard Medical School.

Studies have shown that women with a history of depression run nearly twice the risk of having trouble conceiving. As a result, Dr. Domar and her colleagues at Harvard Medical School have developed a behavior-oriented fertility treatment program. On average, about 44 percent of the women in the program get pregnant—a success

when to see a doctor

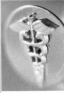
Young couples who have not achieved pregnancy within a year should see a reproductive specialist. There's a good chance that either you or your partner has a physical problem that's going to make getting pregnant a challenge, says Ken Gelman, M.D., a reproductive endocrinologist and clinical assistant professor of medicine at the University of Miami.

If your periods are painful or irregular, or if the bleeding is unusually light or heavy: These are common symptoms of endometriosis, uterine fibroids, pelvic inflammatory disease, or polycystic ovary syndrome, all of which can lead to infertility.

rate that's comparable to women who are in their reproductive prime.

The program stresses stress management, esteem issues, and positive thinking. Some of the most important things women can do include:

Try visualization. A woman might be angry because she had a miscarriage. She might resent her husband for failing to understand her despair, and she'll probably be angry at the doctors who can't "fix" the problem. The more frustration she feels, the more likely she is to have trouble conceiving, Dr. Domar says.

Women need to release their negative emotions—not by venting, which can make them feel worse, but by filling their minds with positive thoughts and images.

Here's an example of how it works. Take a few minutes every day to imagine that a magic carpet has arrived to take you away from your troubles. As you sail through the clouds above mountaintops, mentally place the day's disappointments inside a stone—then gleefully hurl the stone away from you.

This type of imaginative thinking, called visualization, is an excellent way to cope with anger and anxiety and to replace the emotions with feelings of strength and power, says Dr. Domar.

Permit yourself to lie low. Women who are infertile often say that they find it difficult to be around children—or around people who are always asking whether they're making "progress." You can't isolate yourself forever, but you shouldn't feel obligated to maintain a busy social life at times when you'd rather be alone, says Dr. Domar.

Confront destructive ideas. Women who are trying without success to get pregnant often link their self-worth to their ability to have children—and they may blame themselves for having "waited so long" to start a family. Put these feelings behind you, Dr. Domar advises. They distort reality and needlessly cause frustration or fear.

Multiple Births Equal Multiple Diapers

Women who undergo assistive reproduction procedures, such as in vitro fertilization and gamete intrafallopian transfer—which involves the injection of one or more eggs mixed with sperm directly into the fallopian tubes—will have multiple births about 38 percent of the time. Among those who use ovulation-inducing drugs, 20 percent of the children are twins or triplets or other "multiples."

Fertility specialists advise women that multiple births have higher risks of birth defects or delivery complications, especially in older moms.

Then there's the sheer workload. Women who are considering fertility treatments should ask themselves if they have the energy and tolerance that's required, say, for the more than 1,000 monthly diaper changes required by a set of triplet newborns. That comes to three new diapers (one for each of three little bottoms) every 2 hours for an entire month. ■

WHEN BAD THINGS HAPPEN TO HEALTHY WOMEN

She Shed Negative Thoughts—And Conceived Twins

Valerie Gattozzi Mei and her husband, Richard, desperately wanted children. For 6 years, Mei worked with reproductive specialists. She endured tests, surgeries, and side effects from medications—and nothing helped.

"Each year that went by, the desperation and depression became more unbearable," she recalls. "Summers on the beach, which used to be my favorite getaway, became nothing but a torturous reminder that I had no children to watch play in the sand."

Since she had already exhausted most of the medical options, Mei tried a different approach: changing her state of mind.

She enrolled in a 10-week program at the Mind/Body Medical Institute for Women at Harvard Medical Center and Beth Israel Deaconess Medical Center in Boston, where she worked with trained professionals to develop a more positive attitude and reduce her feelings of anger and depression.

In addition, Mei and her husband decided to stop trying to conceive for an entire summer. Rather than feeling the constant pressure, they put all of their energy into enjoying their new boat on the shore.

At the end of a lovely summer, Mei felt ready to pursue one round of in vitro fertilization. "Before I learned how to manage my feelings, the whole idea of in vitro fertilization scared me horribly, so I never considered it," she says.

One month later, she learned that she was pregnant with twins.

Today Mei, 43, is the busy mother of 6-year-old Emily Rena and Olivia Lorraine. She continues to use tools she learned during her long struggle to get pregnant. "I now know that it's pointless to get yourself in a tizzy over nothing," she says. "When I catch myself doing it, I remind myself to stop, think, breathe, relax, and go easier on myself." ∎

Try writing down your thoughts in a diary or talking to a supportive friend or family member. If these techniques don't help, consider talking to your doctor about counseling.

Medical Options

 When you're having trouble getting pregnant, the first order of business is for your partner to see a urologist or fertility specialist, who will probably perform a semen analysis to rule out a low sperm count or sperm abnormalities. You'll want to visit your gynecologist or a fertility specialist, who will ask about your menstrual history and perform a complete physical exam.

Both of you may need further evaluation of your reproductive organs to check for problems such as blocked tubes or scar tissue in the woman.

Infertility often occurs when a woman is ovulating irregularly or not at all. These cases are often easy to correct because for more than half of couples, the use of drugs leads to pregnancy after 6 months if there are no other problems requiring treatment.

Assisted reproduction technologies, such as in vitro fertilization, manipulate eggs and sperm outside the womb to improve the chances of pregnancy. According to the Centers for Disease Control and Prevention, 32 percent of women younger than 35 who used assisted reproductive technologies gave birth. In women over age 40, the success rate was 8 percent.

Women are usually advised to progress from the easiest treatment options to the most aggressive, giving each treatment at least three menstrual cycles to take effect; after six menstrual cycles, it's probably time to move on to another approach.

"It may be important to move more quickly through your options if you feel that your proverbial reproductive clock is ticking," says Dr. Gelman. "Some couples in their forties want to bypass medications and elaborate testing and go straight to in vitro fertilization. It's always an individual choice."

For more information about infertility, visit the Web site of the National Infertility Association (RESOLVE) at www.resolve.org.

24

Polycystic Ovary Syndrome

When ovaries are stimulated by high levels of hormones, they sometimes develop blisterlike growths, called cysts. The cysts themselves are unlikely to cause problems, but the hormones that trigger their growth may cause problems elsewhere in the body.

Some women suffer with lots of tiny ovarian cysts as a result of a condition called polycystic ovary syndrome (PCOS). Women with PCOS may develop unwanted hair growth on the face, torso, chest, and/or buttocks—and thinning of the hair on the head. They may gain weight or develop acne as adults. PCOS can interfere with menstrual cycles and fertility as well.

All women produce a small amount of testosterone, the "male" hormone, but women with PCOS produce relatively high amounts. The extra testosterone disrupts levels of other hormones in the body. It may cause irregular menstrual cycles and stop ovulation. Because of this, the body continues producing estrogen but stops producing progesterone.

Many women with PCOS don't know they have it. All they know is that they're unhappy with the appearance of their bodies—and they often don't suspect that there's an underlying physical reason, says Walter Futterweit, M.D., clinical professor of medicine in the division of endocrinology at Mount Sinai School of Medicine in New York City and an advisory board member of the Polycystic Ovarian Syndrome Association.

In young women, PCOS is the leading cause of infertility. It may not be discovered until a woman tries to conceive but cannot.

Luckily, most women with PCOS can control the symptoms with a combination of medications and home care.

when to see a doctor

If you have a history of skipped menstrual periods that are followed by serious acne outbreaks, make an appointment to see an endocrinologist. This is a classic symptom of polycystic ovary syndrome (PCOS), says Walter Futterweit, M.D., clinical professor of medicine in the division of endocrinology at Mount Sinai School of Medicine in New York City.

If you have hair growth on the face or body and thinning hair on the head: In women this usually means that the balance of hormones has been disrupted, and you could have PCOS.

Lifestyle Strategies

Exercise regularly and keep an eye on your weight. In women who are overweight, testosterone is converted in the fat tissue to female hormones. An effective way to restore hormones to their proper levels is to maintain a healthful weight. Talk to your doctor about appropriate exercise and diet plans. As you lose fat tissue, your estrogen levels will naturally decline.

Nutritional Treatments

Control insulin levels. The majority of women with PCOS develop a condition called insulin resistance. Insulin is the hormone that carries glucose (blood sugar) into cells where it's needed. If the cells become resistant to insulin, the body produces more of it—and this in turn stimulates the production of more testosterone by the ovaries.

There are a number of ways to overcome insulin resistance. In addition to helping to control weight, exercising regularly—it can be walking, bicycling, hiking, or even working in the yard for 20 to 30 minutes most days of the week—will help the body's insulin become more efficient, says Dr. Futterweit. You also may be told to follow a low-glycemic (low-carbohydrate) diet. (For more information on low-glycemic eating, see chapter 15.)

Curb your sugar cravings. Sugar increases your insulin levels, which causes weight gain and aggravates hormone imbalances, says Lila Amdurska Wallis, M.D., clinical professor of medi-

---

THREE THINGS I TELL EVERY FEMALE PATIENT

WALTER FUTTERWEIT, M.D., clinical professor of medicine in the division of endocrinology at Mount Sinai School of Medicine in New York City, advises women with polycystic ovary syndrome (PCOS) to follow these recommendations.

1 REARRANGE THE FOOD GUIDE PYRAMID. The standard for healthy eating, the food guide pyramid recommends getting the bulk of calories from complex carbohydrates, such as whole grains. Women with PCOS, however, should get about 40 percent of calories from lean protein, such as lamb, fish, or legumes. About 30 percent of calories should come from vegetables, and only about 30 percent should come from complex carbohydrates. Some women have even more success when only about 10 to 20 percent of calories come from carbohydrates.

2 GET SERIOUS ABOUT LOSING WEIGHT. Many women with PCOS are obese. The good news is that losing as little as 7 to 8 percent of the weight is often enough to lower excess hormone levels.

3 SEE AN EXPERT. PCOS can be complicated to control. Your family doctor can help, but women with PCOS really need to be under the care of an endocrinologist, an expert on the body's hormones. ■

WHEN BAD THINGS HAPPEN TO HEALTHY WOMEN

She Was Eating All the Wrong Foods

Christine Gray DeZarn had kept her weight at 140 pounds throughout her adult life—so she was understandably alarmed when it suddenly jumped to 200 when she was 27. She responded the way a lot of women do: by going on an ultra low calorie diet. But even when she was getting a skimpy 800 calories daily, she continued to gain weight.

"The doctor I was seeing was convinced I was cheating on my diet, but I was practically starving," she remembers.

At about the same time, she began getting acne along her jaw. She also discovered hair growing on her face and stomach, and when she and her husband tried to have their first child, they had no success after 6 years and 11 trials of expensive assisted reproduction treatments.

DeZarn first heard about polycystic ovary syndrome (PCOS) on an online infertility support group. "I read everything I could get my hands on about metabolism, and how blood sugar and hormones are affected by the different foods you eat. I found out what a mistake I had made by following a low-fat,

high-carbohydrate diet. It doesn't work for people with insulin resistance. I was actually triggering my condition by eating a lot of processed grains and cutting back on protein."

As soon as DeZarn eliminated sugar, pasta, rice, and other high-carbohydrate foods from her diet, the pounds started to naturally drop off. She lost 30 pounds in 3 months, and 50 pounds within the first year. "Within 2 years, I was down to 132 pounds, which is better than where I started," she adds.

As a busy travel industry trainer, DeZarn had to maintain her eating plan while staying in hotels and eating on airplanes and in restaurants. She always eats the same breakfast: scrambled eggs and fresh fruit. Most restaurants serve grilled chicken Caesar salad, and it's also easy to find her favorite snack—celery with blue cheese dressing.

Today, a decade after she was diagnosed, DeZarn, 38, continues to follow a strict diet because it controls her weight and other symptoms of PCOS. "I will eat this way for the rest of my life because it works," she says. ∎

cine at Weill Medical College of Cornell University in New York City and past president of the American Medical Women's Association. Replace sugary treats with foods like grains, fruits, and vegetables. Without those sweets taunting your hormone levels, you'll feel healthier and more energetic.

Eat small amounts at a time. "If you are in the habit of eating two or three heavy meals a day, switch to five to six light meals," Dr. Futterweit advises. Each meal should contain between 250 and 300 calories. That's about all that insulin-resistant cells can handle at one time, he explains.

Enjoy protein or low-carbohydrate snacks. Women are usually advised to enjoy bagels, bread, or other high-carbohydrate foods. For women with PCOS, however, foods that are high in carbohydrates may cause surges in insulin. Better snack choices include protein (such as plain yogurt, string cheese, or nuts and seeds), or low-starch vegetables, such as cucumber or broccoli.

Drink water—but avoid fruit juices. Juices are generally too sweet for women with PCOS. The ideal beverage is water. It's also fine to drink unsweetened almond milk or fat-free or low-fat milk.

Medical Options

Rx Lower insulin with medications. Doctors often advise women with PCOS to take metformin (Glucophage), an insulin-regulating drug that's commonly used to treat diabetes. Women who take it can often nor-malize their menstrual cycles. They also may see a reversal in weight gain or unwanted hair growth, says Dr. Futterweit.

Consider the Pill. Oral contraceptives may be used to restore a normal menstrual cycle and help reduce hair growth and acne. Anti-androgen (male hormones) pills such as spironolactone (Aldactone), which block the effects of testosterone, can also be helpful in conjunction with the Pill.

Shut down the source. When the symptoms of PCOS can't be controlled with other medications, your doctor may recommend that you take drugs called GnRH agonists (such as Synarel), which "turn off" the ovaries. Once the ovaries stop functioning, the troublesome hormones will gradually return to more normal levels. This is not used often in view of the loss-of-bone effect, which may occur after 6 months of use.

For more information on polycystic ovary syndrome, see the Web site of the Polycystic Ovarian Syndrome Association at www.pcosupport.org.

Fibroids

The thought of uterine fibroids—benign growths of the uterine muscle called leiomyomas—is enough to rush many women into action. As a rule, however, if fibroids aren't causing symptoms, they may not need treatment at all.

Between 20 and 25 percent of American women over 35 years of age have fibroids; African-American women are at least twice as likely to have fibroids as other women. You can have one fibroid or a whole cluster. Most fibroids are between the size of a pea and a tennis ball, although they can potentially grow much larger.

It's not uncommon for women with fibroids to be unaware of them. They're often discovered during routine exams, when a gynecologist feels them while pressing on the abdomen.

Most women with fibroids will experience a dull ache in the abdomen, pelvis, or back. Fibroids may also cause abnormal menstrual bleeding.

In many cases, however, they cause no symptoms at all—and doctors advise women to simply get used to the idea that there are harmless guests inside the pelvis.

If you are having symptoms, your doctor may simply advise you to wait: Fibroid growth is stimulated by the female hormone estrogen. Once a woman approaches menopause, and estrogen levels decline, the symptoms will usually disappear, says Sam Jacobs, M.D., a reproductive endocrinologist and associate professor of obstetrics and gynecology at Robert Wood Johnson Medical School in Camden, New Jersey.

In the meantime, you may want to take a few steps to manage fibroids naturally.

Home Remedies

Manage your weight. Excess body fat leads to excess estrogen, which can increase the size of fibroids. The best way to maintain a healthful weight is to get regular exercise. A combination of weight training and aerobic activities—such as running, bicycling, or fast walking—decreases fat tissue and adds muscle, which can help lower excess levels of estrogen in the body. (For a complete guide to maintaining a healthful weight, see chapter 6.)

Ease the ache. Applying heat to the abdomen will often relieve discomfort, especially when you're having your period. Mercedes Cameron, M.D., a family practitioner at the Women's Place at St. Mary's Hospital in Grand Junction, Colorado, advises using a castor oil pack.

Pour 4 ounces of castor oil on a thick piece of cotton cloth. Fold the cloth in half and put it on your abdomen. Cover it with plastic wrap and a thin towel, then put a heating pad or hot-water bottle on top. Leave the pack on your tummy for up to an hour a day, and repeat the treatment daily, says Dr. Cameron.

Nutritional Treatments

Eat less meat. "The estrogenic additives used in the beef industry can disrupt your hormone levels enough to signal fibroids to grow," says Dr. Jacobs.

In one study, Italian researchers compared the diets of 2,400 women. They found that women with fibroids ate more beef, ham, and other red meats than those without fibroids. A plant-based diet is beneficial because fruits and vegetables contain natural plant compounds called isoflavones, which help prevent estrogen from fueling fibroid growth, Dr. Jacobs says.

Alternative Therapies

Try an Eastern remedy. Asian practitioners have many approaches for treating fibroids, including herbal and dietary treatments that are designed to remove excess estrogen in the body. Seaweed has shown to be very effective in treating fibroids. Eating liver or taking liver organ supplements has been shown to be the most effective in removing excess estrogen, reducing fibroids, and regulating the menstrual cycle. In addition, an Asian doctor may advise women with fibroids to perform healing movements, such as tai chi or qigong, which are said to restore healthy circulation to the pelvic area.

THREE THINGS I TELL EVERY FEMALE PATIENT

LYNN BORGATTA, M.D., associate professor in the department of obstetrics and gynecology at Boston University School of Medicine and Boston Medical Center, offers this advice to women with fibroids.

1 **DON'T BE FRIGHTENED.** Fibroids are tumors, but they're benign and won't increase your risk for cancer. They're almost always harmless, and the symptoms (if there are any) will probably be easy to manage, possibly with medications that shrink fibroids, among other options.

2 **BE CONSERVATIVE.** If you need relief from fibroid symptoms and you're planning to have children, talk to your doctor about medication before considering surgical procedures like myomectomy or uterine embolization.

3 **TALK TO YOUR DOCTOR ABOUT HYSTERECTOMY OPTIONS.** If you need a hysterectomy, let your doctor know that you don't want the ovaries and cervix removed along with the uterus unless it's absolutely necessary. A supracervical hysterectomy is less traumatic and healthier in the long run. ■

To find a qualified practitioner, contact the American Association of Oriental Medicine, 433 Front Street, Catasauqua, PA 18032. You can also call the association at (610) 266-1433 or, toll-free, (888) 500-7999. You can log on to the Web site at www.aaom.org.

Medical Options

Fibroids need to be treated when they're causing heavy or abnormal menstrual bleeding, chronic pain, bowel or urinary obstructions, or other symptoms, says Lynn Borgatta, M.D., associate professor in the department of obstetrics and gynecology at Boston University School of Medicine and Boston Medical Center. You'll also need treatment if you're trying to conceive and the fibroids are interfering with pregnancy.

The treatment options include:

- Gonadotropin-releasing hormone (GnRH) agonists (Lupron/Lupron Depot). These are medications that shrink fibroids temporarily. Their main use is to shrink fibroids prior to surgery. The drawback to these medications is that they may cause menopause-like symptoms, such as hot flashes and vaginal dryness. Over time, they can also raise cholesterol levels and increase the risk of osteoporosis, so they are usually not used longer than 6 months.

- Myomectomy. This means removing fibroids surgically. Small fibroids can be cauterized (destroyed) with a laser or electrical needle; larger fibroids are cut away from the uterine wall. De-

when to see a doctor

If your periods are heavier than usual, or you're having irregular bleeding, see your gynecologist. This is often the first symptom of fibroids, says Lynn Borgatta, M.D., associate professor in the department of obstetrics and gynecology at Boston University School of Medicine and Boston Medical Center.

If you're having trouble urinating or moving your bowels: It can mean that fibroids are getting large enough to exert pressure on the bladder or intestine.

If you've been diagnosed with fibroids, whether or not they're causing symptoms: You'll need to have them monitored regularly: 3 months after the diagnosis, and every 6 months thereafter.

pending on the location of the fibroids, surgery may be done through the abdomen or through the vagina. The surgery is usually successful, although there's a small chance that a hysterectomy will be needed to finish the surgery. Also, there's a 30 percent chance that the fibroids will return. Fertility is usually preserved, but pregnancy can sometimes be complicated.

- Hysterectomy. This means removing the uterus. Once the uterus is removed, the fibroids are also gone and won't come back. The problem with hysterectomy is that it's major surgery—there may be a long recovery time. Also, women who have this procedure won't be able to have children afterward. A supracervical hysterectomy is limited to removal of the uterus only, leaving the ovaries and cervix intact.

WHEN BAD THINGS HAPPEN TO HEALTHY WOMEN

Acupuncture Saved Her from a Hysterectomy

After an emergency room visit for abdominal pain, Sharon Saunders, a cookbook writer in Allentown, Pennsylvania, discovered that she had a fibroid the size of a 16-week pregnancy. The fibroid had grown so fast and was causing so much discomfort that her gynecologist recommended a hysterectomy.

Saunders wasn't convinced that surgery was her best option, especially because she knew that fibroids often shrink with the onset of menopause. At 48, she was hoping to find a treatment that would tide her over for a few years.

After reading an article about the use of acupuncture for treating fibroids, she decided to give it a try. She made an appointment with a practitioner of traditional Chinese medicine, who recommended weekly acupuncture treatments, along with medicinal herbs. After 4 months, she checked back with her gynecologist, who reported that the fibroid had shrunk by a third.

"I got to keep my uterus, and the pain went away entirely," says Saunders, who continues to get regular acupuncture treatments. "I go back once a month for what I call wellness maintenance," she says. "It has really helped my allergies, too." ■

■ Uterine embolization. This is a surgical procedure in which the blood vessels that supply the fibroids are destroyed with a bombardment of plastic particles. The advantage of this procedure is that it's less stressful than other forms of surgery, and it's unlikely to interfere with a woman's ability to conceive. It's a relatively new procedure, however, and experts aren't sure how effective it will prove to be over time.

"When medical interventions are necessary, ask your doctor about all your options—the right treatment will be different for everyone," says Dr. Borgatta. There are a lot of considerations to keep in mind, including the severity of symptoms, whether you'll want to get pregnant in the future, and how close you are to menopause. The size of the fibroids and where they're growing can also affect your treatment options as well as your risks, Dr. Borgatta adds.

Endometriosis

The uterus is lined with a spongy tissue called the endometrium, which provides a soft nest for fertilized eggs. Normally, an egg is released each month, and if it isn't fertilized, the endometrium swells, breaks down, and sloughs off, exiting the body as menstrual fluid.

Sometimes, however, the cells that make up the endometrium grow outside the uterus on nearby organs, such as the fallopian tubes or ovaries. The cells also sometimes implant themselves on the outside of the uterus. They can even spread to the lungs, digestive tract, or other parts of the body. This disease is called endometriosis, and it can result in painful, and potentially serious, symptoms.

Because endometrial cells are sensitive to the hormonal changes of the menstrual cycle, the symptoms often flare during the menstrual period. Women may experience severe, even incapacitating pain, fatigue, and many other symptoms. Endometriosis also can result in gastrointestinal symptoms, painful sex, or, during periods, painful urination. More than 30 percent of women with endometriosis also face infertility.

Endometriosis sometimes can be controlled with the use of birth control pills or other hor-

mone-altering medications. Surgery to remove the tissue is another treatment that can help. But for about one in three women, the renegade tissue will eventually come back, says Carolyn R. Kaplan, M.D., a reproductive endocrinologist who practices at Georgia Reproductive Specialists and is an assistant clinical professor of obstetrics and gynecology at Emory University School of Medicine, both in Atlanta.

Doctors aren't sure what causes endometriosis. Evidence suggests that the cells get "scattered" around the pelvis when menstrual blood doesn't effectively make its way out of the body. The immune system should recognize and destroy these errant cells, but for some reason it doesn't, says Dr. Kaplan.

There are a number of treatment options for endometriosis. A good starting place is for women to strengthen their immune systems and do everything possible to keep their hormones in the proper balance, says Deborah A. Metzger, M.D., Ph.D., associate clinical professor of reproductive endocrinology and obstetrics and gynecology at Stanford University and director of Helena Women's Health in San Jose, California.

Some women with endometriosis will require

medical treatment, either to remove the tissue or to manage the monthly flare-ups. In many cases, however, women can control the discomfort with home care.

Home Remedies

Treat yourself to heat. Applying warmth to the lower abdomen is a very effective way to soothe the uterus, says Toni Bark, M.D., director of the department of integrative medicine at Good Shepherd Hospital in Barrington, Illinois, and medical director of the Center for the Healing Arts in Glencoe, Illinois. Taking warm baths or applying a hot-water bottle or a heating pad is the easiest approach. For longer-lasting heat, your doctor may advise you to use a patch that releases heat for long periods of time, such as ThermaCare therapeutic heat wraps, available in drugstores.

Exercise when able. Walking, swimming, and other forms of exercise increase circulation, which helps the body remove excess estrogen from the blood. Exercise also stimulates endorphins, natural chemicals that help reduce pain.

Avoid pollutants. The hormones in a woman's body are exquisitely balanced, but modern society has thrown a wrench into the works. Humans have introduced more than 70,000 industrial chemicals into the environment, and some of them suppress immunity and disrupt the natural balance of hormones, says Dr. Metzger.

Dioxin, for example, a waste chemical that's widespread in the environment, might have profound effects on a woman's hormones. In one 13-

THREE THINGS I TELL EVERY FEMALE PATIENT

TONI BARK, M.D., director of the department of integrative medicine at Good Shepherd Hospital in Barrington, Illinois, and medical director of the Center for the Healing Arts in Glencoe, Illinois, has seen great success when women with endometriosis do the following:

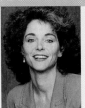

1 TAKE 1 TABLESPOON OF GROUND FLAXSEED DAILY. Flax contains an oil that reduces painful inflammation. It's also high in fiber, which can help remove excess estrogen. "I recommend having it for breakfast every morning," says Dr. Bark. "You can mix it with sunflower seeds, fruit, and almond milk."

2 USE EVENING PRIMROSE OIL. Available as a supplement, evening primrose oil reduces inflammation and often relieves pain within a month, says Dr. Bark. The recommended dose is 500 milligrams twice daily.

3 TAKE A MULTI SUPPLEMENT THAT CONTAINS B VITAMINS AND VITAMIN E. Vitamin E carries oxygen to tissues and helps reduce scar formation in women with endometriosis. The B vitamins are particularly important because they help balance the body's hormones, says Dr. Bark. ▪

year study, female rhesus monkeys were exposed to dioxin, and 79 percent developed endometriosis. These studies were in monkeys, not humans, but something similar may occur in humans. We don't know for sure without more studies, says Dr. Metzger.

An important place to start, according to the Endometriosis Association, is to avoid food that may have high amounts of dioxin in it, but more about that later. Products that have been bleached with chlorine may contain dioxin and other chemical contaminants. Although a survey by the Endometriosis Association did not show a connection between tampon use and endometriosis incidence, some women like to use non-chlorine-bleached tampons and sanitary napkins.

Some people may find it's also helpful to use dioxin-free bathroom tissues (available in health catalogs and stores), cosmetics, and other products whenever possible. Opt for cloth towels and cloth napkins instead of paper.

Nutritional Treatments

 Eat organically. Commercial livestock typically is injected with growth hormones and antibiotics—and women who eat meat may suffer the effects. "In my opinion, an immediate way to protect your hormone balance and immune system is to make sure that you don't eat meat and dairy products that aren't certified as organic," says Dr. Bark.

Filter your drinking water. Use water purifiers that filter out lead, mercury, chlorine, and other hormone-disrupting contaminants, advises Dr. Bark. Check the labels for the specific substances that each type of filter will remove.

Alternative Therapies

Relax as much as you can. Stress management helps to improve immune function and may also decrease pain, says Dr. Bark.

Every woman has her own ways of coping with stress, including meditation, yoga, and relaxation exercises. Or try more creative approaches: Take an art class; do volunteer work; get more engaged with your hobbies. Women

when to see a doctor

 If you have abdominal pain that increases with your period, around ovulation, or with intercourse: There's a good chance that you have endometriosis, and it may get worse without prompt treatment, says Carolyn R. Kaplan, M.D., a reproductive endocrinologist at Georgia Reproductive Specialists and an assistant clinical professor of obstetrics and gynecology at Emory University School of Medicine, both in Atlanta.

If you're having trouble getting pregnant: Endometriosis is a common cause of infertility, says Dr. Kaplan. Endometriosis may cause scarring around the tubes and ovaries that could lead to infertility. If other women in your family have had endometriosis, you have a higher risk of getting it as well, she adds.

WHEN BAD THINGS HAPPEN TO HEALTHY WOMEN

Natural Treatments Gave Her Control

Menstrual periods are rarely as regular as the textbooks would have you believe, but for Karen Susag, they were unusually erratic from the beginning.

"My periods varied greatly. Sometimes I would only get a period every 6 months, and when I did, I'd be immobilized with pain. There also were times that I would end up at the emergency room," says Susag, a community organizer for Communities for a Better Environment in San Francisco.

At one point, the pain was so severe and frequent that she missed an entire semester of college. That's when a doctor finally recognized that her symptoms were caused by endometriosis.

In the next 10 years, she had surgery six times for endometriosis and to remove scar tissue. She also tried a variety of hormone medications, which invariably brought on headaches, nausea, and fatigue.

On the advice of a practitioner specializing in immunotherapy, Susag eliminated dairy, sugar, yeast, alcohol, and caffeine from her diet. In addition to immunotherapy, she underwent acupuncture and took Chinese herbs under supervision of an Oriental medicine doctor. And she did everything possible to reduce the stress in her life.

"I have a whole different way of approaching things," she says. "I listen to my body, and know when I'm pushing myself too hard. If I work late, then I take the morning off."

The treatments have worked, Susag says. Her pain level is way down, and she generally has a lot more energy. "The hardest thing about having endometriosis is knowing that it's a chronic problem. But I've discovered that if you keep your life in better balance, you can keep it in check." ∎

who nurture their creative sides will naturally experience less stress, Dr. Bark explains.

Medical Options

 Consider drug therapy. Gonadotropin-releasing hormone (GnRH) agonists and antagonists, such as leuprolide (Lupron) and nafarelin (Synarel), turn off the signal to ovulate, leading to a reversible "medical menopause," Dr. Kaplan says. This causes estrogen levels to

drop. Menstrual periods stop, and over time the errant endometrial cells will shrink.

Ask your doctor about immunotherapy. A poll of women with endometriosis conducted by the Endometriosis Association found that immunotherapy—a broad-based treatment plan that includes testing for hormone allergies and other allergies and desensitizing for those allergies—was ranked higher for effectiveness than painkillers, hormone medications, or surgical approaches for endometriosis. A literature review on the role of autoimmunity in the development of endometriosis found that endometriosis shares enough characteristics with autoimmune diseases to warrant treatment along those lines.

To find a physician who practices immunotherapy for endometriosis, contact the Endometriosis Association in Milwaukee at (800) 992-3636.

Look into IUDs. Intrauterine devices (IUDs) were once discouraged for women with endometriosis or other pelvic problems, but a new type of IUD, sold under the name Mirena, releases a synthetic hormone called levonorgestrel into the uterus. It appears to suppress endometrial growth, says Dr. Kaplan.

A Finnish study looked at 56 women who were considering hysterectomies to relieve excessive uterine bleeding. Half of them were asked to use the Mirena IUD to see if it helped. Two-thirds of the women experienced enough relief that they decided to cancel the surgery. Although this was only one small study of women who were considering hysterectomies for "excessive uterine bleeding," not endometriosis, the Mirena might be considered an option for endometriosis.

27

Pelvic Inflammatory Disease

If you suspect that you may have contacted a sexually transmitted disease (STD)—symptoms include a foul-smelling discharge, painful urination, and a dull ache in the lower abdomen; pelvic pain; or fever and chills—don't wait to see if it will go away. Call your doctor right away.

You have to act quickly if there's even a hint that you have an STD. That's because untreated STDs can lead to pelvic inflammatory disease (PID), a broad term that refers to infections of the upper genital tract, usually involving the fallopian tubes and sometimes the ovaries and even the lining of the uterus. As with many infections, intensive treatment with antibiotics is necessary to destroy the bacteria that are making you sick. Delays in treatment, on the other hand, can allow the harmful organisms to rage out of control, potentially damaging your reproductive organs beyond repair.

Unfortunately, women don't always see a doctor at the first sign of symptoms. A quarter of PID cases require hospitalization and the use of intravenous antibiotics; in rare cases emergency surgery is needed, to drain infectious fluid from the abdomen or repair organ damage. Because the infection can scar and block the fallopian tubes, PID may result in infertility. Blocked tubes can

also put a woman at higher risk for ectopic pregnancy, a dangerous condition in which a fertilized egg grows in the fallopian tube instead of in the uterus.

About 1 million American women are treated for PID every year. It's a common result from STDs. It doesn't have to be, though; the vast majority of cases can be prevented by taking precautions against sexually transmitted diseases by using condoms, says Sam Jacobs, M.D., a reproductive endocrinologist and associate professor of obstetrics and gynecology at Robert Wood Johnson Medical School in Camden, New Jersey.

Unwelcome Infections

The organism that results in PID is usually chlamydia or, less commonly, gonorrhea (or both). These STDs are especially prevalent among sexually active women with multiple partners.

If you've had unprotected sex and suspect that you may have been exposed to an STD, get tested right away. One reason that STDs are so dangerous is that one in five people infected with chlamydia or gonorrhea doesn't have symptoms. Women can carry the disease for weeks, months, or even years before the infection spreads or results in full-blown PID.

PID isn't always caused by sexually transmitted diseases. Some women may develop infections after childbirth, abortions, or other types of pelvic surgeries. These types of infections are rare, however. In most cases—99.9 percent—STDs are to blame, says Dr. Jacobs.

Regardless of the cause, STDs can be successfully treated with antibiotics. While completing the antibiotic treatment, you can also relieve much of the discomfort with home care.

Home Remedies

Allow yourself some downtime. Your body has taken a beating, and you need time to recover. Drink a lot of fluid, eat lightly, and get some rest.

Avoid sex until the antibiotic treatment is complete—usually after 2 weeks. Otherwise, you could pass the infection to your partner. When you do resume sexual activity, be certain that your partner has been tested and treated for STDs. You don't want to be exposed to the same harmful organisms that made you sick in the first place.

Steam away infection. Sitting in a hot environment—a steamy shower, for example, or a deep bath—increases body temperature, which boosts the activity of the immune system and creates an unfavorable environment for harmful germs. The moist heat will also reduce discomfort in the abdomen and back.

Don't be hard on yourself. Because of the link between PID and sexually transmitted diseases, women often feel guilty, embarrassed, or ashamed. Put the feelings behind you. It's fine to

THREE THINGS I TELL EVERY FEMALE PATIENT

SAM JACOBS, M.D., a reproductive endocrinologist and associate professor of obstetrics and gynecology at Robert Wood Johnson Medical School in Camden, New Jersey, gives the following advice for preventing pelvic inflammatory disease (PID). Women who get PID once have a 15 percent risk of infertility; two infections, 30 percent; and a woman who gets PID a third time has a 50 percent risk.

1 USE PROTECTION. If you and your sexual partner aren't mutually monogamous, or if you haven't both been tested for sexually transmitted diseases, use condoms, even if you're on another form of birth control, says Dr. Jacobs.

2 INTRAUTERINE CONTRACEPTIVES AREN'T FOR EVERYONE. "Although intrauterine contraceptives are an excellent form of birth control, they're not appropriate for women with a history of multiple partners, STDs, or pelvic inflammatory disease," says Dr. Jacobs.

3 DON'T DOUCHE. It pushes bacteria up into the reproductive tract, which can increase the risk for PID, says Dr. Jacobs. ∎

acknowledge that you may have made some mistakes, but it's more important to look forward to the future.

"Stress, anxiety, and negative thoughts will only make the amount of pain and dysfunction worse," says Emmett Miller, M.D., medical director of the Center for Healing and Wellness in Los Altos, California, and author of *Deep Healing: The Essence of Mind/Body Medicine.* "Tell yourself, 'Okay, I got it, and I'm going to take

steps to prevent getting it again.' After that, let it go," he advises.

Alternative Therapies

 Use live-culture supplements. Antibiotics kill beneficial bacteria in the body along with the bad. To replenish "good" bacteria, take probiotic supplements, which contain live cultures of *acidophilus* and *bifidus.* Probiotics improve digestion, assist the immune system, and help prevent yeast infections in women who are taking antibiotics, says Toni Bark, M.D., director of the department of integrative medicine at Good Shepherd Hospital in Barrington, Illinois, and medical director of the Center for the Healing Arts in Glencoe, Illinois.

Dr. Bark advises taking 1 teaspoon of probiotic powder three times daily for as long as you're taking antibiotics. Continue taking the probiotic for an additional 3 weeks.

Look for probiotics that are kept in the refrigerated section of health food stores, she adds. They contain the highest concentration of beneficial bacteria.

Savor spicy stir-fries. The spices ginger, turmeric, and cayenne contain chemical compounds that reduce inflammation, pain, and congestion in the abdomen. Garlic is also helpful because it has powerful antibacterial effects, says Dr. Bark.

Put your mind to work. Some studies have shown that guided imagery, or visualization exercises, in which you form clear mental images of

when to see a doctor

If you have a foul-smelling vaginal discharge, along with a dull ache in the lower abdomen or back, or fever and chills accompanying either of the above, see your doctor **right away.** These are early signs of PID, says Sam Jacobs, M.D., a reproductive endocrinologist and associate professor of obstetrics and gynecology at Robert Wood Johnson Medical School in Camden, New Jersey.

If you develop symptoms after having unprotected sex: You could have chlamydia, gonorrhea, or another sexually transmitted disease, which can increase your risk for PID.

If you have flulike symptoms or a heavy vaginal discharge or bleeding, along with pelvic pain, go to the emergency room. If you have PID, the infection may have reached a serious stage. It's not uncommon for PID to be misdiagnosed as endometriosis, so you may want to ask the doctor about getting your white blood cell count checked and having a pelvic ultrasound, advises Dr. Jacobs; these tests will help differentiate between the two conditions.

the healing powers of your body, can increase immunoglobulins and possibly help infections heal more quickly.

Here's how it works. Twice a day, find a quiet place and relax by taking slow, deep breaths, says Dr. Miller. Create a mental image of your reproductive organs, but with a slight blur over them; the blur represents the infection. Form a picture in your mind of thousands of white blood cells pouring into your organs. As they work, they'll flush out inflammation and clear away the blur, revealing healthy tissue underneath.

Medical Options

Rx **Get prescribed antibiotics immediately.** If you're treated for an STD early enough, a single course of oral antibiotics will cure it for good. PID requires long-term therapy with multiple antibiotics, says Dr. Jacobs.

Finish the prescription. Often a woman with PID who takes antibiotics starts feeling better within 2 days. But the antibiotics aren't done working. You'll need to finish the full prescription—1 to 2 weeks' worth—to eliminate all the bacteria from your body. Women who quit antibiotics too soon may see the infection come right back, says Dr. Jacobs.

Stay in touch with your doctor. You'll want to make an appointment for 2 to 3 days after you begin treatment with antibiotics to ensure that the drugs are working. Make another appointment for when the treatment is done. Your doctor will make sure that the infection is gone and that you don't need an additional round of antibiotics, Dr. Jacobs says.

28

Perimenopause

You may notice typical patterns as your body begins the 4- to 10-year transition out of its reproductive phase and into perimenopause—which ends with the permanent liberation from pads, period alerts, and PMS.

Starting in your early forties, expect your periods to gradually become lighter and your cycles to lengthen or shorten. You can also expect to feel more sensitive to hot and cold temperature changes than you did in your twenties and thirties.

"Women often become concerned about their health when they sense that they are nearing menopause. That can be a good thing because it can motivate them to make healthy lifestyle changes. Women often ask me what they should take for menopause," says Margery Gass, M.D., professor of obstetrics and gynecology and director of the University Hospital Menopause and Osteoporosis Center at the University of Cincinnati College of Medicine. "The good news is that they don't necessarily have to take anything to be healthy—that the transition to menopause is a perfectly natural process. The most important thing is a healthy lifestyle: nutritious food, normal weight, adequate calcium and vitamin D, exercise, and no smoking."

Coping with Change

If your hormone shifts are causing discomfort, remind yourself that perimenopause doesn't last forever. For example, you may experience premenstrual symptoms—such as irritability or monthly bloating—for the first time in your life, but the symptoms will disappear as your hormonal fluctuations settle down, Dr. Gass says. Even hot flashes, if you get them at all, might occur only for a month or two. More typically, they come and go for 2 to 3 years.

Other changes, such as a thinning, less moist vaginal lining, are permanent, but may or may not cause any complications, such as uncomfortable sex or more frequent infections.

If you've fallen behind on healthy habits, your first step to avoiding difficulties is to get back on track by eating well, exercising regularly, and practicing sensible self-care. It's a good idea to cut back on caffeine and alcohol during perimenopause. That's because during this time women often become more sensitive to stimulants, which can disrupt sleep cycles or mood. Additionally, caffeine and alcohol relax the capillaries and promote hot flashes.

How or when to take further action depends entirely on how severely you experience certain changes and to what extent these changes affect your overall quality of life.

MANAGING MENSTRUAL DIFFICULTIES

When you approach perimenopause, you are coming to the end of a lifetime supply of approximately 400,000 eggs. You won't ovulate as regularly as you used to. Although your ovaries are working their way out of the estrogen production business, estrogen sometimes peaks rather than plummets during the transition—sometimes as high as pregnancy levels. Then there's progesterone, which comes and goes according to whether you ovulate. Normal hormone shifts are enough to stimulate premenstrual discomfort, but the dramatic fluctuations that occur during perimenopause explain why some women experience menstrual or premenstrual discomfort for the first time in their lives—and why women who have always had PMS have it more severely.

Menstrual irregularities are also common. Even if your periods were always regular, you may find that they're coming more often, sometimes even twice a month, and then disappearing altogether for a few months. Many women experience unusually heavy menstrual flows as well. To manage menstrual difficulties, here are some strategies you may want to try.

Medical Options

Rx Look into short-term hormone replacement therapy (HRT). Deciding whether or not to take hormones long term is a serious decision, and you must consider all the pros and cons. But in the meantime, your doctor may advise you to undergo HRT on a trial basis. It will quickly ease hormone-related changes while you decide whether or not to continue the therapy once you reach menopause, says Mary Jane Minkin, M.D., clinical professor of obstetrics and gynecology at Yale University School of Medicine.

Supplemental estrogen and progestin provide immediate relief from symptoms such as menstrual difficulties, hot flashes, insomnia, vaginal dryness, or urinary frequency, says Dr. Minkin. "Plus, when you are just taking hormones short term, you don't need to be as concerned about increasing your risk for breast cancer."

Consider birth control pills. Oral contraceptives aren't for everyone. They contain higher amounts of hormones than those used in HRT, which means even greater concerns about stroke, heart attack, and estrogen-sensitive cancers. But as long as you don't smoke or have a history of blood clotting, birth control pills are a reasonable way to resolve menstrual irregularities.

Of course, birth control pills also offer solid protection against a pregnancy that might prove particularly difficult at this stage in life.

Start with progesterone alone. Although the root of irregular cycles at menopause is often hormonal, you don't necessarily have to undergo full-fledged HRT for just this one issue. A small dose of premenstrual progesterone 10 to 12 days before your period might be enough to regulate your cycle and prevent heavy periods due to inconsistent ovulation, says Dr. Gass.

In addition, progesterone can protect your endometrium, the lining of the uterus, from being overstimulated by estrogen, which is a real concern when ovulation is hit-or-miss. Your doctor can prescribe a progesterone tablet or a topical cream. Or you can try an over-the-counter progesterone cream (the type labeled "USP"), available in health food stores. If you choose this option, follow the directions carefully—it is a hormone, after all. Keep your doctor informed of what you are doing. One drawback of using progesterone cream is that there are few studies to indicate proper doses or how many days per month the cream should be used. Wild yam cream has no benefit, Dr. Gass adds, because your body cannot convert the cream to progesterone.

Ask your doctor if hormone treatment is causing bleeding. Healthy women who don't smoke may take oral contraceptives for cycle control and get the added benefits of contraception and treatment of hot flashes. Women can use oral contraceptives or HRT if they are having hot flashes along with their irregular bleeding. But a side effect may be even more erratic periods.

Your doctor may advise you to take a "cyclic dose" of hormones—rather than a "continuous" dose—to allow a more "scheduled" time for bleeding. "HRT is a much lower dose of hormones than oral contraceptives. Sometimes HRT is just not strong enough to control a woman's irregular cycles in perimenopause," says Dr. Gass. Once you are a couple of years beyond menopause, you may decide to switch to "continuous dose" hormones, which shut down the cyclic bleeding completely.

Alternative Therapies

Try black cohosh. An herb, black cohosh appears to interact with the pituitary gland and reduce the production of luteinizing hormone—the hormone that often triggers the aggravating symptoms of menopause. Women who take black cohosh often maintain stabler levels of hormones, which keeps the menstrual cycle on track. There also may be a reduction in menstrual pain.

In a study of 80 menopausal women, researchers found that black cohosh was as effective as HRT at lessening the severity of hot flashes, memory loss, depression, and mood swings, as well as improving the thickness of vaginal tissues. Black cohosh is used instead of—not with—conventional HRT. The recommended dose is usually 20 drops of 1:1 tincture three times daily, for no more than 6 months. (For more information on black cohosh, see the chart on page 66.)

Try this sexy herb. The herb vitex, also known as chasteberry, is well-recognized for regulating levels of progesterone and prolactin. The progesterone boost can smooth out your periods, whether they're infrequent, abnormally long, abnormally short, or unusually heavy or light. The prolactin boost from vitex reduces bloating, improves sex drive, and increases vaginal tone.

The recommended dose of vitex is 60 drops of 1:5 tincture twice daily, or tablets containing 250 milligrams of 4:1 extract twice daily. If you are taking birth control pills, be aware that vitex may counteract their effectiveness. When using vitex, be patient: It often takes several months to bestow the full effects.

OUTSMART HOT FLASHES

When the ovaries are changing over to their less active status at the time of perimenopause, more than 70 percent of women experience what are technically known as "vasomotor symptoms"— nervous system reactions by the part of your brain that regulates body temperature.

A full-out hot flash is unmistakable. Following a feeling of pressure in the head, your pulse quickens, and the skin on your chest, neck, and head feels warm and sweaty as blood rushes to the surface. After approximately 4 minutes, the flushed feeling dissipates, and you feel cold and clammy.

For some women, it feels as if their heart is racing, or they experience vertigo, weakness, or shortness of breath. For others still, the feeling is more a sensitivity to heat than actual sweaty incidents.

Every woman has individual triggers that provoke hot flashes. As you get more experience, you may find yourself recruiting a family member to take things out of the oven or using only the low setting on the hair dryer. Even so, steadying your hormone levels is the only established method to actually treat hot flashes, and even then you may have some symptoms, says Dr. Minkin.

Fortunately, there are plenty of time-tested methods to reduce the discomfort.

Home Remedies

Reduce the heat in your diet. Don't order hot buffalo wings unless you're willing to suffer the consequences. The spices used in Cajun, Mexican, and Eastern cuisines can trigger hot flashes. In the kitchen, you may want

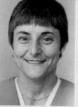

to cut back on salsa, curry concoctions, hot-pepper sauce, and black pepper.

Breathe away heat. Several studies have shown that women who practice a relaxing breathing technique can reduce hot flashes. While sitting in a comfortable chair, close your eyes and relax your muscles as much as possible. Slowly inhale and exhale until you can slow your breathing down to as little as seven or eight breaths a minute. Work to increase the depth of your belly breathing and decrease the depth of your chest breathing. If you practice this technique daily for 10 to 20 minutes, you may find that you're having fewer hot flashes than you did before.

Dress to keep cool. When you're venturing out for the day, think "layers." If you find yourself getting hot, you can start peeling off layers one at a time. "Lots of perimenopausal women find that they are no longer comfortable in turtle-necks and clothes that hug the body," Dr. Gass adds. You may be more comfortable wearing breathable, loose fabrics, such as linen and cotton.

Treat your feet. Research confirms that if you keep your feet cool, you'll have fewer night sweats. Don't wear socks at night. If you do get a hot flash, put your feet in a cold basin of water—it will help cool your entire body.

Nutritional Treatments

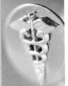 **Take sweat-stopping nutrients.** Research suggests that combining vitamin C and bioflavonoid supplements may strengthen and stabilize capillaries and other small blood vessels, which can prevent hot flashes from occurring. You can find supplements that combine vitamin C with bioflavonoids at most health food stores. Look for a supplement that combines 500 to 1,000 milligrams of vitamin C with 200 to 500 milligrams of bioflavonoids per capsule.

Try vitamin E. Many women report that taking 400 IU of vitamin E daily helps prevent hot flashes. It doesn't work right away, however. You may have to take vitamin E for at least 6 weeks before noticing any effects.

when to see a doctor

If you have abnormally heavy bleeding or spotting between periods, make an appointment to see your doctor. These symptoms are often normal at the time of perimenopause, but they can also be caused by endometriosis, fibroids, or even cancer.

If you experience hot flashes, vaginal dryness, or other perimenopausal symptoms prior to age 40: About one in 100 women between the ages of 15 and 40 will experience premature ovarian failure, also known as "early menopause." You may need medical treatment to protect your bones and maintain fertility.

Alternative Therapies

Try essential oils. In addition to smelling great, essential oils such as rose, geranium, and peppermint have cooling properties, says Jane Buckle, Ph.D., an instructor in the holistic nursing program at the College of New Rochelle in New York and author of *Clinical*

Aromatherapy in Nursing. Put 6 to 8 drops of an essential oil in a water-filled 4-ounce spray bottle. Keep the bottle by the bedside or in your purse, and spray it on your neck, chest, and shoulders when you feel a sweat coming on.

Medical Options

 Add testosterone to HRT. If you are already taking estrogen, your doctor may advise you to combine it with testosterone to reduce hot flashes. A prescription medication called Estratest combines estrogen and testosterone.

Ask your doctor about other medications. Estrogen is the best approach for hot flashes, but some women can't take estrogen for medical reasons. A number of other medications may be helpful, says Dr. Gass. A low-dose progesterone called Bellergal-S, for example, acts on the part of the central nervous system that controls body temperature. Some women get relief from clonidine (Catapres Transdermal), a patch worn to control high blood pressure.

Yet another approach is to take antidepressants. Studies have shown that paroxetine (Paxil), fluoxetine (Prozac), and venlafaxine (Effexor) may reduce the severity as well as the duration of hot flashes.

OVERCOMING VAGINAL AND SEXUAL PROBLEMS

Just as your reproductive organs have a developmental stage at puberty, they also go through changes as you exit your childbearing phase. Your uterus, cervix, and urinary tract slightly decrease in size, and the skin lining your reproductive organs begins to thin.

Declines in estrogen affect the amount of bloodflow to the pelvic area, as well as mucus production in the vagina. It's not uncommon for perimenopausal women to need lubrication, often for the first time, during sex. They also tend to get more vaginal or urinary tract infections.

None of this, however, means that you're going to enjoy sex less over the years. In fact menopause and beyond often bring the best lovemaking because couples grow in intimacy and confidence, says Dr. Minkin.

If you find that sex is compromised—either due to discomfort from physical changes or due to a lower libido—hormone therapy is one of the most powerful remedies. Here are some additional ways to deal with the changes.

Home Remedies

Switch to showers. Taking long baths removes lubricating oils from the skin. Quick showers, on the other hand, will help keep your skin soft and supple.

Use a water-soluble moisturizer. The most effective products you can buy for long-term management of vaginal dryness are labeled as vaginal moisturizers. They act directly on the tissue to make it less dry. Plus, they maintain a healthful acid balance in the vagina, which can help prevent infections. Some examples are Replens and K-Y Long Lasting Vaginal Moisturizer.

Use commercial lubricants. Vaginal lubricants such as Astroglide, Lubrin, and Moist Again

WHEN BAD THINGS HAPPEN TO HEALTHY WOMEN

Yoga Helped Ease the Effect of Perimenopause on Her Breathing Problems

During Corrine Goodman's first career as an overworked hairdresser, she sought out a yoga class to help her deal with job-related stress. Renewed, she went on to start her own cosmetics company.

When she was diagnosed with emphysema in 1989, she again tapped into yoga techniques to manage the life-threatening condition.

By the time perimenopause hit, Goodman, who lives in Cleveland, was working for the American Yoga Association. This time she had even more resources—everything from yoga postures and breathing exercises to meditation—to help her cope with the changes. Even so, she says, perimenopause hit hard.

In addition to the discomfort of hot flashes, she felt her personality start to change. "I was irritable, jumpy, and at times a raving maniac. I never had PMS before, but I guessed that was what a really bad case felt like," she says. To make things worse, her doctor noticed that she was starting to experience bone loss.

"Holding certain postures and slowing down through breath work helped me tremendously to transition into menopause, as it helped me through all the other challenges in my life," she says. To deal with hot flashes, she turned to ancient yoga techniques. She also made it a point to emphasize weight-bearing yoga positions in order to stimulate bone growth.

Goodman connected with other women, many of whom were going through the same changes, in her yoga classes. Along with Alice Christensen, founder of the American Yoga Association, she devised meditations targeted specifically for midlife changes. "We visualized who we were and what we would like to see ourselves doing as mature women," she says. "We talked a lot about self-esteem and about giving ourselves permission to be spontaneous."

After years of being director of curriculum and instruction for the American Yoga Association, Goodman got the chance to truly practice the lessons. She was asked to teach a class herself. At age 62, she found herself leading students one-third her age in the Hatha yoga tradition that has guided her life.

"During the first class, I was amazed at my endurance and strength," she says. "I have to say that I'm stronger now than I've ever been in my life, both physically and mentally." ■

will help prepare mucous membranes for intercourse. Apply the lubricant to your vaginal opening and to your partner's penis. Avoid lotions and oils that aren't marketed specifically for genital health, such as petroleum jelly or cocoa butter. They can actually increase friction and promote infection.

Revive your relationship. It's not uncommon for women to blame their hormones for a decline in libido, when what's really happening is a problem in the relationship, says Dr. Minkin. If the sex itself is a problem, you need to really talk about what will make you more comfortable or aroused. If you're growing apart emotionally, make an effort to invest more time with your partner in order to recapture the fun and intimacy that you shared earlier in the relationship.

Medical Options

Change contraceptives. If you are already using oral contraceptives at perimenopause, your remedy for a flatlined libido may be as simple switching to a different progestin formula, says Dr. Minkin. Certain progestins have "androgenic" effects that boost sex drive; others can depress libido.

Ask your doctor about products that contain androgenic progestins, such as levonorgestrel (Mirena), norethindrone (Aygestin), or ethynodiol (Demulen). Nonandrogenic formulations have norgestimate (Ortho-Cyclen) or desogestrel (Apri) as the key ingredient, Dr. Minkin says.

Consider topical estrogen. Applying estrogen cream, available by prescription, to the vaginal area will help improve tone and comfort. Some products are inserted outside of the vagina; others are designed to treat vaginal dryness and sensitivity—they come in the form of a ring, which is inserted in front of the cervix.

FEEL VITAL AGAIN

Some women have no specific physical complaints during the time of perimenopause but may feel a general plummet in their energy or mood.

"Women at midlife tend to have a lot of irons in the fire," says Dr. Gass. "They're caring for aging parents or taking care of children and grandchildren. I advise women to take a step back and try to see how much stress they're experiencing."

A minority of women may experience depression or anxiety due to hormone shifts, but it's more likely that multiple perimenopausal changes are having a snowball effect on your overall quality of life. Hot flashes, night sweats, and menstrual discomfort, for example, can start a pattern of poor sleeping habits, which in turn can lead to malaise and moodiness, especially if you're too tired to keep up with regular exercise and other healthful lifestyle behaviors.

Before your mood or overall sense of vitality starts going downhill, it's essential to tackle individual symptoms at soon as they appear, says Sadja Greenwood, M.D., assistant clinical professor of obstetrics and gynecology at the University of California, San Francisco.

Home Remedies

Maintain a regular sleep schedule. If night sweats or other perimenopausal complaints are keeping you up at night, you may experience disruptions in your natural sleep cycle. You may find yourself trying to compensate by snoozing late on weekends—but that can make it even harder to get back on track. It's important to go to bed and wake up at the same times every day. Maintaining a regular sleep/wake cycle helps minimize hormonal fluctuations, and you'll also feel more rested overall.

It's fine to enjoy a quick nap in the afternoon, but sleeping more than 15 minutes may make it harder to get to sleep at your usual time. If you find that your sleep cycles have been disrupted, you may have to make a few changes. For example, dim the lights after sundown, says Dr. Greenwood. It will help give your body the signal that it's time to unwind and begin preparing for sleep.

Make sure you're getting enough iron. Symptoms of iron deficiency include weakness, fatigue, and low energy. Women who don't eat meat, or those who are experiencing heavy menstrual bleeding, are prime candidates for iron deficiency anemia. Prevent this energy-draining situation by making sure that your daily supplement contains 100 percent of the Daily Value of 18 milligrams of iron.

In addition, ask your doctor to test your iron levels. If you're bleeding heavily each month, your doctor may recommend that you get even more iron than the recommended daily amount. You don't want to take extra iron unnecessarily, however. Excessive iron can cause just as many problems as too little.

Keep a worry book. Every day, take a few moments to write down frustrations and concerns that may be keeping you from getting all the rest you need. Just jotting them down may relieve some of the emotional pressure. So will outlining possible solutions—such as "get organized tomorrow."

Take a progesterone supplement. The body's production of progesterone declines as a woman approaches perimenopause. This can be a problem because progesterone has a calming effect. When levels decline, women may experience irritability or insomnia. In fact, natural forms of progesterone were used as sedatives in the 1930s.

Unfortunately, the synthetic progestins in HRT and contraceptives might have the opposite effect and trigger anxiety and mood swings. One solution is to take a natural progesterone supplement, available in health food stores and pharmacies. Follow the instructions carefully and make sure that you purchase a product that contains pharmaceutical-grade progesterone—look for "progesterone USP" on the label. Your doctor can also prescribe a natural progesterone-containing gel called Crinone.

Medical Options

Rx **Have your thyroid tested.** Low levels of thyroid hormones can drain your energy and lead to depression, while an overactive thyroid can produce feelings of anxiety and panic. Make sure that you are getting your thyroid levels screened every year.

Since thyroid hormones and estrogen affect one another, it's likely that you'll need to have your thyroid medication adjusted at perimenopause, especially if you're undergoing HRT, says Steven Petak, M.D., associate professor at the Texas Institute for Reproductive Medicine and Endocrinology in Houston and clinical assistant professor at the University of Texas–Houston Medical School.

29

Menopause

We think of estrogen as affecting mainly the ovaries and uterus. But our bodies are really soaked in this reproductive hormone.

Blood vessels throughout the body contain estrogen receptors, molecular docking sites that allow estrogen to be delivered to the various tissues. Estrogen helps regulate cholesterol levels, blood pressure, even the metabolism of certain nutrients. Estrogen and other sex hormones play a role in the part of brain chemistry responsible for cognitive function, the sleep/wake cycle, and moods. And estrogen—or the lack of it—determines whether bones are strong or weak.

At menopause, reproductive hormone levels plummet. We have less than half of the estrogen that we had in our reproductive years, and the progesterone that once was released from the ovaries is nearly phased out. How can a woman survive without estrogen and progesterone when nearly every tissue and organ in the body is affected by reproductive hormones?

Actually, women do just fine. Even those who undergo hormone replacement therapy (HRT) are not actually replacing all of their sex hormones. They're only supplementing a small fraction of what used to circulate in their premenopausal bodies.

Menopause is a natural transition in a woman's life, says Margery Gass, M.D., professor of obstetrics and gynecology and director of the University Hospital Menopause and Osteoporosis Center at the University of Cincinnati College of Medicine. The reason the ovaries stop putting out massive quantities of estrogen and progesterone is that the hormones are no longer needed for reproductive functions. After all, progesterone's main purpose is to service the uterus—either to stimulate a monthly period or to nurture a growing baby. If there aren't any more eggs, it's logical for progesterone levels to diminish.

After menopause, estrogen and other sex hormones continue to affect parts of the body that aren't involved with reproduction. That's why the ovaries and adrenal glands continue to produce maintenance levels of sex hormones—between 10 and 50 percent of the amounts that were produced in the reproductive years.

If the body needs additional estrogen, it can produce extra amounts by recycling other hormones. Fat cells produce "backup" estrogen as well.

Of course, if illness or surgery has disabled your ovaries or adrenal glands, you will need to take supplemental hormones to maintain bone mass, healthful cholesterol levels, and the like. For everyone else, it is a personal decision if you want to give your hormones a little help.

The decision to take supplemental hormones isn't a small one. Nor are the various questions surrounding the use of HRT easy to sort out. In the following pages, we'll take a look at the issues involved with hormone management. And since more than just hormonal changes occur at menopause, we'll guide you in maximizing your personal fulfillment and all-around wellness.

Making the Mental Shift

There are good reasons that the body is programmed to reduce the production of hormones at the end of ovulation. In anthropological terms, menopause is of profound value to society, says Sadja Greenwood, M.D., assistant clinical professor of obstetrics and gynecology at University of California, San Francisco.

In primitive cultures, such as the Hadza tribe of Northern Tanzania, postmenopausal women bring in 70 to 80 percent of the food for the tribe while their daughters are busy nursing babies and rearing children. "Even women in their sixties and seventies are doing hard labor, digging up tubers and carrying water for miles," Dr. Greenwood says.

Similarly, American women are busier than ever at menopause. Apart from grandmothering their children's children, they're often caring for older parents. This is also a time when careers and creativity are often are at their peaks.

"One of the reasons that women make such valuable contributions to society after menopause is that they develop a sense that there's more to life than the daily grind," says Dr. Greenwood. "They want to connect with nature and other people in a more profound way than ever."

Here are a few ways to make the most of this exciting time.

Rise above ego. Statistically, many middle-age men are interested in dating 20- and 30-something women. Some women find that they become invisible to men around the time of menopause, says Dr. Greenwood.

This is no reflection of your own attractiveness or value. Instead of working harder to look younger, allow your self-worth to flow from within. You will find yourself needing less validation from others, and you'll be more satisfied on a spiritual level when you pay attention to your heart's longings and inner guidance. Join the trend of women going back to college at midlife, start the business that you always talked about, or discover an entirely new personal passion, Dr. Greenwood advises.

Strengthen and renew female bonds. Girlfriends make every rite of passage more meaningful. When physical or emotional difficulties arrive, women have a special way of forming a circle of safety and love. If you catch yourself deprived of quality girlfriend time, you're never too old to organize a slumber party, or sign up for a women's retreat where you stay up late putting on skits, singing, drumming, and telling stories of your life.

Volunteer. You don't need grandkids to experience the life-affirming gift of sharing decades' worth of wisdom and talents. Not only does volunteering make life meaningful, but research shows that people who have a lot of human connections live twice as long as those who don't. Whether you're interested in comforting shelter animals, reading to second graders, or offering history tours of your town, you'll find plenty of volunteer opportunities. Check your local newspaper. Or contact the Volunteers of America, headquartered in Washington, D.C., at (800) 899-0089. The Web site is www.voa.org.

Focus on good posture. Due to the natural loss of muscle tone that happens with age, your abdomen *will* protrude more than it did in younger years, even if you exercise diligently, says Dr. Gass. Hormone shifts and a downshifting of metabolism also encourage fat storage.

Yes, you need to watch how much you eat, and regular exercise is important, but you also need to accept that your figure is designed to change with age. In fact, some postmenopausal women find it life affirming to decorate their homes with artwork that reflects the human figure in all shapes and sizes.

Whatever figure you have, good posture will make you look and feel more youthful. Make an effort to keep your head level, pull your shoulders back, and walk tall. Rounded shoulders and a stooped back call attention to stomach imperfections and steal vitality.

Rethink Your Hormone Status Annually

If you were taking oral contraceptives during perimenopause to manage premenstrual discomfort or erratic menstrual bleeding, once you hit menopause the birth control pill is no longer necessary to shut off your system. Rather than oral contraceptives, you may wish to switch to lower doses of hormones in HRT. It will prevent problems that don't go away after menopause, such as vaginal dryness.

Whether you have any bothersome symptoms or not, menopause is a call for every woman to evaluate her hormone management plan, says Steven Petak, M.D., associate professor at the Texas Institute for Reproductive Medicine and Endocrinology in Houston and clinical assistant professor at the University of Texas–Houston Medical School.

"When your doctor first confirms that you are menopausal—and every annual period-free anniversary after that—you're going to want to decide if hormones help you meet your current health goals, especially the key areas like bone density and heart protection," he says.

About a third of menopausal women choose HRT as an integral part of their long-term health goals. Another third decide that HRT is not nec-

when to see a doctor

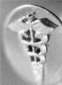

If you've started HRT and are experiencing breast pain, nausea, bloating, or other side effects, call your doctor right away. Lowering the dose or switching to a different hormone may be all that's needed to resolve the problem.

If you're having breakthrough bleeding: It's common when women start HRT that combines estrogen and progesterone—but it can also be caused by endometriosis or uterine cancer. You'll need a comprehensive exam by your doctor to make sure that you're healthy.

essary and conflicts with their health goals. The remaining third haven't really thought about supplement hormones and forgo treatment with HRT, says Dr. Gass.

If you aren't taking HRT, you may want to reconsider. Compelling research suggests that postmenopausal women who take HRT live longer than those who don't, says Dr. Petak. It's not clear, however, if the hormones themselves are improving long-term health or if women who choose HRT tend to be more proactive about taking care of their health generally.

"Whatever you choose to do in the area of hormone management, be as informed as possible, and be specific about your needs. If you do that, you and your doctor are more likely to make the best decision for you," says Dr. Gass.

The following steps are essential for making educated decisions about managing your hormones.

Review your current health status with your doctor. You have to determine your most pressing long-term health concerns. You can then match your goals with the current data on what hormones offer. In order to be specific, you'll need to complete the following:

- A complete physical
- Personal and family health history, particularly concerning cancer and cardiovascular disease
- Baseline bone mineral density scan
- Complete lipid profile—total cholesterol, HDL (high-density lipoprotein), LDL (low-density lipoprotein), and triglycerides
- Pap test
- Mammogram
- Test for thyroid-stimulating hormone (TSH)

Rule out risks. The next specific question to ask is whether hormones are any kind of a threat, either because of a family history of certain illnesses or because of red flags in your current health reports. You need to abstain from taking HRT, or be closely monitored, if you have the following conditions.

Hormone Replacement Strategies

If you are considering hormone replacement therapy (HRT), keep in mind that it can take some trial and error to find the regimen that works best for you.

Brian W. Walsh, M.D., director of the Menopause Clinic at Brigham and Women's Hospital in Boston and assistant professor of obstetrics and gynecology at Harvard Medical School, offers the following advice.

Give it a short-term trial. Even though HRT is meant to be taken long term, there's nothing wrong with trying it for about 3 months to see if side effects will be an issue, says Dr. Walsh. In addition, if new health information changes your thinking about HRT, you can stop at any time.

If you quit, quit gradually. Women who abruptly discontinue HRT may be faced with hot flashes, excessive menstrual bleeding, vaginal dryness, or difficulties sleeping. If you decide to phase out HRT, work with your doctor to reduce the dosage gradually. ■

- Breast and endometrial cancers, gallbladder disease, or other illnesses commonly triggered or aggravated by estrogen

- A blood-clotting disorder

- Bleeding from the uterus that hasn't been evaluated

- Hypertension

- Migraine and other headaches that are aggravated by hormones

- Smoking

Compare forms and dosages. When researching the pros and cons of taking hormones, keep in mind that generalizations about the effects of estrogen and progesterone are often meaningless. Every formulation of hormones has different effects; how the hormones are taken makes a difference; and the dosage can have a significant impact. (To compare the subtle differences among hormone formulations, see the chart on page 295.)

"If you are leaning toward taking HRT, then it's necessary to be flexible and adopt the spirit of experimentation while you sample different forms and see what affects you best," says Dr. Petak.

For example, "natural hormones"—those designed to more closely approximate the body's own chemistry—are reportedly less symptomatic in terms of mood changes, menstrual discomfort, and headaches than the more synthetic brands and formulations that most doctors use. (Don't be confused by the terms "natural" and "synthetic": Both types are created in laboratories.)

Doctors don't always recommend natural hormones, also known as custom formulations, because they haven't been as well-studied as other products and they tend to cost more. For some women, however, they're the only way to go. Other women actually fare better on synthetic versions—perhaps because the dosages and formulations may be more consistent than the natural formulations.

Weigh the Pros and Cons

Taking hormones isn't a guaranteed insurance package for your health. Whether or not you should take hormones, and the types of hormones that you take, will always be an educated guess on the part of you and your doctor. But the more educated you are, the less guessing you'll have to do. Hormone management requires well-rounded, careful research. The following review takes an in-depth look at what we currently know about what hormones can and cannot offer.

HORMONES AND CANCER RISKS

Excessive stimulation of an organ by hormones can result in tumor formation, and estrogen is particularly active in breast tissue and the uterus.

In fact, estrogen stimulates the lining of the uterus to grow so actively that it can increase the risk of endometrial cancer threefold. However, if you take progesterone along with estrogen, you don't have this to worry about. By helping the uterine lining to thin out, progesterone actually has the opposite effect.

The risk of colon cancer is reduced when you take HRT. Research shows that taking estrogen lowers your risk by as much as 40 percent.

On the other hand, the risk of breast cancer is a very real concern. A large-scale study monitored women's breast cancer rates over a 10-year period. Women who stayed on HRT the whole time had almost double the rate of breast cancer as those who stayed on HRT for a shorter time.

In an analysis of more than 50 medical studies, the risk of breast cancer increased by 2.3 percent each year in women using HRT. This review is one of several that have led experts to make the general conclusion that estrogen causes a "moderate" increase in breast cancer risk—essentially changing the risk from 10 women out of 10,000 per year to 13 women out of 10,000 per year.

Another landmark study from the Women's Health Initiative was abruptly halted when its results revealed breast cancer risk to be higher than previously estimated—for every 10,000 women, there were 8 more cases of breast cancer among those on HRT than among those who took placebos.

Each study is worth considering, but experts try to base recommendations on the pool of data as a whole. To put the risk in perspective, remember that the majority of women who get breast cancer are not taking hormones. Not taking estrogen is no assurance that you aren't going to get cancer, says Dr. Petak. Breast cancer has genetic causes and all sorts of other triggers besides estrogen.

The kind of breast cancer that is associated with HRT tends to be the most treatable kind, Dr. Petak adds. In addition, research shows a correlation between the length of time on HRT and breast cancer risk. You have some control over your risk by limiting the number of years that you take HRT.

"You'll see all kinds of numbers, but we have enough to go on for general recommendations," says Dr. Petak. To balance your hormones and also protect against breast cancer, here's what doctors advise.

Limit HRT. The "moderate" risk for breast cancer that appeared in the studies didn't clearly show up until women had been taking hormone replacement therapy for 10 years or longer, says Mary Jane Minkin, M.D., clinical professor of obstetrics and gynecology at Yale University School of Medicine. If you want the benefits of HRT, such as strengthening bones, but want to minimize your risk for breast cancer, giving yourself a limited time on HRT is a reasonable compromise.

Don't focus only on breast cancer. While long-term HRT increases the risk for breast cancer, it can reduce the risk for other serious conditions.

When you're considering whether or not to take HRT, it may be helpful to list all of the benefits—such as bone protection, fewer hot flashes, better sexual health, and possibly the prevention of colon cancer and Alzheimer's disease—on one side of a sheet of paper. On the other side, list the potential risks. If a moderately increased risk of breast cancer is the only downside, you may decide that the potential benefits of HRT make it worth doing.

Look deeper into family history. It's true that if you have the genetic mutation for breast cancer, your risk for getting the disease rises 50 percent, even without taking estrogen. But don't assume that your risk for cancer is unusually high just because your female relatives got it. What really matters is when they were diagnosed, says Dr. Minkin.

Women who develop breast cancer before

WHEN BAD THINGS HAPPEN TO HEALTHY WOMEN

Breast Cancer at Menopause Sent Her Back to Church and School

Eileen Moore-Simmons got breast cancer and menopause as a package deal. At the age of 42, she began to experience painful, irregular menstrual cycles. At about the same time, she discovered a lump in her breast.

Her doctors explained that there was no connection between the cancer and painful periods. But the chemotherapy that followed accelerated the perimenopause stage, and she soon stopped getting periods for good.

Because of the cancer, Moore-Simmons, of Philadelphia, was not eligible for hormone replacement therapy (HRT). She opted for topical estrogen cream to help maintain her vaginal tone. A three-pack-a-day smoker, she also gave up the habit for good. But her life was just beginning to change.

"Between cancer and the reminder that I was entering midlife, I became acutely aware of my own mortality," she says. "I thought to myself that I had lived for 40 years and hadn't fulfilled too many of my dreams."

After not having entered a church for 20 years, she found herself one day at a worship service around the corner from her house. "I

was moved, and I came back for more," she says. "My faith grew, and I developed a closeness with God that I had never felt before."

When the minister asked her to help with Sunday school, she realized that one of her lifelong ambitions had been to teach. She got her high school GED, then enrolled at community college. She got straight A's, which earned her admission to Philadelphia's Temple University.

In addition to education courses, Moore-Simmons took classes in acting and writing. She and her daughter took turns buying seasonal passes to the theater, ballet, and opera.

More than 10 years passed. Moore-Simmons, now 53, has a potential teaching job lined up. Her college professors are encouraging her to attend professional acting auditions, and she recently purchased her first house. "I'm so happy I could burst," she says. "I rediscovered my faith. I rediscovered my dreams. I've always been fairly happy, but this midlife 'crisis' has truly proved my philosophy that something good comes out of even the worst situations." ■

menopause are more likely to have a genetic predisposition to the disease, she explains. If the women in your family developed breast cancer at an early age, that might be an argument to forgo HRT.

Reduce progestin. While the progestin component of HRT has a protective effect against cancer of the uterus, recent evidence indicates

that combined estrogen–progestin therapy may raise the possible risk for breast cancer more than taking estrogen alone. To get the uterus-protecting benefits of progestin while preventing the double risk factor of estrogen plus progestin, ask your doctor about taking progestin less frequently, says Dr. Minkin. With "intermittent cyclical dosing," you may be advised to take progestin every other month—or even every 3 months—while taking estrogen daily.

Watch your alcohol intake. In the large Iowa Women's Health Study, researchers noted that the women who took hormones and consumed "substantial" amounts of alcohol had an elevated risk for breast cancer. "Substantial" is defined as 5 grams or more of alcohol daily—equivalent to 2/3 ounce of whiskey or 3 ounces of wine. Whether or not you're on HRT, *Prevention* magazine advises limiting alcohol intake to two to three drinks weekly.

Step up your breast screenings. The slightly elevated breast cancer risk that occurs when taking HRT is an important reason to keep up with monthly breast self-exams, as well as with annual mammography (starting at age 40 with a baseline mammogram) and clinical breast exams (starting at age 20). Keep in mind that HRT sometimes makes the breasts feel lumpier. HRT can also make it difficult to get an accurate mammogram reading; the treatment contributes to a denser concentration of cells in some women's breasts. Be sure that all of your doctors (and mammography technicians) know that you're taking HRT.

HOW HORMONES AFFECT YOUR HEART

Protecting the heart has been a major justification for taking supplemental hormones after menopause. When the National Institutes of Health (NIH) issued its sweeping new cholesterol guidelines last spring, however, one of the most surprising recommendations was that women at risk

for heart disease should take one of the cholesterol-lowering drugs known as statins rather than HRT for heart protection after menopause. Since then, the American Heart Association has issued similar guidelines. And several recent studies support the view that HRT won't help all female hearts.

"It's not that HRT isn't valuable," says Margo A. Denke, M.D., associate professor of internal medicine at the University of Texas Southwestern Medical Center in Dallas and a member of the NIH panel. "It eases menopausal symptoms and can protect bones during and shortly after menopause. But it just doesn't appear to prevent heart disease as well as we had hoped." On the other hand, a significant body of research shows that statin drugs do cut cholesterol and prevent heart attacks.

If you're already taking HRT, should you switch to a statin? Here's how to tell.

- Stick with HRT if you want relief from menopausal symptoms, if your cholesterol is normal, and if you're concerned about bone health.

- Add a statin if you fit the description above but you have high cholesterol that hasn't responded to dietary changes. Adding a statin drug will get your cholesterol under control.

- Switch to a statin if you have high cholesterol, if you're postmenopausal, and if you're taking HRT just for heart protection.

HOW HORMONES AFFECT YOUR BONES

About 25 million Americans suffer from the bone-thinning condition called osteoporosis, and about 80 percent of them are women. It's no coincidence. Estrogen has a tremendous effect on the strength of the skeleton. It helps the intestines absorb calcium, and it helps the kidneys hoard this important mineral. It also stimulates the production of vitamin D, which helps the bones take up calcium.

Estrogen also plays a key role in bone remodeling—the process by which the bones rebuild themselves over time. When estrogen levels decline at menopause, the bones begin to lose density and mass at an accelerated rate. By age 60, women can lose 15 to 30 percent of peak bone mass. This decline starts around age 30 but becomes much more aggressive at menopause. Women can lose 3 to 5 percent of their bone mass annually.

The diet and exercise recommendations in chapter 17 are essential for bone protection. But HRT is one of the most important strategies. In fact, bone protection is the main reason that women 60 years and older take supplemental hormones.

But you may want to begin HRT sooner. British researchers evaluated HRT studies and found that a reduction in bone fractures was found only in women who started HRT before age 60.

If you already have osteoporosis or have a high risk for developing it, your doctor may advise treatments other than hormone replacement therapy. But for most women, HRT may offer valuable benefits for bone protection. Other steps to protect your bones include:

Get the best tests. There are several ways to measure bone mineral density. Those heel or wrist scans provided at local health fairs are a good place to start—but keep in mind that the most serious injuries are hip and spinal fractures. If you're menopausal or have high risk factors for osteoporosis, you'll want to have tests that measure bone density at the hip, spine, and wrist. An x-ray test called DEXA (dual energy x-ray absorptiometry), which can detect bone loss at an early stage, is your best choice.

Combine treatments for additional benefits. If your bones aren't getting stronger with HRT, your doctor may advise combining estrogen with alendronate (Fosamax). The drugs are more effective when used in tandem rather than singly, and the combination is entirely safe, says Dr. Minkin.

Injectable parathyroid hormone, which may be available in 6 months to a year, represents the new wave of therapy for osteoporosis, Dr. Minkin says.

Consider adding testosterone to HRT. Estrogen may not be the only sex hormone that helps protect the bones. Higher levels of testosterone in the body have been linked to higher levels of bone density. One study that compared the use of estradiol (a kind of estrogen) with estradiol plus testosterone found significantly greater increases in bone density in those using the combined therapy.

"We're not certain if the testosterone itself is benefiting the bones, or if testosterone is converting to estrogen," says Dr. Petak. Experts don't recommend adding testosterone to HRT just for bone health. Because long-term safety hasn't been proved, testosterone isn't recommended for routine use. But if you have other health issues, such as depressed libido, the addition of testosterone to HRT may boost testosterone levels to a more normal female range.

Take ipriflavone as a fallback. It's a laboratory-derived version of isoflavones, bone-protecting compounds that are found in soy foods. Ipriflavone can strengthen bones without exerting hormonelike effects on the breasts and uterus.

Some small studies point to ipriflavone's ability to prevent bone breakdown and increase bone density. "The benefit is likely equivalent to taking a very small dose of estrogen," says Bruce Ettinger, M.D., an ipriflavone researcher in Oakland, California.

The recommended dose is 600 milligrams daily, combined with 1,000 milligrams of calcium. It's safe, though you may experience bloating, diarrhea, or stomach irritation. Ipriflavone is available at health food stores and some pharmacies.

Keep up with exercise. In a 5-year study, women who did high-impact, weight-bearing exercise three times weekly gained or maintained bone density while also building muscle and improving balance. Women in the same study who didn't follow the exercise recommendations lost bone density.

For the best bone protection, combine regular exercise with HRT, says Mona Shangold, M.D., director of the Center for Women's Health and Sports Gynecology in Philadelphia. "It has been shown that the combination of resistance exercise and estrogen therapy leads to a greater improvement in bone density than either one alone," she says.

Feeling Good Overall

The potential benefits of HRT are wide-ranging. It may play a role in boosting libido, preventing middle-age weight gain, maintaining memory, and improving overall vitality, says Dr. Gass.

Hormones are hardly a fountain of youth, she adds. While some women experience an extra "glow" when taking supplemental hormones, not everyone does.

So far, HRT has been proven to do only three things: improve hot flashes, relieve vaginal dryness, and improve bone density. While hormones may provide other benefits, women always have to weigh the potential downsides, such as the increased risk of blood clots or breast cancer.

As long as the potential benefits of HRT add up to a happier, healthier life, it's certainly worth considering. But it's not a panacea, and there are times it's not the best choice. For example:

- If your main health concern is improving cholesterol, other medications, such as the statins, should be your first choice.

- If you already have osteoporosis, consider medications such as alendronate, risedronate, raloxifene, or calcitonin, not hormones.

- If you already have heart disease, don't turn to HRT.

Your Guide to Menopause Management Options

At one time, medications like Premarin or Prempro were the only forms of hormone replacement that women and their doctors had to choose from when it came time to decide whether to use HRT. Today there are dozens of types of estrogen, progesterone, or testosterone, in various forms, dosages, and combinations. So if one doesn't suit you, another might. This at-a-glance guide, created exclusively for *Prevention* magazine, can help you sort through your options with your physician.

Oral Estrogens

Product	Main Roles	Unique Benefits	Potential Disadvantages
Estradiol (Estrace) **Esterfied estrogen** (EstraTab, Menest) **Estropipate** (Ogen, Ortho-Est) **Conjugated equine estrogens** (Premarin) **Synthetic conjugated estrogens** (Cenestin)	Relieve hot flashes Relieve vaginal dryness Relieve urinary complaints Increase bone mass	Raise beneficial HDL cholesterol and lower LDL Some studies suggest lower risk for Alzheimer's disease and diabetes Might prevent gum disease and improve skin tone	Most common side effects include bloating, breast tenderness, headaches, nausea, and irregular bleeding Risk of blood clots Risk of breast and uterine cancers Raise triglyceride level

Estrogen Injections

Product	Main Roles	Unique Benefits	Potential Disadvantages
Custom formulations	Same as oral formulations	Same as oral formulations	Erratic hormone levels make them unpopular form of ERT

Transdermal Estrogen Patches

Product	Main Roles	Unique Benefits	Potential Disadvantages
Estradiol (Alora, Climara, Estraderm, FemPatch, Esclim)	Relieve hot flashes Relieve vaginal dryness Relieve urinary complaints Increase bone mass	May help control blood pressure and blood vessel constriction More even hormone levels than oral forms Less frequent reported side effects such as headache, nausea, and mood swings Shown to reduce depression in clinically depressed, post-menopausal women	Most common side effects include bloating, breast tenderness, headaches, irregular bleeding (blood clot risk not as high as with oral forms) Can irritate skin at site of application Patch can fall off

continued

Topical Estrogen Formulations

Product	Main Roles	Unique Benefits	Potential Disadvantages
ESTROGEN CREAMS: **Estradiol** (Estrace) **Estropipate** (Ogen) **Dienestrol** (Ortho) **Conjugated equine estrogens** (Premarin)	Relieve vaginal dryness and vaginal atrophy	Faster vaginal symptom relief than with oral and patch estrogens Less breast and uterus cell proliferation than with oral and patch forms Estradiol products may also protect against urinary infections	Can be messy Not approved for hot flash relief or for bone and heart protection benefits
ESTROGEN RING: **Estradiol** (Estring)	Relieves vaginal dryness and vaginal atrophy Prevents and treats urinary infections	Low-fuss method that doesn't require daily routine of oral and vaginal methods Doesn't have to be used with progesterone	Isn't approved for hot flash relief

Custom Estrogen Formulations

Product	Main Roles	Unique Benefits	Potential Disadvantages
Estriol/estrone/17-beta estradiol combination (Tri-Est) **Estriol cream**	Same as other oral and transdermal estrogens	Generally more recommended by natural health care practitioners for having fewer side effects and health risks Estriol cream doesn't need to be accompanied by progesterone to protect the uterus	Custom formulations lack thorough testing and assurance of reliability Prescription can be filled only at pharmacy specializing in compounding Insurance may not cover

Synthetic Progestins

Product	Main Roles	Unique Benefits	Potential Disadvantages
Medroxyprogesterone acetate (Amen, Cycrin, Provera) **Norethindrone** (Micronor, Nor-QD, Activella) **Norethindrone acetate** (Aygestin) **Norgestrel** (Ovrette) **Levonorgestrel** (Norplant) **Levonorgestrel IUD** (Mirena)	Protect uterus from overstimulation from estrogen Relieve estrogen-dominated conditions, including fibrocystic breasts, endometriosis, ovarian cysts, and uterine fibroids	Norgestimate and norethindrone can help reduce breakthrough bleeding	Associated with mood changes, depression, and anxiety Side effects include fluid retention, headaches, breast tenderness Counteract beneficial cholesterol effects of estrogen replacement therapy

"Natural" Progesterone

Product	Main Roles	Unique Benefits	Potential Disadvantages
Progesterone USP (Prometrium) **Progesterone IUD** (Progesasert)	Protect uterus from overstimulation from estrogen May relieve estrogen-dominated conditions, including fibrocystic breasts, endometriosis, and ovarian cysts	Fewer side effects reported than with synthetic progestin formulations Don't disrupt beneficial HDL cholesterol Associated with feelings of natural calm and reduced depression and anxiety May also promote sound sleep, fluid balance, libido enhancement, bone mass preservation, improved fat metabolism, and protection against breast cancer	Can cause drowsiness (unless taken before bed) May encourage more breakthrough bleeding than with synthetic progestins Prometrium prescriptions can be obtained only from pharmacies specializing in compounding
Progesterone vaginal gel (Crinone)	Relieves hot flashes Normalizes menstrual cycle Relieves PMS complaints in peri-menopausal women	Sufficient progesterone to protect uterus from estrogen stimulation Reports of "emotional boost" benefit Decrease in headaches, depression, and mood swings when compared with synthetic progestins Doesn't produce messy discharge	Can cause drowsiness

Combination Estrogen/Progesterone Products

Product	Main Roles	Unique Benefits	Potential Disadvantages
Estradiol/ norethindrone acetate (CombiPatch) **Conjugated equine estrogen/ medroxyprogesterone** (Premphase, Prempro)	Relieve hot flashes Relieve vaginal dryness Relieve urinary complaints Increase bone mass Protect uterus	Simpler regimen than with separate products	Most common side effects include bloating, breast tenderness, headaches, mood changes, and nausea Breakthrough bleeding more common in combined products

continued

Androgens ("Male Hormones")

Product	Main Roles	Unique Benefits	Potential Disadvantages
Methyltestosterone (Estratest)	The only androgen-containing product approved by the FDA for treatment of hot flashes in women who aren't helped by estrogen alone Increased sexual desire, arousal, and general sexual enjoyment	Offers some protection against bone loss May also increase energy, improve mood, and help manage weight Helpful for maintaining lean muscle mass after menopause	Inappropriate doses can lead to male features (body hair, lower voice, muscle weight gain), acne, and feelings of aggression, agitation, or depression Can severely disrupt cholesterol levels
17-alkylated androgens **Oral micronized testosterone** **Sublingual testosterone** (Cyclodextrin) **Transdermal matrix testosterone patch** (under development)	Similar benefits to those listed above, when taken with estrogen and in proper doses	Similar benefits to those listed above Transdermal patch promising for most closely approximating pre-menopausal testosterone levels	Same dangers as those listed above, but more likely because of unregulated dosages 17-alkylated androgens associated with liver toxicity Inconclusive data on bioavailablity, side effects, and effectiveness

Osteoporosis Drugs

Product	Main Roles	Unique Benefits	Potential Disadvantages
SELECTIVE ESTROGEN RECEPTOR MODULATORS (SERMS): **Raloxifene** (Evista) **Tamoxifen**	Spine fracture preventative Treatment for osteoporosis Act as estrogens in some tissues and anti-estrogens in others	Produce favorable changes in blood lipids that can protect against cardiovascular disease; don't stimulate the breasts and the uterus (common with estrogens); may reduce breast cancer risk; don't need to be accompanied by use of progestins	Increased risk of blood clots (also common with estrogens) Generally not beneficial for treating hot flashes and other symptoms that estrogen relieves
BIPHOSPHONATES: **Alendronate** (Fosamax) **Risedronate** (Actonel)	Proven to reduce risk of spine and hip fracture Treatment for osteoporosis	The only drugs proven to specifically reduce hip fracture risk	No effect on hot flashes or other symptoms
SPRAY OR INJECTION: **Calcitonin** (Miacalcin)	Slows bone loss, increases spinal bone density, and relieves pain associated with hip fractures	Favored for women 5 or more years past menopause, particularly women who want to reduce spinal fracture risk	Injection of calcitonin can cause allergic reaction, flushing of face and hands, urinary frequency, nausea, and skin rash; calcitonin spray can cause runny nose No effect on hot flashes or other symptoms or hormone-related health risks

Over-the-Counter Hormone-Regulating Products

Product	Main Roles	Unique Benefits	Potential Disadvantages
Black cohosh (Remifemin and various other herbal product brands)	Hot flash relief, vaginal dryness treatment, hormone-related mood swing relief, and menstrual cycle regulation	Not associated with risks of estrogen-sensitive cancer May protect against age-related memory decline May enhance sex life	Recommended only for 6-month intervals and without the use of HRT; potency and reliability not regulated by FDA; may produce gastrointestinal side effects
Phytoestrogen/ isoflavone supplements (Promensil, Estroven, and various other brands)	Recommended by FDA to lower cholesterol and reduce risk of cardiovascular disease May help relieve hot flashes and vaginal dryness	Act similar to body's own estrogen and may provide protection against bone loss, heart disease, and breast cancer	Not proven safe to use in conjunction with HRT Effectiveness and long-term safety not established Overconsumption may stimulate breast and uterus; similar cancer risks as HRT
Soy foods (soy nuts, soy milk, tofu, various brands)	Recommended by FDA to lower cholesterol and reduce risk of cardiovascular disease; may help relieve hot flashes and vaginal dryness	Act similar to body's own estrogen and may provide protection against bone loss, heart disease, and breast cancer	Effectiveness and long-term safety not established Overconsumption can stimulate breast and uterus, creating similar cancer risks as HRT
7-isopropoxy-isoflavone ("Natural Ipriflavone," various brands)	Mild bone loss prevention and bone density increase	May lower cholesterol and offer cancer protection; does not appear to have hormonelike effects on the breasts and uterus	Bone protection milder than prescription options
Progesterone (wild yam or soy cream, various brands)	Hot flash relief; regulates menstrual cycles; protects uterus when estrogen is used	None	Potencies and reliability not regulated by FDA
Vitex	Relieves vaginal dryness, improves libido in women with elevated prolactin levels, and curbs PMS in perimenopausal women	Can enhance progesterone while reducing prolactin hormone	Potency and reliability not regulated by FDA
DHEA	Converted by body to testosterone to improve libido, general vitality	None	Same risk as with prescription androgens Efficacy and ability of body to absorb DHEA unclear

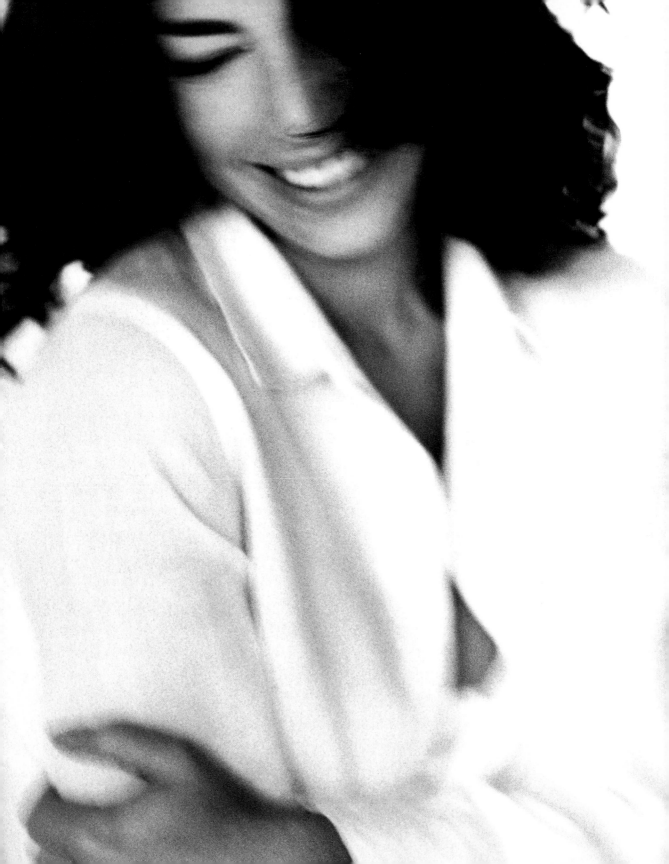

PART FIVE

DOCTORS'

BEST

SYMPTOM

SOLVERS

abdominal fat

When most women think of ways to flatten their stomachs, images of zillions of crunches flash through their minds, and they may feel defeated before they've even begun.

That's probably needless mental torment, though. Leading weight-loss and fitness experts agree that some lifestyle changes, along with simple exercises and everyday activities such as walking, gardening, and playing tennis, can lead to a leaner waistline because they help decrease overall body fat.

"If a woman takes in more calories than she's expending, she will gain weight and store fat in certain areas of her body, such as the abdomen," explains Ellen Glickman, Ph.D., professor of exercise physiology and coordinator of the exercise science program at Kent State University in Ohio.

"Women are genetically predisposed to store fat in the abdominal area because it's nature's way of protecting the childbearing area of our bodies," she explains. "Extra calories get stored as fat around the abdomen and hips to protect a baby against trauma."

When it comes to abdominal fat, genetics may dictate that women have an uphill climb, but that doesn't mean it's not worth the effort. A firm tummy looks great in everything from bathing suits to jeans. In addition, research continues to demonstrate that having a trim middle can protect against life-threatening diseases, such as breast cancer, heart disease, and diabetes. Fat inside the abdomen is more likely to release fatty acids into the liver than fat elsewhere on the body. As a result, excessive amounts of cholesterol and insulin seep into the bloodstream, contributing to the development of disease.

"Women with large bellies also complain of back pain," says Dr. Glickman. "Back pain is often caused by weak abdominal muscles, so strengthening these muscles helps your back support your body and takes pressure off the back. Where there's less pressure, there's less pain and discomfort."

Here are some strategies to make your belly bulge less noticeably or lose it entirely.

Immediate Solutions

home remedies

Drink up. For premenstrual bloating, drink lots of water. This will actually help flush away excess fluid, not increase it. And avoid carbonated drinks and those with lots of sugar, which can blow your belly up like a balloon.

Skip the chips. Salt makes you retain water, especially before your period. Processed and canned foods tend to be high in sodium.

Ditch the chewing gum. Chewing gum can cause you to swallow excess air, which may "inflate" your stomach.

Get some java "to go." If you're feeling overdue for a bathroom session, studies show that a cup or two of coffee can get things moving.

Stand up straight. Imagine a string with one end attached to the top of your head and the other tied to the ceiling. Pretend it's tugging you upright, and your belly will instantly look flatter.

Don't slump. Sitting in a slump accentuates your stomach. To improve your posture, check your chair. If the seat is too high to let your feet touch the floor without making you slump, use a footstool about 4 inches high, or place a pillow at the small of your back to help move you forward in your chair.

Shape up underneath. Body shapers—high-waisted spandex waist slimmers and panties—can take off an inch or more. The more spandex (Lycra) they contain, the more control you'll get.

Wear black. "Wearing black makes women of all shapes and sizes look thinner and taller," notes Dr. Glickman.

Keep your outfits monochromatic. Wear the same color top, skirt or pants, and shoes for an elongating effect.

Choose belly-slimming fabrics. Rayons, silks, knits, and nonclingy matte jerseys generally work best.

Accessorize. Choose eye-catching earrings and necklaces or colorful scarves. They'll draw attention away from your belly and toward your face.

Long-Term Solutions

home remedies

Aim for at least 30 minutes of exercise most days of the week. To do that, set a specific time to work out, and stick to it. "Women are increasingly taking on more roles, and they tend to put themselves last," notes Dr. Glickman. "We put our jobs, children, and house before our own health and wellness. We claim to have less and less time to be physically active and do daily exercise.

Stay Calm and Trim Your Middle

According to research, stubborn flab called stress fat can pad a woman's midsection when levels of the stress hormone cortisol are high—even if she's thin. When researchers checked how well 59 premenopausal women adapted to laboratory stress tests, they found that those with bigger bellies performed more poorly on the tests, and secreted significantly more cortisol, than those without tummy bulges. In addition, while overweight women with belly fat gradually adapted to stress (their cortisol levels dropped), lean women with bellies didn't (their cortisol levels stayed high).

Researchers suspect that large amounts of cortisol can increase visceral fat, a particularly dangerous type of fat that's associated with increased risk of diabetes and heart disease.

To help balance levels of cortisol, practice this quick stress reducer. Find a quiet, comfortable place to sit. Next, take several slow, deep breaths to help clear your mind. Continue breathing deeply and repeat the word *one* to yourself as you exhale. (If you get distracted, just bring your focus back to the word *one*.) Practice this for 5 to 10 minutes once or twice a day. ■

"Most women in this country expend a lot of time and effort counting fat grams and calories," she points out. "But what they need to realize is that exercise combined with a reduction in calorie intake is the best way to a flat tummy because you reduce your overall body fat while maintaining lean muscle tissue."

Start at the top. "When you do upper-body weight lifting or resistance exercises, your lower body, especially the abdomen, will work to stabilize the body," says Dr. Glickman.

Another bonus: Building upper-body muscles, such as those in your arms and shoulders, can make your waistline *look* smaller. Dr. Glickman recommends starting out slowly, then working your way up to at least three sets of 12 repetitions.

Sign up for a few Pilates classes. Dancers have used this series of stretching-type exercises done on the floor and on special equipment for decades. Now hundreds of others, including many celebrities, attribute their tight abs to this low-impact form of exercise. For a list of studios and instructors near you, contact the Pilates Studio at (800) 474-5283.

Give kickboxing a whirl. Aerobic kickboxing is more than just a great fat-burning, cardiovascular workout. All those arm thrusts and high kicks firm the abs, too. To learn kickboxing, pick up a videotape from a library or video store. Or contact a local gym, hospital, or community center and ask about kickboxing classes.

Do a clean sweep. Does the sidewalk or garage need sweeping? Grab a broom (not the push type) and get to it. The back-and-forth motion is a great ab toner. And don't forget the dustpan: Bending over works the abs, too, mostly when you exhale.

(continued on page 310)

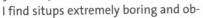

WHAT WORKS FOR ME

ELLEN GLICKMAN, PH.D., *professor of exercise physiology and coordinator of the exercise science program at Kent State University in Ohio, talks about how she stays in shape.*

I find situps extremely boring and obnoxious. That's why I refuse to do them. People say, "God—your stomach is so flat." But I haven't done any situps.

My approach is to combine an aerobic exercise program with an anaerobic one. For the aerobic workout, I jog 4 miles every day. For the anaerobic exercise, I lift weights three times a week, focusing on my upper body. I do lat pulldowns and a lot of triceps work. The tummy gets flat naturally because while doing the upper-body workout, the abdominal muscles are contracting to stabilize the body, and they become more toned.

I'm conscious of my calorie intake in the sense that I make a mental note of how many calories I take in each day. I read labels, and I eat basically the same foods, so I've memorized how many calories each food has. For example, I eat bananas all the time, and I know that each one has about 100 calories. I also eat low-fat, high-complex-carbohydrate meals such as pasta dishes or broiled salmon. ∎

Shoot for Strength

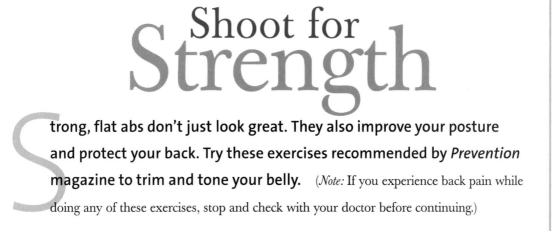

Strong, flat abs don't just look great. They also improve your posture and protect your back. Try these exercises recommended by *Prevention* magazine to trim and tone your belly. (*Note:* If you experience back pain while doing any of these exercises, stop and check with your doctor before continuing.)

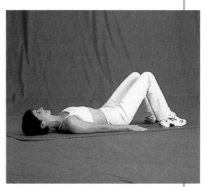

Pelvic Tilt

Lie on the floor with your arms at your sides, knees bent, and feet flat on the floor. Press your lower back to the floor so that your pelvis tilts upward. Straighten your legs by slowly sliding your heels along the floor, and stop when you can no longer hold a full tilt position; hold for a count of six. Next, move one leg at a time back to the starting position, maintaining the pelvic tilt throughout. Hold the starting position for six counts, then relax.

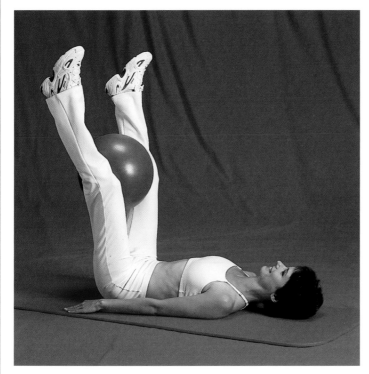

Leg Raise

Lie on the floor and raise your legs straight up. Place an exercise ball between your knees, then do a slight pelvic tilt from the hips. Squeeze the exercise ball for 1 second, then relax.

continued

Shoot for Strength

continued

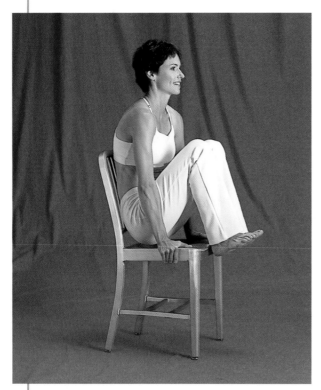

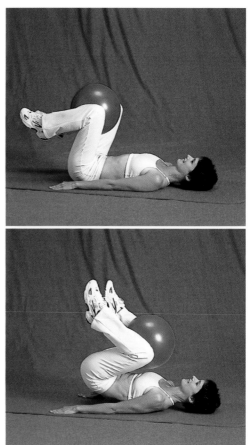

Seated Body Lift

Sit erect in a firm, armless chair and place your hands on the sides of the chair in front of your hips. Tighten your abs and support yourself with your hands as you slowly pull your knees up toward your chest. Keep your lower back against the chair back. Hold and then slowly lower. (This move is more easily performed without shoes.)

Hip Raise

Lie on the floor and place an exercise ball between your bent knees (top). Lift your hips off the floor, and bring your knees toward your chest (bottom). Squeeze the ball for 1 second, then relax.

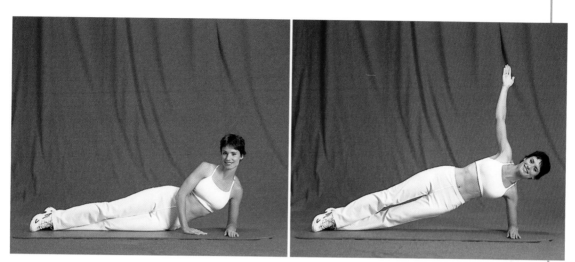

Side Body Lift

Lie on your left side, supporting your upper body on your left elbow, forearm, and hand. Your elbow should be directly under your shoulder (left). Slowly lift the rest of your body off the floor so only your forearm and feet are on the floor (right). (Use the other arm for balance. For an advanced move, hold that arm straight up in the air.) For maximum effect, keep your body as straight as possible. Hold for as long as is comfortable or until you can no longer maintain good form, then slowly lower and relax. Repeat on the other side.

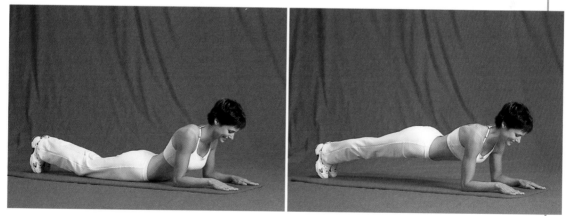

Front Body Lift

Lie facedown on the floor, supporting your upper body on your elbows, forearms, and hands (left). Slowly lift the rest of your body off the floor until you're balanced on your toes (right). Keep your body straight, and hold for as long as is comfortable, then slowly lower and relax.

Be Posture Perfect

The following exercises will strengthen your shoulders, chest, and back so you can stand tall and minimize the appearance of your belly.

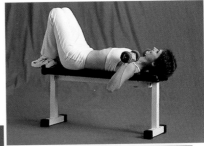

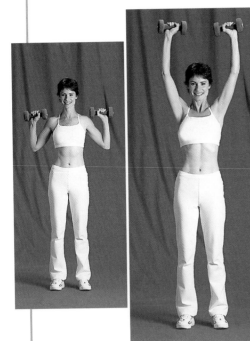

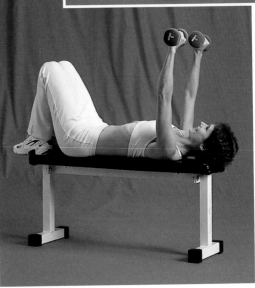

Shoulder Press

To target your shoulder muscles, stand erect with your feet firmly on the floor, holding a dumbbell in each hand at shoulder height, palms facing forward (left). Slowly press both dumbbells straight up until your arms are fully extended (right). Don't arch your back. Hold, then lower the weights.

Bench Press

This exercise works your chest muscles. First, lie on the floor or an exercise bench with your knees bent and your feet flat on the floor or the bench. Hold two dumbbells or a barbell at chest height with your hands slightly more than shoulder-width apart (top). Slowly press the weights straight up until your arms are fully extended and your elbows almost locked (bottom). Hold, then lower the weight.

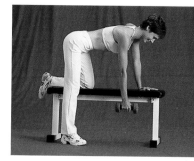
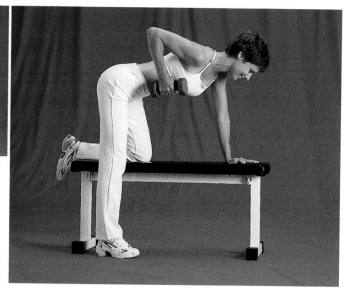

One-Arm Row

This is a great way to strengthen the muscles of your mid and upper back. Put your left knee and left hand on a bench or a chair, keeping your back flat. Hold a weight in your right hand with your right arm straight and the weight hanging toward the floor, parallel to the bench (left). Raise the weight, keeping it close to your body, until it's even with your waist; your elbow should be pointed toward the ceiling (right). (The movement is like starting a power lawn mower, only slower and smoother.) Hold, then slowly lower the weight. Switch sides.

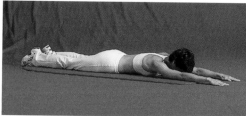
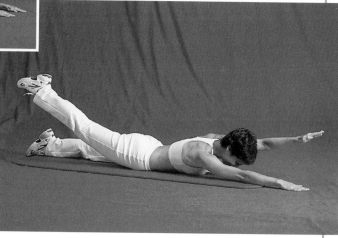

Back Strengthener

Lie facedown with your legs extended straight behind you, toes pointed and arms extended straight over your head. Keep your chin up off the floor at a comfortable level (above). Slowly raise your left arm and your right leg at the same time until they are both a few inches off the floor (right). Hold, then slowly lower them back to the starting position.

Get out and garden. Gardening involves bending, lifting, pulling, pushing, and digging. The spinal twisting and abdominal contractions you do while digging are a particularly good ab workout.

Go for a walk. According to a Harvard study, women who walked regularly were 16 percent less likely to gain inches at the waist than those who didn't. "Walking is an outstanding exercise for overall weight reduction for women of all body shapes, all ages, and all weight ranges," says Dr. Glickman. "It's the safest form of exercise, with a very low risk of injury. Research shows that it helps to maintain the integrity of bone, which will reduce the chances of developing osteoporosis."

Try tennis. As you play a few sets of backhand and forehand, you'll feel it around your middle. Each time you turn to make a stroke, you strengthen the oblique muscles on either side of your abdomen.

Go for a swim. A vigorous crawl stroke can tighten abs. Since you must breathe in and out forcefully as you swim, your abdominal muscles contract constantly. The reaching forward and pulling back in the butterfly stroke also tones the abs.

Play a few holes. Swinging a golf club shapes up the oblique muscles on the sides of your abs. Playing 9 or 18 holes is a real workout. (For an aerobic workout, skip the cart.)

Don't smoke, and skip the alcohol. Both increase levels of the stress hormone cortisol, which in turn can increase abdominal fat.

Eat more fiber. Not only is fiber great for overall weight loss (it fills you up so you don't eat as much), but it also prevents constipation, which can cause a tummy bulge. To stay regular, aim for 20 to 35 grams of fiber a day by eating more whole grains, fruits, and vegetables, or try a fiber supplement such as Metamucil.

THREE THINGS I TELL EVERY FEMALE PATIENT

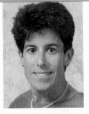

ELLEN GLICKMAN, PH.D., professor of exercise physiology and coordinator of the exercise science program at Kent State University in Ohio, offers this special advice for keeping in shape.

1 DO SOMETHING AEROBIC EVERY DAY. Walking is great because it will help you lose overall body fat, including abdominal fat.

DO SOMETHING ANAEROBIC THREE TIMES A WEEK. Weight lifting is really helpful. "I emphasize upper-body workouts that include lat

pulldowns and triceps pullbacks because they not only help flatten the tummy; they also strengthen the part of the body that's used a lot," says Dr. Glickman. "As we get older, the activities that we're engaged in most often—such as getting out of a bathtub, getting off the commode, getting out of a car—rely on upper-body strength."

2

3 ENJOY WHAT YOU'RE DOING. If you do, you'll be more likely to stick to your exercise program. ∎

anemia

Every time you take a breath, oxygen is picked up by hemoglobin, an iron-rich protein in red blood cells, and carried to tissues throughout the body. Women who have insufficient levels of hemoglobin or red blood cells can't get all the oxygen they need. This condition, called anemia, can result in weakness, fatigue, headaches, heart palpitations, difficulty concentrating, and other symptoms.

Anemia rarely causes serious health problems for women, but doctors take it seriously because something is causing hemoglobin or red blood cells to decline. Heavy menstrual bleeding or insufficient iron in the diet is often to blame. There could also be internal bleeding—due to ulcers, for example, or some forms of cancer, says Barbara Goff, M.D., associate professor of obstetrics and gynecology at the University of Washington School of Medicine in Seattle. Even hemorrhoids can result in anemia if they bleed profusely.

Women who are vegetarians sometimes get anemia because the iron in plant foods isn't as easy for the body to absorb as the iron found in meats. Pregnancy also affects iron levels, which is why women are often advised to take iron-containing prenatal supplements when they're expecting.

Most cases of anemia are caused by insufficient iron in the diet, but there are other forms of this condition as well. A deficiency of vitamin B_{12} can result in a decrease in red blood cells that may lead to anemia. This nutrient is found only in animal foods, so strict vegetarians may not get enough. Pernicious anemia, which often affects elderly adults, is caused by the lack of a stomach protein that's needed to transport vitamin B_{12} from the stomach to the small intestine—the inability to produce the stomach protein leads to inadequate absorption of vitamin B_{12}.

Anemia always needs to be checked out by a

when to see a doctor

If you have heavy menstrual periods and you're also suffering from constant fatigue, see your doctor right away. The odds are very good that you have iron deficiency anemia, says Scott A. Fields, M.D., vice chairman of family medicine at Oregon Health Sciences University in Portland. You'll probably need to get extra iron in your diet, and your doctor will want to ensure that the bleeding is normal and that there isn't an underlying problem.

If your energy is low and you're a strict vegetarian: You could have low levels of vitamin B_{12}, which is found only in animal foods. If you avoid eggs and dairy foods as well as meats, you may need to take B_{12} supplements. The Daily Value is 6 micrograms.

If your stools appear black or tarry: Bleeding from the gastrointestinal tract is a common cause of anemia, and it always needs to be investigated by a physician.

doctor—but once you have the okay from your doctor, there are a variety of home care options that can offer effective treatment.

For Immediate Relief

home remedies

Increase your iron intake. The Institute of Medicine recently revised the guidelines for iron intake. Women between the ages of 18 and 50 are advised to get 18 milligrams of iron daily; during pregnancy, your doctor will increase the amount to 27 milligrams. Women 51 years and older need only about 8 milligrams of iron daily.

Eat lean red meats. They help prevent—or reverse—anemia in two ways: They're rich in dietary iron; and the form of iron that they contain, called heme iron, is easy for the body to absorb.

Enjoy iron-rich greens. Spinach, chard, turnip greens, and spirulina (seaweed) are good sources of iron. The one problem with these foods is that they contain a type of iron called nonheme iron, which is somewhat harder for the body to absorb than the heme iron found in meats.

Put beans on the menu. Pintos, navy beans, and lentils are good sources of iron. Half a cup of navy beans, for example, provides about 2.3 milligrams of iron, while ½ cup of lentils provides about 3.3 milligrams.

Drink orange juice with meals. Or finish off your meals with a few slices of orange or grape-

THREE THINGS I TELL EVERY FEMALE PATIENT

SCOTT A. FIELDS, M.D., is vice chairman of family medicine at Oregon Health Sciences University in Portland. He sees a lot of women who suffer from anemia, and he always offers this advice.

1

DON'T TREAT IT ENTIRELY ON YOUR OWN. Many women know the signs of anemia— such as fatigue around their menstrual periods—and they assume that getting extra iron is all that they need to do. Iron will certainly improve your levels of red blood cells, but it won't correct the underlying problem, says Dr. Fields. It's essential that you see your doctor, who will run laboratory tests to determine what's causing your symptoms.

2

TELL YOUR DOCTOR IF IRON SUPPLEMENTS ARE CAUSING SIDE EFFECTS. Many women with anemia quit taking iron supplements because they can't handle the diarrhea, nausea, or other disagreeable digestive symptoms that sometimes occur when taking them. "We may try different types of supplements that you'll be able to digest more easily," says Dr. Fields. "Or we might be able to manage your symptoms with dietary management."

3

BE PATIENT. "It usually takes weeks or months for supplemental iron—either from foods or supplements—to correct anemia," says Dr. Fields. "In the meantime, rest when you feel tired—and take comfort in the fact that we've found an explanation for your symptoms." ∎

fruit. Citrus fruits are very high in vitamin C, which enhances iron absorption. This is especially important when you're eating plant foods that contain difficult-to-absorb nonheme iron.

Save the coffee for later. Along with tea, coffee reduces the body's absorption of iron. It's fine to enjoy these beverages as long as you have them a few hours after meals.

Take advantage of breakfast cereals. If you find that you're eating less meat in order to reduce the amount of fat in your diet, you'll have to make an effort to find other sources of iron in the diet. Fortified breakfast cereals, which contain added iron, are good choices. A cup of regular instant oats, for example, provides only about 1.6 milligrams of iron. A cup of fortified oats, on the other hand, may provide more than 8 milligrams.

Take multi supplements. Multi supplements will help your body keep pace with the normal iron losses that take place during menstruation, according to *Prevention* magazine. Premenopausal women should take a multi containing 100 percent of the Daily Value of iron. Postmenopausal women should take a "senior" multi supplement with 9 milligrams of iron.

Don't take iron supplements without checking with your doctor first.

medical options

Ask your doctor about the Pill. Some women lose so much blood during menstruation that they're almost always anemic. Your doctor may recommend that you go on the Pill: It will normalize your periods and help prevent excessive blood loss, says Dr. Goff.

Report strange cravings. It doesn't happen very often, but women will sometimes develop powerful, nearly overwhelming cravings for unsavory substances, such as dirt, clay, laundry starch, or even cigarette ashes. This condition, known as pica, is often a sign of iron deficiency anemia.

Doctors aren't sure if iron deficiency causes pica or if it's the other way around—that pica causes iron deficiency anemia because women eat so much of the nonnutritious substances that they don't get enough wholesome foods in the diet.

In either case, be sure to report unusual cravings to your doctor. If you're suffering from pica, taking supplemental iron will often cause the cravings to disappear, sometimes in as little as 24 hours.

arthritis

To many women, the word *arthritis* brings to mind an image of a snowy-haired grandmother leaning on a cane or an elderly aunt struggling to open a jar with stiff fingers. Actually, although the incidence increases with the years, arthritis can affect women at any age, including during childhood. Nearly three out of every five people with arthritis are under age 65.

According to the Centers for Disease Control and Prevention (CDC), arthritis is the number-one cause of disability in the United States, affecting 43 million men and women. The CDC predicts that by 2020, that number will rise to 60 million, and more than 11 million will be disabled.

The term *arthritis* (literally, "joint inflammation") actually refers to a group of more than 100 diseases and conditions that can cause pain, stiffness, and swelling in the joints. If not diagnosed and treated, arthritis can cause irreversible joint damage. With treatment, however, women with arthritis can minimize the discomfort and avoid permanent damage.

The two most prevalent forms of arthritis are osteoarthritis, which is the focus of this chapter, and rheumatoid arthritis. (For more information on rheumatoid arthritis, see page 463.)

The pressure of gravity and the wear and tear of everyday life cause some kinds of osteoarthritis, which was once called degenerative joint disease. Genetic predisposition also plays a role in developing osteoarthritis. The resulting damage to the joints and surrounding tissues leads to pain, tenderness, swelling, and decreased function.

Osteoarthritis primarily affects the cartilage, the slippery tissue that covers the ends of both bones in a joint. Healthy cartilage is thick enough to let the bones glide smoothly over each other and absorb energy from the shock of physical movement. In osteoarthritis, the cartilage breaks down, wears away, and becomes thin, so the bones rub together and cause pain, swelling, and stiffness. Over time, the joint can lose its normal shape. Small, bony growths called bone spurs can form on the edges of the joint, and bits of cartilage can break off and float inside the joint space, causing more pain and damage.

In its early stages, osteoarthritis may cause swelling, but its onset is subtle and gradual, usually involving only one or two joints, such as the knee, hip, and hand. Pain is the earliest symptom.

For Women, Osteoarthritis Is Most Common

Osteoarthritis affects more than 20 million people, according to the Arthritis Foundation. It is the most common type of arthritis that affects women, mostly after age 45. The risk increases with age, especially if there's a family history of the disease.

"Often a woman's mother, grandmother, or aunt had osteoarthritis," says Jeffrey R. Lisse, M.D., head of clinical osteoporosis research, associate chief of the Arizona Arthritis Center, and professor of medicine at the University of Arizona College of Medicine in Tucson. "We now know that there's a genetic component to it. It tends to run in families."

A woman in her fifties, for example, can begin to feel pain and stiffness in her knee, then recall a

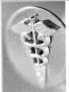

when to see a doctor

If you have severe pain or disability that interferes with normal activities, contact your physician right away. Many remedies take at least 8 weeks to start working, so it's best to get an early, accurate diagnosis.

sports injury or accident when she was a young adult. Being overweight can also cause damage. Obese adults tend to wear out their joints more quickly than do those at a healthy weight.

Fortunately, having arthritis doesn't have to mean the beginning of the end of playing golf, cooking gourmet meals from scratch, or doing anything else that you love. Here's how you can ease the pain if you already have arthritis, and possibly lower your risk of developing it if you don't.

For Immediate Relief

home remedies

Broil a salmon for dinner. The omega-3 fatty acids in fish oil may ease arthritis pain by providing anti-inflammatory building blocks. "Fish oil has a mild anti-inflammatory effect by decreasing prostaglandins, which cause inflammation," says Dr. Lisse. Good food sources of omega-3s include salmon, tuna, sardines, and mackerel. *Prevention* magazine suggests eating them two or three times a week. Fish oil is also available in supplements. Three grams, or 3,000 milligrams, a day of EPA and DHA (omega-3 fatty acids found in fish oil) is the suggested dose.

Eat your other vegetables. Research has shown that people with high intakes of vitamin C and beta-carotene had a reduced risk of knee pain and disease progression. To be sure that you get enough of these nutrients (as well as other plant-based protective compounds, such as lutein and lycopene), eat lots of carrots, sweet potatoes, broccoli, spinach, tomato sauce and tomato juice, oranges, kiwifruit, and strawberries.

Take some E and D. In studies, vitamin E eased arthritis pain better than a placebo (inactive substance) or a nonsteroidal anti-inflammatory drug (NSAID) such as aspirin or ibuprofen. To get the amount of vitamin E that most experts recommend, you'll need a supplement containing 400 IU.

The research also showed that osteoarthritis progression was three times higher in people with low levels of vitamin D, so taking a multivitamin/mineral supplement that supplies 100 percent of the Daily Value for D (400 IU) is a good idea.

Walk away pain. "Walking is great exercise for women with arthritis because it helps keep muscles warm and flexible, which eases pain," says Dr. Lisse. "Start slowly, then build up to walking for at least 30 minutes 3 to 5 days a week."

Concerned that you might do more harm than good? In several studies involving people with osteoarthritis of the knee, none has shown any harm from 30 to 45 minutes of moderately brisk walking on a good walking surface while wearing well-designed shoes. If walking does cause pain, try walking more slowly, or use some type of shoe insert or orthotic. And take a good look at your walking shoes: It may be time for a new pair. If the pain continues, stop the brisk walking and contact your physician.

Long-Term Solutions

home remedies

Apply heat. "For chronic arthritis pain, place a heating pad on the painful site for 10 to 15 min-

(continued on page 320)

Warm Up to Water Walking

When you have arthritis, warm-water exercise can encourage stiff joints to become more flexible and can relax tight muscles. The buoyancy of the water supports the joints.

A warmup is essential to prevent pain and injury for all exercisers, but especially for people with arthritis. *Prevention* magazine recommends starting with the following set of full-body range-of-motion exercises on this and the following spread, done in a pool, to increase flexibility. Do these before and after the water walking routine described on page 319.

The warmup: Walk into the water to chest height. (The body part you're working on should be underwater. You'll need to go deeper or crouch down to get your shoulders underwater when doing the first exercise.) Do all of these moves slowly, and never stretch to the point of pain or discomfort. Do at least three repetitions of each, but depending on your individual needs and condition, you can do as many as 10 reps of any move to help loosen a stiff joint. Repeat the entire set of exercises to cool down after your water-walking workout.

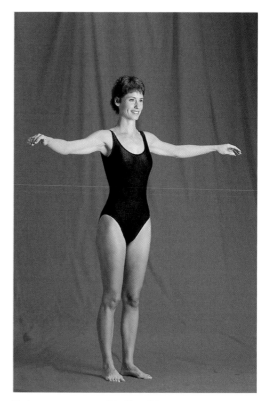

Swing your arms out to the sides.

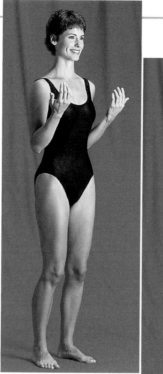

Bend your elbows.

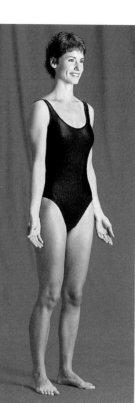

Straighten your elbows.

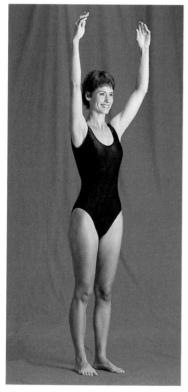

Lift your arms over your head.

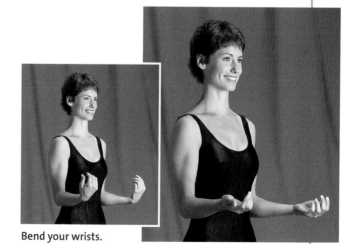

Bend your wrists.

Straighten your wrists.

continued

Warm Up to
Water Walking

continued

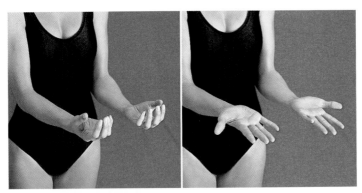

Hold each hand in a loose fist with fingers bent.

Straighten your fingers.

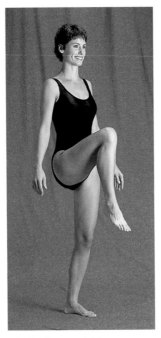

Take high steps, lifting your raised knee toward your chest.

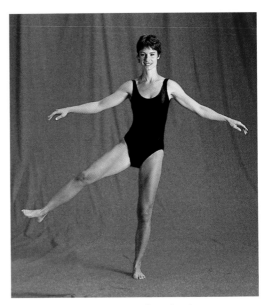

Standing on one leg, swing the other leg out to the side; then switch sides.

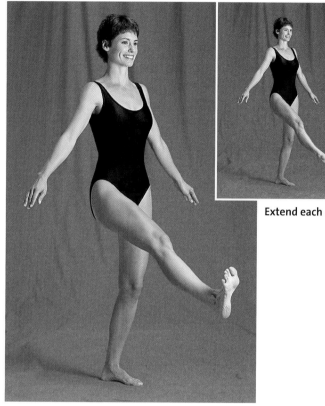

Flex each ankle.

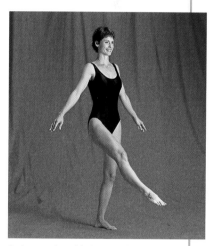

Extend each ankle.

Swing each ankle in a circle.

The exercise: After completing the warmup routine shown in this photo series, you're ready to exercise. Standing in water that's between hip and waist deep, start walking and swinging your arms. Start slowly, then pick up speed and work up to a comfortable, brisk pace. Start with 5 minutes, then gradually increase the time until you feel it could be rated as moderate, which the Arthritis Foundation describes as anywhere from "still light but starting to work" or "still comfortable but harder" to "getting to be somewhat hard." Do the workout three to five times a week. For more information, check at a YMCA for water-walking classes designed for people with arthritis.

utes three times a day," says Dr. Lisse. "Heat can be very soothing for sore, stiff muscles and joints. It relaxes them so they move more freely."

Go for glucosamine. Glucosamine is a natural substance that furnishes the building blocks needed to make and repair cartilage. In a Belgian study that followed two groups of people over age 50 who had mild to moderate osteoarthritis, one group received 1,500 milligrams of glucosamine daily, while the other was given a placebo. After 3 years, the group taking the glucosamine showed little or no joint deterioration. That group also reported improvement in their symptoms, such as pain, and in joint function. The placebo group's joint deterioration worsened, and they did not feel that their symptoms improved.

The Arthritis Foundation recently changed its position on glucosamine based on this study and concludes, "There is emerging evidence to suggest that glucosamine is an appropriate treatment for people with arthritis of the knee."

Though the study focused on arthritis of the knee, Nancy Lane, M.D., codirector of clinical rheumatology at San Francisco General Hospital and one of the National Institutes of Health investigators, says, "If it's going to work on the knee to reduce pain, it may work for other joints." The experts aren't sure exactly how glucosamine

THREE THINGS I TELL EVERY FEMALE PATIENT

JEFFREY R. LISSE, M.D., head of clinical osteoporosis research, associate chief of the Arizona Arthritis Center, and professor of medicine at the University of Arizona College of Medicine in Tucson, offers this special advice.

1 USE A CREAM. "I have some luck with capsaicin cream with my patients," says Dr. Lisse. Capsaicin is a substance found in hot peppers, and in this topical analgesic cream, it acts on nerve endings to ease arthritis pain. The cream doesn't work instantly, so repeated applications are key. Also, it produces a burning feeling when you first apply it, but this side effect diminishes over time. Follow label directions carefully, and thoroughly wash hands after each application to avoid stinging if you accidentally contact your eyes or other sensitive areas later. Capsaicin cream is available at drugstores.

2 EXERCISE. "It's important to exercise daily to keep the joints and muscles flexible and moving. If you stay physically active, you'll see an improvement in symptoms," says Dr. Lisse.

3 KEEP YOUR WEIGHT DOWN. "Obese women have more problems with arthritis because extra weight puts pressure on the joints. Keeping weight within the normal range may lower the risk of developing osteoarthritis," says Dr. Lisse. "For the woman who already has arthritis, keeping her weight in check will reduce the pressure, which eases pain. If you're overweight and can't lose on your own, talk to your doctor. He can put you in touch with a dietitian who can design a weight-loss program tailored to your tastes and needs." ■

works. Made from extracts from crab, lobster, and shrimp shells, it contains the chemical building blocks the body needs to make and repair cartilage.

In addition, some research shows that glucosamine soothes knee pain as well as ibuprofen does, but without the stomach upset, bleeding, or ulcers that long-term use of high doses of NSAIDs can cause. Studies also show that it can slow cartilage loss, although it may work only for mild to moderate arthritis. "Glucosamine may prevent further wear and tear on the joints by maintaining the integrity of cartilage," says Dr. Lisse. *Prevention* magazine recommends 1,500 milligrams a day in two or three doses. You should take it for at least 8 weeks before deciding whether it works for you.

Try SAM-e. Some experts believe this supplement may improve joint mobility and relieve the pain of osteoarthritis by boosting levels of an amino acid, adenosine triphosphate (ATP), and supporting cartilage production. Some studies have shown that SAM-e may help relieve mild osteoarthritis pain almost as well as NSAIDs, but without digestive discomfort. *Prevention* recommends a dose of 200 to 400 milligrams three times a day.

medical options

Ask about new medicines. If taking NSAIDs causes gastrointestinal problems, ask your doctor to prescribe a different medication. COX-2 inhibitors such as celecoxib (Celebrex) and rofecoxib (Vioxx), for example, are prescription drugs that block pain and inflammation but cause less stomach irritation than NSAIDs do.

For more information: Contact the Arthritis Foundation (1330 West Peachtree Street, Atlanta, GA 30309; 800-283-7800; www.arthritis.org) or the National Institute of Arthritis and Musculoskeletal and Skin Diseases (1 AMS Circle, Bethesda, MD 20892-2350; www.nih.gov/niams).

asthma

Contrary to what many people may believe, feeling rotten doesn't have to be part of living with asthma.

"The American Lung Association did a study of 1,300 families and found that people with asthma think that waking up in the middle of the night with symptoms, getting out of breath, not participating in sports, and going to the ER and being hospitalized are absolutely normal. But this is not normal," says Linda B. Ford, M.D., past president of the American Lung Association and an allergist in Omaha, Nebraska. People with asthma who find themselves having "events" or curtailing their normal activities need to be more aggressive about getting the appropriate treatment, she says.

For one thing, studies have shown that allergy shots, or immunotherapy, may prevent asthma, and regular injections can also help after you've been diagnosed.

For others, a host of medications—either inhaled or taken as a pill, or a combination—can keep asthma under control. "With proper diagnosis, treatment, education—and close monitoring—the vast majority of people with asthma can lead normal lives," says Bill Berger, M.D., clinical professor in the division of allergy and immunology at the University of California, Irvine; vice president of the American College of Allergy, Asthma, and Immunology; and author of *Allergies and Asthma for Dummies*. "The key is to take control of the disease and not let it control you."

Asthma causes what doctors call twitchy lungs, which overreact to stimuli that are harmless to many people. Anxiety, animal dander, dust mites, and even your monthly menstrual cycle can trigger asthma episodes or worsen existing symptoms. When asthma flares, the muscles around your bronchial tubes squeeze tightly, causing the airways to narrow. Then the inflamed bronchial tubes swell even more and produce thick mucus.

Although the exact cause is not known, if you have episodes of wheezing and coughing, you probably inherited from a parent the propensity to have asthma. Then, with repeated exposures to your environment, sensitivity develops and symptoms begin. Doctors also know that childhood allergies increase the risk of developing asthma and that children of women who smoked during pregnancy are also more likely have it. "One study showed that 50 percent of babies delivered to mothers who smoked went on to develop asthma. That increased risk was only from the exposure the baby received in utero," says Dr. Ford.

Here are some strategies that can help you calm your twitchy lungs and breathe easier.

For Immediate Relief

home remedies

Know the signals. Most asthma attacks start slowly, and you can often stop an episode in its tracks by using medication. Anyone with asthma should learn the warning signs, which include wheezing, faster-than-normal breathing, an itchy or sore throat, tightness in your chest, shortness of breath, coughing, or a drop in your peak flow rate, measured by a device called a peak flow meter. When you blow into this device, a mechanism that moves a small pointer along a scale measures how well your lungs are able to expel air, which is known as the peak flow rate. At the first sign of an attack, the best advice for most people is to take their medication and rest.

Relax and breathe. During a mild attack, "sit down and take a few sips of a warm beverage," Dr. Ford advises. Concentrate on breathing slowly. If those steps don't work, use your reliever inhaler. You and your doctor should have previously decided on an "asthma action plan" for attacks, so follow it now. "If you don't have one, ask your doctor for one," Dr. Ford says. The asthma action plan should include self-assessment either with peak flow monitoring or symptom monitoring and self-management prescribed by your doctor, which should include what to do if you have acute asthma symptoms and when to call the doctor or 911.

Long-Term Solutions

medical options

Have an allergy test. To change your asthma, you must change your environment. "In asthma, prevention—and avoidance—is really the key," says Monica Kraft, M.D., director of the Carl and Hazel Felt Lab of Adult Asthma Research and associate professor of medicine at the National Jewish Medical and Research Center in Denver.

"One of the worst mistakes that people make is not finding out what their triggers are, so they arbitrarily get rid of the cat, or whatever. The answer is to be tested for allergies," adds Ira M. Finegold, M.D., assistant clinical professor of medicine at Columbia University and chief of the division of allergy and clinical immunology and director of the R. A. Cooke Institute of Allergy at St. Luke's–Roosevelt Hospital Center, both in New York City.

home remedies

Reduce your exposure. If you discover that you are allergic to your cat, for example, and you can't bear to get rid of the animal, keep her outdoors or in the basement. At the very least, keep her out of your bedroom. To reduce dander, wash your pet at least two or three times a month with a shampoo recommended by your veterinarian.

THREE THINGS I TELL EVERY FEMALE PATIENT

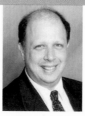

RAN ANBAR, M.D., associate professor of pediatrics and director of pediatric pulmonary medicine at the State University of New York Upstate Medical University in Syracuse, offers this special advice.

TAKE YOUR MIND TO A RELAXING PLACE. Imagine yourself somewhere that's delightful, peaceful, and especially meaningful to you, such as a quiet beach. Do you smell the fresh ocean spray? Can you hear the roar of the surf as it crashes against the sand and feel the warm water on your skin? "The more senses you imagine using, the more relaxing it is," Dr. Anbar says.

CREATE A HYPNOTIC SUGGESTION. Each time you mentally travel to your special spot, touch one thumb with the forefinger of the same hand. Remind yourself that whenever you touch your fingers in this way, you'll be able to relax and breathe more easily. You can use this suggestion as you use your rescue medicine, or try using self-hypnosis first, then see if you still need to use your medication, Dr. Anbar says. He adds: "The average adult needs more practice than the average kid. Kids are incredibly imaginative."

FIND A PRO. Dr. Anbar recommends that beginners work with a hypnotist certified by the American Society of Clinical Hypnosis, a professional group that requires significant training for certification. ■

Rake with care. Stirring up those colorful leaves can expose you to *Alternaria alternata*, one of the most common autumn molds in the United States, and put you at risk for severe asthma attacks and allergic reactions.

If you must rake, take your medication first. Better yet, have a relative or friend take over the chore, or hire someone to do it. Avoid leaf blowers—even those used by lawn-care companies—because they spit mold into the air at full force.

To keep mold out of your home during leaf cleanup, close the windows and leave them closed for at least an hour.

Check the medicine cabinet. Some medicines—such as the beta-blockers propranolol (Inderal) and metoprolol (Lopressor) used to treat heart disease, high blood pressure, and migraines—can worsen asthma.

In addition, 10 to 20 percent of all people who experience asthma are sensitive to common over-the-counter painkillers such as aspirin and ibuprofen, and acetaminophen can also trigger asthma attacks.

So make doubly sure that any doctor who prescribes medication for you knows that you have asthma.

Breathe easy with a cup of joe. According to one large study, men and women with asthma who drank two to three cups of coffee each day reported 25 percent fewer attacks than those who didn't go for java. Caffeine, a chemical cousin of the anti-asthma drug theophylline, relaxes the smooth muscles of the bronchial tubes and keeps airways open.

mind-body techniques

Help yourself with hypnosis. People with asthma and others with chronic diseases can calm their symptoms with self-hypnosis, says Ran Anbar, M.D., associate professor of pediatrics and director of pediatric pulmonary medicine at the State University of New York Upstate Medical University in Syracuse.

Dr. Anbar once worked with a 12-year-old girl with very severe asthma. After learning self-hypnosis, she was able to wean herself off rescue medicine, which she had been using five times a day, and dramatically cut back on oral steroid medications that she had been taking for 8 years.

"I want patients to know they have the power themselves, and they can tap into it," he says.

medical options

Take care of monthly problems. Some women notice that their asthma worsens just before and during their periods.

"Check your peak flow readings and see if lower levels are tied to your cycle," advises Harold S. Nelson, M.D., an immunologist and codirector of clinical research at the National Jewish Medical and Research Center in Denver. "If you notice changes, talk to your doctor about changing your maintenance medicines."

Be prepared for emergencies. People who have food allergies as well as asthma are especially susceptible to a life-threatening allergic reaction called anaphylaxis.

"We tell all patients who have both food allergies and asthma to carry Benadryl (an antihistamine) and an EpiPen (a form of lifesaving epinephrine) with them at all times, even if they've never had an anaphylactic event," says Hugh A. Sampson, M.D., director of the Elliot and Roslyn Jaffe Food Allergy Institute at Mount Sinai School of Medicine in New York City.

For more information: Contact the American Lung Association (1740 Broadway, New York, NY 10019; www.lungusa.org) or the American Academy of Allergy, Asthma, and Immunology (800-822-2762; www.aaaai.org).

back problems

The next time you're walking down the street or shopping at the mall, take a look around you—eight out of 10 people that you see will experience back troubles at some time in their lives.

"Back pain can come on suddenly and drop you to your knees, or it can be a chronic, long-term condition," says Stephen Hochschuler, M.D., clinical instructor at the University of Texas Health Science Center in Dallas, founder and chairman of the Texas Back Institute in Plano, and author of *Treat Your Back without Surgery*.

It's not surprising that back problems are as common as they are. The back is subjected to enormous amounts of stress. Whether you're sitting, standing, bending over, lifting bags and boxes, or simply turning to look behind you, the muscles, ligaments, and bones in the spine feel the strain. The lower back, called the lumbar region, is especially vulnerable because it supports a tremendous amount of weight. That's why it's the most injury-prone area of the entire spine, says Dr. Hochschuler.

Men and women suffer from back pain equally, but women have some special risks. After menopause, when a woman's estrogen

levels decline, the bones begin to lose calcium at an accelerated rate. This makes them thinner and weaker than they should be. This condition, called osteoporosis, increases the risk of spinal fractures. Osteoporosis affects both men and women, but women with osteoporosis greatly outnumber men.

when to see a doctor

 If you've hurt your back and the pain hasn't improved after 3 days, make an appointment to see your doctor. You may have suffered nerve or tissue damage that won't improve without medical treatment, says Deborah Saint-Phard, M.D., a physiatrist at the Women's Sports Medical Center at the Hospital for Special Surgery in New York City.

If the pain is excruciating and nothing you do seems to help: You may need prescription drugs to reduce pain, muscle spasms, or inflammation.

If you've lost bowel or bladder function, or if you're having numbness, tingling, or a loss of muscle strength: You could have suffered nerve damage that may require surgery or other medical treatments.

Another problem is the design of the spine itself. The bones of the spine, called vertebrae, are separated by shock-absorbing disks that are somewhat similar in structure to jelly doughnuts: They have a tough outer coating that surrounds a soft center. Over the years, the disks lose moisture and flexibility. They literally shrink and lose some of their ability to absorb shocks or impacts. In some cases, the disks actually rupture, or herniate: The soft material in the center leaks out and puts pressure on tissues in the spine, including the spinal nerves.

"As women start getting into their thirties and forties, the early signs of degenerative disk disease can begin," says Deborah Saint-Phard, M.D., assistant attending physiatrist at the Women's Sports Medical Center at the Hospital for Special Surgery in New York City. As women get older, their risk of developing osteoporosis rises—and the bones themselves become increasingly susceptible to damage. "Even if there's very little stress put on the back, compression fractures are common in women with osteoporosis," she says.

For men and women, extra weight is among the main risk factors for back problems. Even if you're only a few pounds over your ideal weight, those extra pounds are supported by the back. Year after year, they put unnecessary stress on the spine. Even if your disks hold up and your bones remain strong, the muscles and ligaments in the back will feel the strain.

Keeping your back strong requires a combination of strategies, including getting enough calcium in your diet, watching your weight, and keeping the muscles and ligaments strong and flexible.

Even if you do everything right, there's a good chance that you'll eventually suffer a bout of back pain. Most back problems are "self-limiting," which means they'll get better on their own. In the meantime, of course, the pain can be excruciating. Here are a few ways to quickly ease the discomfort of minor backaches and strains—and some long-term strategies for keeping your back strong and healthy.

For Immediate Relief

home remedies

Ice the pain. "Right after you hurt your back, the first thing you should do is apply ice to the area," says Dr. Hochschuler. "Ice will constrict the blood vessels, which reduces bloodflow and decreases swelling."

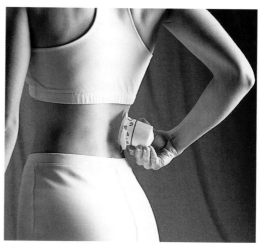

Icing an injury reduces bloodflow and inflammation, which reduces pain as well as the risk of long-term damage.

Ice works best within the first 48 hours after an injury, Dr. Hochschuler adds. If you don't have an ice pack at home, you can wrap a washcloth or dish towel around some ice cubes. Apply the pack for only 5 to 10 minutes at a time. Or fill a few paper cups with water and freeze them. Peel back the paper and apply the ice directly to the sore spots, in a circular motion, for no more than 5 to 10 minutes at a time.

Follow ice with heat. When you've hurt your back, most of the swelling occurs within the first 2 days—which is why applying ice is the best initial treatment. After 2 days, however, you want to *increase* bloodflow to the area, which will help the damaged tissues heal.

"Put a heating pad on the area for 20 minutes at a time, using a lower setting in order to avoid a burn," says Dr. Hochschuler. Another option is to lounge in a hot bath several times a day. "Standing in a hot shower will also help relieve the pain," says Dr. Saint-Phard.

Take anti-inflammatory drugs. Over-the-counter pain relievers are among the best treatments for back injuries because they inhibit the body's production of prostaglandins, chemicals that excite nerve endings and cause pain. Aspirin, ibuprofen, naproxen, and acetaminophen all can be helpful, says Dr. Hochschuler.

Get some rest—immediately. Back pain is your body's way of telling you that you've done something wrong. Don't ignore the message: Stop whatever you've been doing, and give your back a chance to recover.

If you hurt your back playing golf, stop

THREE THINGS I TELL EVERY FEMALE PATIENT

DEBORAH SAINT-PHARD, M.D., a physiatrist at the Women's Sports Medical Center at the Hospital for Special Surgery in New York City, advises her back patients to do the following:

CHANGE POSITIONS OFTEN. Whether you've recently hurt your back or simply want to avoid problems later, don't spend too much time in any one position. It's especially important not to sit for extended periods because it increases pressure on the spine.

BE CONSCIOUS OF HOW YOU MOVE. "Little stresses accumulate to cause back problems," says Dr. Saint-Phard. "Bend your knees when lifting objects—even if you're just picking up a feather. Just because you don't feel pain doesn't mean that you're not creating abnormal stress on the back."

FIND EXERCISES THAT WORK FOR YOU. Regular exercise is among the best ways to manage—and prevent—serious back problems, but there isn't a one-size-fits-all exercise plan. "What works to relieve back pain for one woman may cause it in another," says Dr. Saint-Phard. "If you try a new exercise and have a backache the next day, move on to something else." ∎

playing and take a break in the clubhouse. If you've been working in the yard, put down the rake and take the rest of the day off. Staying active when the muscles and ligaments are irritated will only increase the damage—and increase the risk of long-term damage.

"Even if the pain is severe enough to warrant bed rest, limit it to 2 days," Dr. Hochschuler adds. "Staying inactive for longer than 2 days will cause the back muscles to weaken and become stiff and inflexible."

Walk it off. "If you can tolerate it, go for a short walk," says Dr. Hochschuler. Walking is a gentle aerobic activity that gets the blood moving and stretches out stiff muscles. "It can also relieve some of the tension that could be contributing to your back pain," Dr. Hochschuler adds.

Try water walking. "If walking on hard surfaces is too painful, try walking in a pool (if you have access)," says Dr. Hochschuler. "It's less painful because the water creates an environment of near weightlessness. Start out slowly, and as it becomes easier, walk faster."

Long-Term Solutions

home remedies

Change positions often. It's not unusual for back problems to persist for weeks or even months. One of the best ways to relieve stiffness and also prevent future problems is to change positions frequently. This is especially important if you spend a lot of time sitting, which puts a tremendous amount of stress on the lower spine, says Dr. Saint-Phard.

"Every 20 minutes, take a break and change your position," she advises. If you tend to get so focused on your work that you lose track of time, set an alarm or the beeper on your watch. When you hear the alarm, get up and walk around. Do some stretching exercises. Or simply stand up for a while. The change in position will prevent muscles and ligaments in the spine from "locking" into position.

Lift with your knees, not your back. "It's of paramount importance that women use their knees and hips to bend down and pick up kids or groceries," says Dr. Saint-Phard. Whether you're picking up something light, like a piece of paper, or something heavy, like a large carton, bend your knees and get in a squatting position. "The back should remain fairly erect while the knees bend, as opposed to bending forward at the waist," she explains.

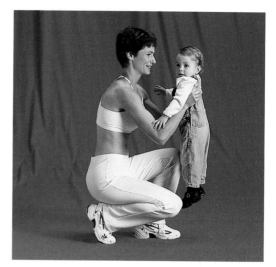

When lifting, always bend your knees and not your back. It's among the best ways to prevent back pain.

(continued on page 334)

Strengthen
Your Back Muscles

People who stay in shape don't necessarily have a lower risk for back pain, but they do tend to recover more quickly from back attacks than those who are sedentary and out of shape, says Stephen Hochschuler, M.D., clinical instructor at the University of Texas Health Science Center in Dallas, founder and chairman of the Texas Back Institute in Plano, and author of *Treat Your Back without Surgery*. One of the best exercises for your back is also the simplest. It's called opposite arm and leg lift, and it strengthens the abdominal muscles as well as those in the back. It protects the spine and also improves your posture.

When doing the exercise, try to complete eight to 12 "lifts" with each arm and leg. Rest a moment, then repeat the series again. Doing the exercise two or three times a week will keep your muscles strong and limber.

Opposite Arm and Leg Lift

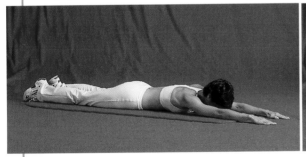 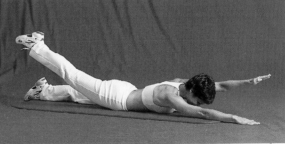

Lie facedown with your legs extended straight behind you, toes pointed and your arms extended straight over your head. Keep your chin up off the floor at a comfortable level.

Slowly raise your left arm and your right leg at the same time until they are both a few inches off the floor. Hold, then slowly lower them back to the starting position. Repeat on the other side.

The Best Exercises for Preventing Back Pain

You need to strengthen your abdominal and back muscles in order to support and protect the spine. It's also important to stretch the hamstrings (the muscles in the back of the thighs) and hips. The following exercises will go a long way toward keeping your back strong and pain-free.

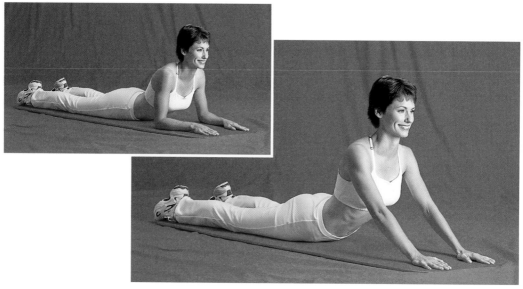

Back Extension

Lie on your stomach. Keeping your hips on the floor, prop yourself up on your forearms and raise your chest (left). Hold the stretch for a few seconds, then raise your upper body as far as you can by straightening your elbows and arching your back (right). Go as far as you comfortably can, hold the position for 10 seconds, then relax.

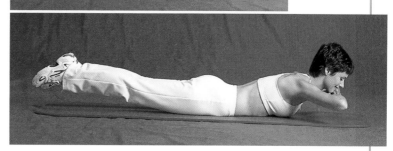

Chest Lift

Lie on your stomach with your hands under your chin (top). Lift your head and feet about 1 to 2 inches off the floor; don't arch your back too much (bottom). Hold the position for a few seconds, then lower yourself.

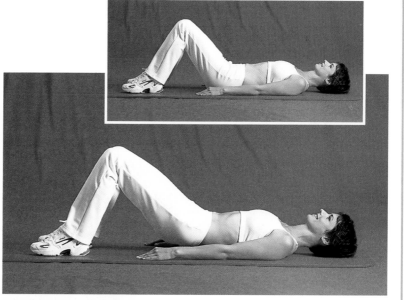

Bridge Lift

Lie on your back with your knees bent and your arms at your sides (top). Slowly lift your pelvis and buttocks off the floor (bottom), hold for about 5 seconds, then lower yourself.

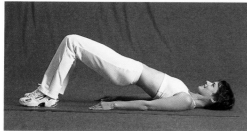

As you get stronger, try to lift your torso until there's a straight line between your knees and shoulders.

continued

The Best Exercises for Preventing Back Pain

continued

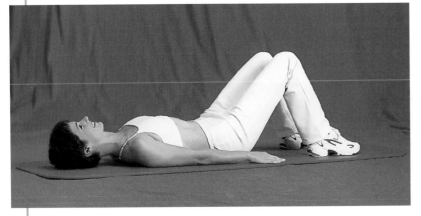

Pelvic Tuck

Lie on your back with your knees bent. Tighten the abdominal muscles and tilt the pelvis upward until the small of your back presses against the floor. Hold for 5 seconds, then relax.

Mini-Crunch

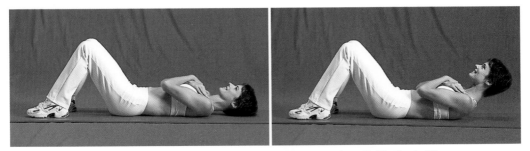

Lie on your back with your knees bent and your arms crossed on your chest (left). Slowly lift your head and shoulders until your shoulder blades come off the floor; don't bend your neck (right). Hold the position for a few seconds, then lower yourself.

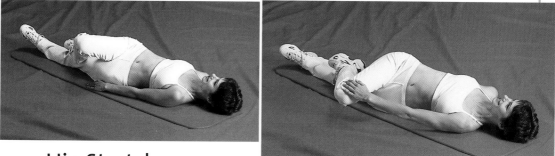

Hip Stretch

Lie on your back with your legs straight. Bend your right leg so it crosses over the left, keeping your foot near your left knee (left). Using your left hand, gently press your right knee toward the floor until you feel a stretch in your right hip and buttocks (right). Hold the stretch for 10 to 30 seconds, then relax. Repeat the exercise with the left leg.

Hamstring Stretch

Lie flat on your back with your legs bent and both feet on the floor. Loop a towel or rope under the arch of your left foot. While keeping a slight bend at the knee, straighten and raise your left leg off the floor and gently pull your leg toward your chest as far as is comfortable. Hold for 10 to 30 seconds, then relax. Repeat on the other leg.

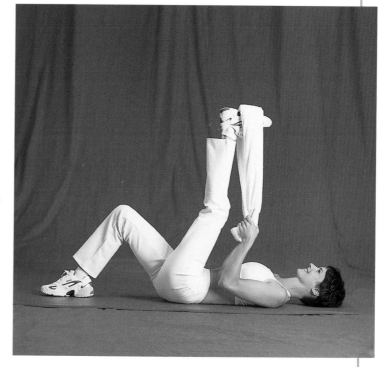

Bend your knees when you sleep. One reason that people often wake up with stiff backs is that they sleep on their stomachs. This causes the back to arch, which puts a lot of pressure on the muscles and ligaments.

"If you have back pain at night or in the morning, it's a good idea to sleep with the knees bent," says Dr. Saint-Phard. "Lie on your side, and put a pillow between your legs. If you're lying on your back, place the pillow beneath the legs."

Try not to twist. "The spine does not like to be bent or twisted, especially when you're lifting things, says Dr. Saint-Phard. Remind yourself to keep your spine straight whenever possible, she advises.

Plan before you move. A lot of back injuries occur when people are doing simple, everyday ac-

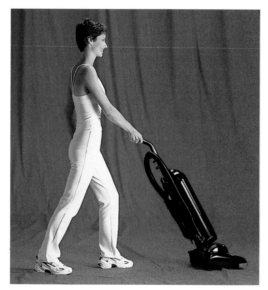

It's always better to bend your knees than to bend your back. Bending your knees slightly and using the hip, leg, and butt muscles can dramatically reduce strain on the lower back.

tivities—but doing them the wrong way. When you're vacuuming or making the bed, for example, do you bend forward at the waist? If so, you're putting a lot of unnecessary pressure on the back.

"Use your leg, hip, and butt muscles to move the vacuum cleaner," Dr. Saint-Phard advises. When you're making the bed or unloading the dishwasher, bend your knees or even kneel down. Your goal should always be to keep your back as straight as possible.

Try to relax. Anxiety and stress cause your muscles to tighten, and tight muscles often lead to back pain. If you already have back problems, emotional stress invariably makes the pain worse. That's why back specialists advise their patients to do everything they can to reduce the tension in their lives.

One technique that often helps is progressive relaxation, says Dr. Hochschuler. It's very easy to do. While you're sitting or lying down, focus on your muscles one at a time. Start with the muscles in your toes; tighten them for a few seconds, then relax. When you're done with your feet, move upward to your legs, hips, back, and chest. It takes 10 to 20 minutes to tense and relax all the muscle groups. When you're done, you'll find that a lot of the tension and stress in your body—and your mind—will have melted away.

alternative therapies

Give willow bark a try. Aspirin is among the most effective remedies for back pain, but it may cause stomach irritation or other side effects. An alternative is to use the herb willow bark, which contains a compound called salicin—the same active ingredient that's found in aspirin. For long-term back pain, willow bark may be superior to aspirin because it's less likely to cause side effects. Health food stores sell a variety of willow bark remedies. Look for products containing 250 milligrams of white willow bark, along with 200 milligrams of white willow bark extract that's been standardized to contain 15 percent salicin. The recommended dose is two to four capsules daily.

Willow bark is safe for most people, but those who are allergic to aspirin or other over-the-counter pain relievers may be allergic to willow bark as well.

medical options

Ask your doctor about PENS. If you've had long-term back pain, your doctor may recommend a procedure called PENS, short for percutaneous electrical nerve stimulation. Acupuncture-like needles are inserted into the soft tissues and muscles surrounding the bones. A small electrical current passes through the needles, which interrupts pain signals.

Researchers at the University of Texas Southwestern Medical Center in Dallas found that back patients treated with PENS required smaller amounts of painkillers. They also slept better and reported feeling better overall.

For more information: Visit the Web site of the National Institute of Neurological Disorders and Stroke at www.ninds.nih.gov.

blemishes, pimples, and breakouts

The teenage years are the prime time for acne, but even women in their thirties, forties, and beyond can suffer from occasional breakouts. The only difference is that teenage acne is mainly guided by heredity; adult women can often blame hormonal fluctuations for unsightly cyclic blemishes.

Even women who never had acne when they were young may have flare-ups in later years—either in conjunction with the menstrual cycle or with the onset of menopause, says Leslie Baumann, M.D., director of cosmetic dermatology at the University of Miami Cosmetic Center.

Treatments for acne have gotten increasingly sophisticated in the past few decades. You can't prevent the occasional pimple from popping up, but with a combination of medications and home remedies, it's usually easy to keep acne flare-ups under control.

For Immediate Relief

home remedies

Use benzoyl peroxide. A topical antiseptic, it kills the bacteria that cause the inflammation, swelling, and discomfort of acne. Available over the counter in cream gel or lotion form, benzoyl peroxide (such as Clearasil) may be the only treatment that you need.

After washing your face, spread a thin layer of benzoyl peroxide over the affected areas. Individual dosages and product formulations vary, so follow your doctor's advice. Generally, benzoyl peroxide should be used once a day at first; as your skin gets used it, gradually increase to six or eight times daily or as needed during outbreaks.

Try salicylic acid. Another over-the-counter remedy, salicylic acid (which is similar to the active ingredient in aspirin), reduces inflammation and loosens the bonds between dead cells, allowing them to shed more easily.

Clean your skin thoroughly, then apply a thin layer of salicylic acid (such as Stri-Dex) to the acne pimple areas. This medication may cause drying of your skin. Dosage varies for each individual and product, so it's best to follow your doctor's instructions. Usually, you start with one application per day and gradually increase to three applications per day as needed.

alternative therapies

Apply a clay paste. Clay has been used for centuries for deep-cleaning oily complexions and removing impurities from the skin. To prepare a poultice for blemishes, combine $\frac{1}{2}$ teaspoon of cosmetic clay (available at health food stores and some cosmetics counters and from online stores) with $\frac{1}{2}$ teaspoon of water. You may need to prepare more of the mixture if you have a larger area to treat or if you want to use it as a facial mask. Mix well, then apply a thin layer over the entire face for deep cleaning, or just on the blemishes, and let the clay dry. If the area you're treating is small, you can leave the poultice on for several hours or overnight, then wash it off. Masks need to be rinsed off thoroughly immediately after the clay dries. Repeat the poultice treatments as needed once daily. Use the clay mask only once a week to avoid overdrying your skin.

Use essential oil of lavender. It makes pimples less painful, and because it has antibacterial and anti-inflammatory properties, it may help

when to see a doctor

If your acne is accompanied by menstrual irregularities, thinning hair, weight gain, or visible facial hair, call your doctor. You might need blood tests to check for excess androgens, "male" hormones that can cause acne outbreaks, says Teresa Soriano, M.D., assistant professor of dermatology at UCLA School of Medicine.

If you have acnelike bumps on your face, especially on the mid-face (forehead, nose, cheeks, and chin) and facial redness and you can also see broken blood vessels, which resemble threads, through the skin: You could have a condition known as rosacea, sometimes called "adult acne." Rosacea may require treatment with antibiotics or other medications.

If the acne doesn't get better with home care: Your doctor may recommend medications, including birth control pills, oral antibiotics, and other drugs to get the outbreaks under control.

eliminate them as well. Apply 1 or 2 drops of lavender oil to pimples as needed.

Ask your dermatologist about facial peels. Unlike the mild salicylic acid that's used in home preparations, your dermatologist may recommend treating acne with a highly concentrated form containing 20 to 30 percent salicylic acid. It removes the surface layer of skin and can improve or eliminate acne within 2 to 4 days, says Dr. Baumann.

Try tretinoin. Available by prescription, it's a derivative of vitamin A. It reduces oil production in the skin, taking away the "fuel" that triggers acne. Applied once daily, tretinoin (Renova) will help eliminate pimples that are already present, and it may help others from forming.

Ask about isotretinoin. This is among the most powerful acne remedies, and it's used only for severe inflammatory acne and when simpler (and safer) treatments don't work. Isotretinoin (Accutane) is very effective, but it may cause ad-verse effects such as itching, headaches, photo-sensitivity, or hair loss, which may persist in some women. More serious possible side effects include elevations of blood fats, abnormal liver enzymes, inflammatory bowel disease, and hearing impairment. The most significant potential adverse effect is that it can cause birth defects if taken during pregnancy. Your doctor will prescribe this medication only if you're absolutely sure that you won't get pregnant while using it.

For Long-Term Relief

Keep stress under control. Emotional stress doesn't cause acne, but it can trigger outbreaks in some women by changing hormone levels and increasing oil gland secretion. If you notice that your complexion tends to get worse during emotionally difficult times, take it as a sign that it's time to unwind—by exercising more, working less, and practicing relaxation techniques such as meditation, deep breathing, or yoga.

breast pain and tenderness

Cramps, minor mood changes, and food cravings are just a few of the signs that a menstrual period is pending. Many women also experience breast pain. The pain usually starts midway though the menstrual cycle, may get progressively worse until the onset of the period, then dissipates. For some women, it can be severe enough to interfere with normal activities.

"Cyclic breast changes occur in response to fluctuating levels of the hormones estrogen and progesterone during the menstrual cycle," says Eric Whitacre, M.D., a surgeon at the Breast Center at Mercy Medical Center in Baltimore.

"The breasts may swell and become tender or painful, which may be due to hormonal changes."

Breast pain, called mastalgia, can have many other causes and affects women of all ages. But because breast tenderness is generally linked to the menstrual cycle, it's much more common in younger women than in those who are post-menopausal. However, any woman may experience pain due to breast tissue changes.

These changes, referred to as fibrocystic conditions, may cause occasional fluid retention in the breasts. The fluid exerts pressure on breast tissues, which in turn may cause pain, says Dr. Whitacre. In addition, some women develop tiny fluid-filled sacs, called cysts, in the milk glands. These cysts are harmless, but they can make the breasts tender for a few days.

Any type of lump or discomfort in the breasts should be brought to the attention of your doctor right away. In most cases, however, you won't have anything to worry about—and it may be possible to relieve the discomfort with a few simple strategies.

when to see a doctor

If you've just started experiencing breast pain, regardless of the time of month, make an appointment to see your doctor. It might be due to normal menstrual changes, or it could be related to medications you're taking, such as birth control or supplemental estrogen or other hormones, says Eric Whitacre, M.D., a surgeon at the Breast Center at Mercy Medical Center in Baltimore.

If there's a lump in or near the breast or in the underarm area; a spontaneous nipple discharge, especially if it's bloody; persistent changes in the breast skin, such as puckering or indentations (called dimpling), redness, or scaliness of the breast skin or nipple; pain in the nipple or the nipple turning inward; or a "funny" feeling, such as itching or tingling in the skin of the breast or the nipple: These are potential symptoms of breast cancer, and your doctor will probably advise you to have a mammogram or sonogram, says Dr. Whitacre.

For Immediate Relief

home remedies

Wear an exercise bra. It will give the breasts extra support. This is one of the best ways to reduce tenderness and pain. You can wear the bra any time it helps you with the discomfort—even while you sleep.

Take an analgesic. Aspirin and ibuprofen can provide fast-acting relief from monthly breast pain. They inhibit the body's production of prostaglandins, chemicals that cause pain and swelling.

For Long-Term Prevention

home remedies

Get less caffeine. Found in coffee, tea, caffeinated sodas, chocolate, and some over-the-counter medications, caffeine stimulates breast tissue, which may cause an increase in monthly pain, says Dr. Whitacre.

Take vitamin E. There's some evidence that vitamin E may reduce breast pain associated with the menstrual cycle as well as the discomforts of fibrocystic breast conditions. "We're not really sure why it works, but it's worth trying," says Dr. Whitacre.

He advises women with monthly breast pain to take 400 to 800 IU vitamin E daily. Try it for 3 months to see if it helps, he advises.

Try evening primrose oil. Found in over-the-counter supplements, it's rich in gamma linolenic acid, which can inhibit the action of prostaglandins. Evening primrose oil can also reduce painful inflammation. The research is inconclusive about its effectiveness in treating the discomforts of fibrocystic breast conditions. Although doctors aren't sure how it works, evening primrose oil supplements have been shown beneficial as a treatment for mastalgia associated with the menstrual cycle.

"At our clinic, we advise women to start with a minimum of 1,500 milligrams of evening primrose oil per day," says Dr. Whitacre. If that dose doesn't help, you can increase the amount to 3,000 milligrams daily. "Sometimes you have to start out high, then gradually taper off," Dr. Whitacre adds. "We've found that you have to take it for 2 or 3 months to see if it will be beneficial." It's advisable to take 1,000 to 2,000 milligrams of fish oil daily along with the evening primrose oil in order to provide a balance of omega-6s and omega-3s.

Keep a food diary. Breast pain is sometimes caused by foods or beverages in the diet. If you keep track of what you're eating and drinking, you may find that pain occurs, or gets worse, only when you eat certain foods.

"One of my patients was consuming large amounts of soy," says Dr. Whitacre. "Soy contains plant estrogens, and estrogen is implicated in breast pain," he explains.

cataracts

Imagine looking at the world through smudgy glasses, or trying to see the countryside through a windshield that's never been washed. You can probably see fairly well, but things simply aren't as clear as they should be.

"A significant number of people with cataracts don't know they have a problem until they are told during a routine eye exam," says Robert Abel Jr., M.D., clinical professor of ophthalmology at Thomas Jefferson University School of Medicine in Philadelphia and author of *The Eye Care Revolution.*

Cataracts occur when proteins clump together in the normally clear lenses of the eyes. They can cause blindness in some cases, but more often they make vision a little blurry or decrease your ability to see in dim light.

"It may be possible to keep recently formed cataracts stable and less likely to cause problems," says Dr. Abel.

For Immediate Relief

Drink plenty of water. The lenses of the eyes don't have their own blood supply. They depend on a tiny trickle of fluid, called aqueous humor, to get the nourishment they need. "You can't believe how much better people will see when they drink enough water," says Dr. Abel. At a minimum, drink six full glasses of water daily, he advises.

Eat blueberries. They contain chemical compounds called anthocyanosides, which strengthen blood vessels in the eyes and also prevent damage from free radicals, harmful oxygen molecules that often damage tissues in the eyes.

"Periodically go outside and look at the stars," Dr. Abel advises. When you've been eating $1/2$ cup of blueberries daily (or drinking bilberry tea, which has the same active compounds), within 3 days the stars should appear sharper and more distinct.

Give up cigarettes. The smoke unleashes enormous numbers of free radicals. If you're not ready to quit, at least take a vitamin C and B-complex vitamin supplement: It will help protect eye tissues from toxins in smoke, says Dr. Abel.

Consider eye surgery. Operations to remove cataracts are extremely satisfying for doctors as well as patients because they're quick, safe, and nearly pain-free, says John D. Hunkeler, M.D., clinical professor of ophthalmology at the University of Kansas School of Medicine in Kansas City.

The surgery is done as an outpatient procedure. More than 95 percent of those who have cataracts removed will have significant improvements in their vision.

For Long-Term Prevention

Put on your sunglasses. Researchers at Johns Hopkins School of Medicine in Baltimore found that the risk of cataracts was 57 percent higher in people who had the most sun exposure, compared with those who had the least.

"Every time you go out without adequate protection, you're increasing your risk," says Sheila K. West, Ph.D., professor of ophthalmology at Johns Hopkins University. Plastic lenses are slightly better than glass at blocking the sun's cataract-causing rays, she adds.

Eat brightly colored vegetables. Broccoli, carrots, sweet potatoes, and other fruits and vegetables with vivid hues are loaded with

when to see a doctor

If you're experiencing changes in vision that are affecting your daily life, get your eyes examined by an ophthalmologist: You could be developing cataracts or another type of eye disease, says John D. Hunkeler, M.D., clinical professor of ophthalmology at the University of Kansas School of Medicine in Kansas City.

If your vision has abruptly gotten worse: There could be a vascular problem that's affecting circulation to the eyes.

carotenoids, pigments that block the eye-damaging effects of free radicals.

One study of more than 50,000 women ages 45 to 67 found that eating five servings of spinach a week reduced cataract formation by 39 percent.

Don't forget the asparagus. Along with onions, eggs, and lean red meats, asparagus is rich in cysteine, an amino acid that's converted in the body to glutathione. Glutathione is a powerful antioxidant that protects the eyes from free radical damage.

Take a vitamin E supplement. People who supplement their diets with vitamin E are up to 56 percent less likely to get cataracts than those who don't. Dr. Abel recommends taking 400 IU vitamin E daily. "Take it with meals," he adds. "It's a fat-soluble nutrient, and taking it with a little fat will increase your body's ability to absorb it."

Get extra vitamin C. It concentrates in the eyes and helps prevent cataracts from getting worse, says Dr. Abel, who recommends taking 1,000 milligrams daily.

For more information on cataracts: Visit the Web site of the National Eye Institute at www.nei.nih.gov.

colds

There's a good reason that colds are called "common." Doctors estimate that men, women, and children alike get 1 billion colds every year. On any given day, nearly one in four young women is reaching for the tissue box, swabbing her eyes, and counting the days until the miserable infection runs its course.

So far, there isn't a cure for the common cold, and there isn't a lot you can do to prevent them. Vaccines don't help because colds are caused by more than 200 viruses, each of which is constantly changing and adapting to whatever medical science throws at it. In addition, cold viruses are everywhere—on your hands, in the air, and on doorknobs, washcloths, and toothbrushes.

Colds are rarely serious, of course, and most people start feeling better within a week. But if you act quickly, you may be able to reduce much of the discomfort and even shorten the duration of the illness. Here's what experts advise.

For Immediate Relief

home remedies

Breathe some steam. It provides quick relief by thinning mucus in your nose, chest, and sinuses and making it easier for the body to expel. When you take your morning shower, run the water a little hotter than usual, and luxuriate while the hot, moist air enters your airways.

Here's another way to take advantage of soothing steam: Fill a cooking pot about a quarter of the way with water. Bring the water nearly to a boil, then add a few drops of eucalyptus oil. Remove the pot from the heat and place it on a protected table or counter. Drape a towel over your head, lean over the pot, and breathe the steam. Be careful not to burn yourself. The eucalyptus thins the mucus and will help you breathe a little easier. Look for eucalyptus oil at a health food store or pharmacy.

Take advantage of chicken soup. It's a traditional cold remedy, and there's some evidence that it helps. Apart from the fact that the heat and steam will make you feel better, the onions and garlic in chicken soup contain antiviral compounds that will help eliminate the virus, says Mary L. Hardy, M.D., medical director of the Integrative Medical Group at Cedars-Sinai Medical Center in Los Angeles.

Add some hot spices. To make chicken soup even more effective, season it with cayenne or chile peppers, suggests Dr. Hardy. Both spices contain a fiery compound called capsaicin, which will quickly clear mucus from the nose and sinuses.

Take plenty of fluids. When you're sick, the body requires extra water to replace fluids that are "burned off" by fever, and also to flush the body of accumulated toxins. Drinking a lot of water, juice, or tea also may thin respiratory secretions, says Kay A. Bauman, M.D., professor of medicine and associate dean at the John A. Burns School of Medicine at the University of Hawaii in Honolulu.

Clear congestion with salt water. Over-the-counter nasal sprays make it easier to breathe, but they often have a "rebound" effect—the congestion gets worse as soon as you quit using them. An alternative is to spritz your nose with salt water. It works nearly as well as over-the-counter sprays, and it won't cause an increase in congestion later.

To make a spray, mix $\frac{1}{8}$ to $\frac{1}{4}$ teaspoon of salt in 8 ounces of water. Suck the solution into a nasal aspirator and give a quick spray. The solu-

WHAT WORKS FOR ME

ANNE L. DAVIS, M.D., *is a pulmonologist and associate professor of medicine at New York University School of Medicine and an attending physician at Bellevue Hospital, both in New York City. She spends most of her days caring for patients with respiratory illnesses—and over the years she has come up with her own strategies for dealing with the common cold.*

I drink hot tea and soups, especially chicken soup, which some studies have shown is particularly beneficial for relieving cold symptoms. I drink a lot of orange juice, both for the vitamin C and to increase my fluid intake. For my throat, I gargle with warm salt water, and I also take honey and lemon, which are very soothing.

I'm not convinced that nasal decongestants can reduce the length or severity of cold symptoms. But when I'm really stuffed up or can't sleep, I'll take a single dose of an over-the-counter decongestant at night. If I have the opposite problem and am sneezing my head off, I'll take an antihistamine. ■

tion is entirely safe, so you can repeat the spray as often as necessary to get relief.

Take acetaminophen. It's the best over-the-counter remedy for reducing muscle aches, fever, head pain, and other cold symptoms. Unlike aspirin, it's unlikely to cause stomach upset. (It's also safer for children and teenagers, who may experience harmful reactions when they take aspirin or aspirin-like drugs.)

Reduce congestion with medications. Pharmacy shelves are packed with products that relieve nose and chest congestion. Over-the-counter decongestants won't cure a cold, but they will make it easier to sleep at night. Antihistamines are also effective. Products such as diphenhydramine (Benadryl) and chlorpheniramine (Chlor-Trimeton) often cause drowsiness, but they tend to be more effective at easing coughs and nasal congestion than nonsedating antihistamines.

alternative therapies

Boost immunity with yarrow. A medicinal herb, yarrow contains compounds that appear to stimulate the immune system's ability to battle colds, says Douglas Schar, Dip.Phyt., an herbalist in London and Washington, D.C., who specializes in disease prevention with herbal medicine. Yarrow also appears to reduce swelling of the mucous membranes and increases their resistance to viruses.

The best way to use yarrow is to take, three times daily, 20 drops of a 1:1 tincture or 1 teaspoon of a 1:5 tincture.

Fight fever with boneset. Another traditional herbal cold remedy, boneset is especially helpful at combating the aches and pains associated with a cold or the flu. Pour a cup of boiling water over ½ teaspoon of boneset. Let it steep, covered, for 30 minutes before drinking.

Shake the On-the-Job Attitudes That Can Make You Sick

Your attitude on the job could affect your odds of getting a nasty cold or flu this winter, a current study suggests.

When researchers tracked more than 200 workers over a period of 3 months, they found that those who had control over how they did their work but either lacked confidence or tended to blame themselves when things went wrong on the job, were more likely to catch the sniffles, flu, or other infections.

The reason behind this? For starters, people who lack confidence or tend to self-blame are more stressed on the job. "And the evidence is increasing that stress can lower your immunity, leaving you more susceptible to infections, particularly to upper respiratory infections," explains lead researcher John Schaubroeck, Ph.D., professor of management at Drexel University in Philadelphia. ■

when to see a doctor

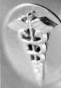

If your cold symptoms last more than 2 weeks, see your doctor right away. Persistent nasal congestion, sore throat, or coughing could mean you have sinusitis, a more serious bacterial infection that requires antibiotics or other medical treatments, says Anne L. Davis, M.D., a pulmonologist and associate professor of medicine at New York University School of Medicine and an attending physician at Bellevue Hospital, both in New York City.

If your mucus is tinged with yellow or green: This often means that the initial cold infection, caused by a virus, has been replaced with a secondary bacterial infection. You may need treatment with antibiotics.

Take zinc lozenges. Doctors still aren't sure if the mineral zinc can shorten the duration of colds. Some studies have shown that it may shave 3 to 4 days off colds, while others have found no such benefits. Until the science is sorted out, it's fine to give zinc a try. Suck on zinc lozenges every 2 to 3 hours during the first few days of a cold. Let the lozenges dissolve completely in your mouth; this allows the mineral to come into direct contact with irritated tissues in the throat.

Use echinacea. Research has shown that the herb echinacea may cut the duration of colds and also reduce the severity of symptoms. It increases levels of a body chemical called properdin, which activates the part of the immune system that fights viruses.

You can make echinacea tea with fresh or dried herb, but it's easier to just take dried root tablets, available in health food stores. The recommended dose is two 500-milligram tablets three times daily. If you prefer a tea, use $\frac{1}{2}$ teaspoon of the dried root added to 2 cups of boiling water. Boil it down to 1 cup and drink 1 cup four times a day.

Try elderberry syrup or tincture. According to herbalists, elderberry (*Sambucus nigra*) can reduce the duration of colds by 30 to 40 percent—and it tastes a lot better than over-the-counter remedies. Look for elderberry syrup and tinctures at your health food store. Take 1 teaspoon of syrup or 1 teaspoon of 1:5 tincture three times a day.

Get extra vitamin C. It strengthens immune cells and also helps block the effects of histamine, the body chemical responsible for causing watery eyes and runny noses. At the first sign of cold symptoms, take 2,000 milligrams of vitamin C daily: Divide it into several doses and take it throughout the day.

For Long-Term Prevention

home remedies

Wash your hands often. One reason that colds are so difficult to prevent is that the viruses spread widely every time you sneeze or blow your nose. Invariably, some of the viruses survive on the hands—and on doorknobs, light switches, and towels—and then find their way into the body. Washing your hands often—every few hours is best—is among the best ways to prevent colds from coming back.

cold sores

There are a few things that every woman should know about cold sores. Despite the name, they have nothing to do with the common cold. They're painful, but not serious; they will clear up on their own in a week or two. If you're lucky, you'll never have more than one outbreak, but you can't count on that: The virus that causes cold sores lives in the body forever.

Fifty to 80 percent of adult Americans are infected with a virus called herpes simplex virus 1 (HSV-1), which is typically contracted during childhood. During the initial outbreak, the virus can cause a variety of symptoms, such as fever, blisters in and around the mouth, and enlarged lymph nodes. Once the infection is done, the virus retreats into the body's nerves, where it lies dormant. In most cases, it never causes another symptom. But for a minority of those infected, the infection periodically springs back to life, triggering painful sores that usually appear on the edge of the lip. A tingling, burning, or itching sensation on the skin usually precedes an outbreak.

You can't get rid of the virus once you have it, but there are ways to prevent outbreaks—and to help the sores heal more quickly.

For Immediate Relief

home remedies

Apply an anesthetic. Cold sores can be intensely painful, especially when you're eating or drinking. One solution is to apply an over-the-counter benzocaine cold sore gel, such as Colgate Orabase B Topical and Oral Anesthetic Gel, which contains a mild anesthetic, says Teresa Soriano, M.D., assistant professor of dermatology at UCLA School of Medicine.

If the pain is unusually intense, you may want to ask your doctor to prescribe a stronger numbing agent. Dr. Soriano suggests a 2 percent viscous lidocaine solution, which can be swished around in the mouth and then spit out. This treatment is especially helpful in reducing pain when it's used before meals, she says.

Speed the healing time. An over-the-counter cream that contains docosanol (such as Abreva) can reduce the duration of cold sore attacks by 1 to 2 days, says David H. Emmert, M.D., a family physician in Lancaster, Pennsylvania, who published a study about the treatment of cold sores. As soon as you notice tingling, burning, or other cold sore symptoms, apply the cream five times daily, and keep using it until the sore has healed, he advises.

Prescription antiviral pills such as acyclovir (Zovirax) or valacyclovir (Valtrex) are also effective in shortening the duration and severity of outbreaks, says Dr. Emmert. Ask your doctor about these medications, especially if you suffer from frequent outbreaks.

alternative therapies

Use lemon balm. German researchers have found that people who apply lemon balm cream to cold sores four times daily heal faster and have less discomfort. You can buy lemon balm creams and ointments in health food stores. To reduce pain and speed healing, apply the cream for up to 10 days.

Reduce pain with lavender. It won't eliminate cold sores, but essential oil of lavender slows nerve impulses and may help relieve the pain of your sores. The oil also inhibits bacteria, which can reduce the chances of infection. You can apply a few drops of the oil to cold sores several times daily.

For Long-Term Relief

home remedies

Coat the sore with petroleum jelly. It traps moisture and prevents the sore from drying or cracking. Coating cold sores with petroleum jelly also speeds the healing time, says Dr. Emmert.

Avoid cold sore "triggers." Research has shown that exposure to wind, cold, or excessive sunlight may trigger attacks in some people. If you're prone to cold sore attacks, it's worth using a lip balm that will protect the lips from the environment, says Leslie Baumann, M.D., director of cosmetic dermatology at the University of Miami Cosmetic Center. Select a lip balm that has an SPF of 15 or greater and reapply it every hour.

Apply an antibacterial ointment. Triple antibiotic ointments such as Neosporin and Betadine don't kill viruses, but they can help ensure that you don't develop a secondary bacterial infection in the open sore, says Dr. Emmert. If you're using an antiviral cream at the same time, be sure to apply it before using the antibacterial ointment.

THREE THINGS I TELL EVERY FEMALE PATIENT

DAVID H. EMMERT, M.D., a family physician in Lancaster, Pennsylvania, who has studied cold sores, offers this advice for women who get frequent outbreaks.

1

THINGS WILL GET BETTER. The herpesvirus tends to reemerge from nerve cells at times of physical or emotional stress—but for most people, the severity and frequency of the attacks diminish over time.

ALWAYS USE LIP BALM. The sun's ultraviolet rays are among the most common triggers of cold sores. If you spend a lot of time outside, always use a lip balm that contains sunscreen. Be sure not to share lip balm with others—the virus is contagious and could be spread this way.

2

WASH YOUR HANDS OFTEN. The virus particles in cold sores are highly contagious. If you touch the sores—and almost everyone does—the infection can be spread to other people or to other parts of your body. Touch the cold sore as little as possible, and wash your hands frequently until the sore has healed. ■

3

conjunctivitis

Women's eyes are constantly exposed to the environment—which includes dry air, pollution, the sun's burning rays, and potentially harmful viruses and bacteria. Anything that irritates the eyes can result in redness and pain. When the irritation affects the conjunctiva, the membrane that lines the eyelids and the white portions of the eyes, it's known as conjunctivitis. One type of bacterial conjunctivitis is known as "pinkeye."

It's not always easy to pin down the precise causes of conjunctivitis. If the redness and irritation last longer than a day, you may need to see an ophthalmologist, who will examine your eyes under a microscope. Other symptoms to watch out for are itching, excessive tearing, blurred vision, discharge, and pain.

"If you wake up in the morning and your eyes are crusted together, you probably have bacterial conjunctivitis," says Sandra Belmont, M.D., associate professor of ophthalmology at Cornell University in New York City. "If your eyes are itchy, burning, and red, it may be allergic conjunctivitis. If you have swollen glands, or you've just gotten over an upper respiratory illness, you may have viral conjunctivitis."

Conjunctivitis usually clears up on its own, although bacterial infections need to be treated by a doctor. To relieve the discomfort right away, here's what doctors advise.

For Immediate Relief

home remedies

Use artificial tears. Available in pharmacies, artificial tears do the same job as natural tears: They moisturize the eyes and relieve itching and irritation. You can use them six to eight times a day until your eyes are feeling better.

For additional relief, keep artificial tears in the refrigerator. The coolness is very soothing, says Stephanie Marioneaux, M.D., assistant professor of ophthalmology at Eastern Virginia Medical School in Norfolk.

When using the drops, don't let the tip of the bottle touch your eye, Dr. Belmont adds. If you

when to see a doctor

If eye irritation or redness persists for more than 24 hours, see your doctor right away. Conjunctivitis doesn't always require treatment, but sometimes it does—and acting quickly can prevent potential eye damage, says Sandra Belmont, M.D., associate professor of ophthalmology at Cornell University in New York City.

If there's a discharge coming from one or both eyes, or if your vision is suddenly getting worse: Some forms of conjunctivitis, including those caused by bacteria, can cause permanent vision loss if they aren't treated promptly.

have viral or bacterial conjunctivitis, the harmful organisms can get on the tip and reinfect you later.

Apply a cool compress. Moisten a washcloth, put it in the freezer until it's cold, then apply it to your eyes several times a day, suggest Dr. Marioneaux. Don't use the cloth to rub your eyes, however, which can make the problem worse.

Avoid over-the-counter drops that "get the red out." These products, referred to as redness relievers, whiten the eyes by constricting blood vessels. The drops aren't harmful, but they don't treat the underlying causes of conjunctivitis—and when you quit using the drops, your eyes may be redder than ever, says Dr. Marioneaux.

medical options

Ask your doctor about medications. There are a number of prescription eyedrops that can be used to treat conjunctivitis. If the infection is caused by bacteria, your doctor will write a prescription for antibiotic drops. For eye irritation caused by allergies, you may need drops that contain antihistamines or anti-inflammatories, says Dr. Marioneaux.

For Long-Term Relief

home remedies

Prevent recontamination. Anything that touches your eye when you have conjunctivitis, including contact lenses and makeup applicators, can potentially be contaminated with harmful organisms. Avoid using eye makeup until after the infection is healed. Your doctor may advise you to discard your old contact lenses as well.

Wash pillowcases, sheets, and towels. The viruses and bacteria that cause conjunctivitis can survive on almost any surface. To prevent yourself from getting reinfected—and to protect other members of the family—be sure to wash bedding, towels, or other linens that may have come into contact with your eyes.

Pillowcases—or anything else that may be exposed to fluids from the eyes—should be washed daily as long as the infection lasts, Dr. Belmont adds.

Wash your hands often. And scrub any surface that you've touched—doorknobs, computer keyboards, and even the steering wheel in your car—with a mild bleach solution, suggests Dr. Marioneaux.

constipation

Grandma got many things right, but when it came to bowel habits, the family matriarch missed some vital information.

All that castor oil she made you swallow on the days you missed a bowel movement definitely wasn't what the doctor ordered.

"A generation ago, people were in the habit of giving children laxatives or enemas if they didn't go every day. But now we know that having a bowel movement anywhere from three times a week to three times a day is normal," says John W. Popp Jr., M.D., clinical professor of medicine at the University of South Carolina School of Medicine in Columbia.

Another common fallacy is that our bodies absorb waste, and our health is threatened as a result.

Constipation generally refers to stools that are infrequent, dry and hard, or difficult to pass. As a general rule you're constipated if you have fewer than three bowel movements a week. There is, however, no "right" number of daily or weekly bowel movements. If you're constipated, the bowel movements may be painful. Some patients also complain of feeling sluggish, bloated, and uncomfortable.

The hormonal changes of pregnancy are one common culprit of constipation. Also, when the growing uterus compresses the intestines, sluggish bowel movements can result.

Multiple sclerosis, lupus, Parkinson's disease, scleroderma, and stroke all can cause constipation. So can diabetes, an underactive or overactive thyroid, and spinal cord injuries. Some medicines trigger constipation, too. The most common medications that may produce constipation are antidepressants, antihistamines for allergies, drugs for Parkinson's disease, diuretics (often called "water pills"), and antacids containing calcium or aluminum. Pain medications, antispasmodic drugs, iron supplements, and anticonvulsants used for epilepsy can also slow your bowel movements.

THREE THINGS I TELL EVERY FEMALE PATIENT

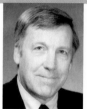

JOHN W. POPP JR., M.D., clinical professor of medicine at the University of South Carolina School of Medicine in Columbia, who has written about constipation for the American College of Gastroenterology, says that patients with bowel problems take their bowel movements very, very seriously.

"I've had patients come in with photographs of their stool," Dr. Popp says with a chuckle. Yet going to the bathroom doesn't have to trigger anxiety. Here's some advice he gives his patients.

1 **DON'T THINK OF HAVING A BOWEL MOVEMENT AS A COMPETITION.** "The key is what's normal for you," Dr. Popp says.

2 **ESTABLISH A BATHROOM ROUTINE.** Set aside a regular time each day—after breakfast or when you've finished dinner—for a visit to the bathroom. Make sure you're not disturbed. "Every morning after breakfast, sit down, but don't become upset if you don't score the perfect-10 BM," Dr. Popp says.

3 **ADD FIBER GRADUALLY.** If you're currently eating 5 to 7 grams of fiber each day and set a goal of 25 grams, don't adjust your diet overnight. "It's a huge mistake to take too much too soon," Dr. Popp advises. "Always start with a very low dose. And make simple substitutions. Replacing a serving of white rice with brown rice will give you triple the amount of fiber." ■

Older adults are more likely to report problems with constipation than young people. That's because they're more likely to take constipating drugs, and they're less likely to exercise, eat adequate amounts of fiber, and drink enough fluids.

Constipation in older women may also be linked to pelvic muscles weakened as a result of pregnancy and childbirth.

Yet too little fiber is often the main cause of constipation. The average woman eats about 12 grams of fiber each day, well under the 25 to 35 grams *Prevention* magazine recommends.

You don't have to eat a regular diet of sawdust to ease your discomfort from constipation. Try these tips from doctors who specialize in the treatment of bowel disorders.

For Immediate Relief

home remedies

Answer nature's call. Yes, the kids are clamoring for breakfast—*now*. That doesn't mean it's prudent to ignore your urge to have a bowel movement. People who ignore the need to go to the bathroom may eventually stop feeling the urge—and that can lead to constipation. If you're already constipated, don't sit and strain. It's better to wait until you feel the urge to go, and then try.

Try a home remedy. Craig Rubin, M.D., professor of internal medicine and chief of the geriatrics section at the University of Texas Southwestern Medical Center in Dallas, suggests mixing $1/2$ cup of unprocessed bran, available in most supermarkets, and $1/2$ cup of applesauce with $1/3$ cup of prune juice. Refrigerate. Take 2 to 3 ta-

blespoons of the mixture after dinner, and then drink a tall glass of water. If needed, increase your dosage to 3 to 4 tablespoons. The mixture will keep for about 2 weeks in the refrigerator.

Find flax. Two tablespoons of nutty-tasting flax each day may offer enough insoluble fiber to keep you regular. To make a flax-rich breakfast smoothie, combine 1 cup of orange juice, one banana, and 2 rounded tablespoons of ground flaxseed (317 calories, 11 grams of fat, 12 grams of fiber). Always refrigerate ground flaxseed.

Consider a little extra help. Metamucil and other over-the-counter fiber supplements may help ease symptoms. Miralax, a laxative that doctors prescribe, has been found to be effective. "If other remedies haven't helped, your doctor may suggest that you try Miralax," Dr. Rubin says.

Analyze your routine. Have you changed your diet, workouts, work schedule? Any deviation from your routine can trigger a change in your bowel habits. Are you taking any medication that might be constipating? Ask yourself these questions to determine if you are truly constipated: Do I have a hard time passing stools? Am I having fewer bowel movements than I normally have each week? Do I have pain during bowel movements? Do I have other problems, such as bleeding? If the answers are yes, you're probably constipated.

mind-body techniques

Consider biofeedback for serious cases. Some patients suffer from abnormalities in the structure of the rectum and anus, conditions doctors call anorectal dysfunction or anismus. Women with anismus cannot relax the anal and rectal muscles used during bowel movements. Some people with these disorders may get relief by using biofeedback to retrain their muscles after they receive instructions on the procedure from their doctors.

For Long-Term Relief

home remedies

Drink when you're dry—and then some. Juices and other liquids such as water may help make bowel movements softer and easier to pass. Aim for eight 8-ounce glasses each day.

Fill up on fiber. "Fiber is very important, and a lot of people will say, 'But I eat bran cereal,' and mistakenly think they're getting a whole day's worth," says Dr. Popp. "I tell my patients a good minimum number to aim for is 20 grams," adds William J. Snape Jr., M.D., director of the Bowel Disease and Motility Center at Long Beach Medical Center and clinical professor of medicine at the University of California, Irvine.

If you replace your cup of Rice Krispies (zero gram) with just ½ cup of Fiber One cereal, you start the day with 14 grams of fiber. Add a couple of apples after lunch and dinner (4 grams apiece), snack on an ounce of dried whole almonds in the late afternoon (3 grams), and down 1 cup of chopped, cooked broccoli at dinner (5 grams), and you'll easily exceed your daily goal.

Don't forget to eat your vegetables. Brussels sprouts, carrots, potatoes, and sweet potatoes with their skins are especially helpful to people with constipation.

Get physical. Doctors aren't sure why, but regular exercise might help your system stay, well,

when to see a doctor

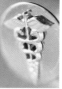

If you've had any change in your usual bowel habits, or if you notice blood in the stool, call your doctor right away. It's probably nothing serious, but these and other changes could be a sign of cancer or other grave illnesses.

"Blood in the stool, a change in bowel habits, a thinning of the stools—all are red flags to call your physician, especially if they occurred out of nowhere," says William J. Snape Jr., M.D., director of the Bowel Disease and Motility Center at Long Beach Medical Center and clinical professor of medicine at the University of California, Irvine.

Yet some patients procrastinate, fearing the truth—and the medical tests, says John W. Popp Jr., M.D., clinical professor of medicine at the University of South Carolina School of Medicine in Columbia. "Patients will say, 'The doctor is putting a lighted tube *where*? No way.' The biggest fear is the fear of the unknown."

Several other symptoms should send you to a doctor, too. They include weight loss, severe abdominal pain, and a change in your bowel pattern, in either the frequency or the consistency of your bowel movements.

Sometimes straining to have a bowel movement causes a small amount of the intestinal lining to protrude from the rectal opening in a condition known as a rectal prolapse. Mucus staining on the undergarments is a symptom.

Abdominal pain and bloating, combined with constipation, could signal an intestinal obstruction.

regular. If you have heart disease, emphysema, or any chronic illness, ask your doctor before you start exercising or change your routine. Even if you are healthy, don't think you have to be a marathon runner. A 20- to 30-minute walk, every day, should be adequate.

Use laxatives prudently. The key words are *temporarily* and *occasionally*. "If you're taking a con-stipating drug like an antihistamine or have an acute illness that causes constipation, it's perfectly acceptable to take a laxative," Dr. Popp says. When you finish the drug or recover from your illness, drop the laxative or else risk becoming dependent. "The more you use laxatives, the more your bowel depends on them, and eventually the bowel may stop working," Dr. Popp says.

cough

Oxygen isn't the only thing that enters the airways when women breathe. There's pollen. Dust. Hair spray. Dander from dogs and cats. These and other environmental particles and toxic or irritant gases or vapors are like sand in the sheets—they're itchy and bothersome, and your body tries to get rid of them with a good cough.

If you have allergies or a cold, of course, the problem comes from within. Buildups of mucus make it harder to breathe, and coughing is your body's way of getting rid of it.

There are two main types of coughs: "dry" coughs, which are usually caused by simple irritation, and mucus-filled, "productive" coughs, which are often a sign of colds or other upper respiratory infections or inflammation occurring for noninfectious reasons, says Anne L. Davis, M.D., a pulmonologist and associate professor of medicine at New York University School of Medicine and an attending physician at Bellevue Hospital, both in New York City.

Some coughs are chronic and persistent, depending on the cause and treatment (or lack of it) received.

A persistent cough—one that lasts more than 3 weeks—and certain temporary coughs may be caused by a number of serious illnesses. A medical examination and laboratory tests may be necessary for diagnosis and specific therapy.

Coughs associated with a specific episode, such as a respiratory infection or a brief exposure to a toxic environmental substance, may also require medical treatment. They usually clear up on their own, but they can make women miserable in the meantime. Here are a few ways to soothe them fast.

For Immediate Relief

home remedies

Get plenty of fluids. Doctors usually advise drinking at least eight 8-ounce glasses of water, juices, or other nondehydrating fluids daily when you have a cough that produces secretions. The extra fluids thin mucus so it's easier to expel. Dr. Davis often recommends that women drink fruit juices that are rich in infection-fighting vitamin C, such as orange, grapefruit, or pineapple juice. To reduce the amount of sugar you're getting, dilute the juice by half or stir a small amount into a glass of water. Plain water is fine, too, adds Dr. Davis.

Suck on hard candy. The juices will coat irritated cough receptors at the back of the throat, which can help suppress dry coughs. Over-the-counter throat lozenges also may be soothing.

Add garlic to your menu. Raw or very lightly cooked garlic helps suppress viruses and bacteria that are often responsible for coughs. Garlic also acts as an expectorant: It thins the mucus and makes coughs more efficient. Incorporate four to eight cloves into your daily diet until the cough is gone.

Breathe some steam. Humidification may help if your house is very dry or if you have to breathe through your mouth because of a stuffy nose. It decreases the viscosity of mucus, which makes it easier to cough up. The easiest way to steam your airways is to enjoy a long shower or bath. At night, plug in a vaporizer or humidifier until you feel relief. The moist air will soothe your airways while you sleep, says Dr. Davis. Some people, however, may find it more difficult to breathe in a humid atmosphere, so experiment to see what works for you.

alternative therapies

Try an herbal soother. Some herbs contain mucilage, a slippery substance that coats irritated tissues in the throat. Two of the best are

THREE THINGS I TELL EVERY FEMALE PATIENT

WILLIAM J. HALL, M.D., is president of the American College of Physicians–American Society of Internal Medicine in Philadelphia and chief of general medicine of the geriatrics unit, professor of medicine, pediatrics, and oncology at the University of Rochester School of Medicine in New York. He advises women with pesky coughs to do the following:

1 TRY TO AVOID DECONGESTANT NOSE SPRAYS. Even though they can reduce coughs caused by postnasal drip, they often increase symptoms as soon as you quit using them.

2 USE COUGH SUPPRESSANTS SPARINGLY. People who use these medications for long periods of time may experience high blood pressure, increased heart rate, or other side effects. Don't take them longer than 2 to 3 days without a medical examination.

3 DON'T INSIST ON ANTIBIOTICS. If you have a bacterial infection, your doctor will prescribe them—but most coughs are caused by viruses, which aren't affected by antibiotics. ■

when to see a doctor

 If your coughs are accompanied by blood in the mucus or by symptoms such as chest pain, wheezing, or shortness of breath, or if they persist or get worse, call your doctor right away. You could have a serious infection or other problem that won't clear up without proper diagnosis and medical treatment, says Anne L. Davis, M.D., a pulmonologist and associate professor of medicine at New York University School of Medicine and an attending physician at Bellevue Hospital, both in New York City. Bacterial infections will require treatment with antibiotics. Just a few of the serious conditions that can cause long-term coughing are asthma, heart disease, and lung cancer.

If you're coughing a lot and also have persistent heartburn: A condition called esophageal reflux, in which stomach acid splashes into the esophagus, often causes chronic coughs, says Dr. Davis.

If you've been coughing for more than 3 weeks: You may have a chronic cough caused by certain drugs you're taking, such as angiotensin-converting enzyme (ACE) inhibitors. Coughs may also be caused by nervousness or emotional and psychological problems.

marshmallow root and slippery elm, which can be brewed into teas. Pour ½ cup of boiling water over 1 teaspoon of powdered herb. Sip throughout the day. You can also buy slippery elm lozenges at pharmacies and health food stores.

Use a natural expectorant. Some herbs are nature's equivalent of over-the-counter expectorants. Herbal supplements and teas that may be helpful include horehound, thyme, and eucalyptus. Make thyme tea by steeping 2 teaspoons of the herb in 1 cup of water for 10 minutes. Drink this three times a day. If you want to try eucalyptus leaf, three times a day take 6 drops of a 1:1 tincture or 30 drops of a 1:5 tincture.

medical options

Choose the right medicine. If you have a productive cough, you can speed it on its way by taking an over-the-counter expectorant that contains guaifenesin (such as Robitussin). To suppress a dry cough, doctors usually recommend products that contain dextromethorphan (like Triaminic DM) or codeine.

dandruff

f it weren't for dark fabrics, few people would give dandruff a second thought. It isn't itchy or contagious. The only way you even know you have it is from the telltale sprinkling of white specks that may appear on jackets, sweaters, and blouses.

Dead skin cells are constantly flaking from the surface of the scalp, only to be replaced with new, identical cells. In those with dandruff, the cells proliferate at an abnormal rate, which is what produces the visible accumulation of white flakes.

About 20 percent of adults have dandruff.

Doctors still aren't sure what causes the skin cells to go into overdrive. One factor appears to be a fungus called *Pityrosporum ovale*, which is thought to irritate the scalp and cause an increase in flaking, says Steven Mays, M.D., assistant professor of dermatology at the University of Texas–Houston Medical School.

There isn't a long-term cure for dandruff, but most people can control the flakes with a few simple strategies.

For Immediate Relief

home remedies

Wash your hair daily. It's fine to use your regular shampoo at first. Frequent washing doesn't eliminate dandruff, but it will remove flakes before they have a chance to accumulate and become visible, says Dr. Mays.

One problem with frequent washing is that it may damage the hair shafts. This is especially true for African-Americans because their hair fractures easily. If you can't wash your hair daily, do it three or four times a week, Dr. Mays advises.

Wash with cool water. Hot water dries the scalp. This doesn't cause dandruff, but it does encourage dead skin cells to flake away and become visible.

Keep your blow-dryer at a distance. Hold it at least 10 inches from your hair, and use the low setting. The reduction in heat allows skin cells to stay moist, which makes them more likely to stay out of sight, on the surface of the scalp.

Switch to a medicated shampoo. If you can't control dandruff with a regular shampoo, use a dandruff shampoo. These products contain one of six active ingredients: ketoconazole, coal tar, sulfur, pyrithione zinc, or selenium sulfide, which help eliminate dandruff-causing fungi from the scalp; or salicylic acid, which breaks up clumps of skin cells and makes them easier to remove.

Dr. Mays recommends starting with a shampoo that contains ketoconazole. "It is over-the-counter, and it's very effective."

Give shampoos time to work. It takes time for the active ingredients in medicated shampoos to soak into the surface of the scalp. When you take a bath or shower, lather your hair right away, then wait 1 to 3 minutes before rinsing out the shampoo.

Apply warm oil. Before you go to bed at night, massage 8 to 10 drops of olive oil or mineral oil on your scalp. "The scales are so thick

when to see a doctor

If dandruff persists for several weeks even though you're using several medicated shampoos, see a dermatologist. "You'll probably need a prescription steroid solution to control scalp inflammation," says Steven Mays, M.D., assistant professor of dermatology at the University of Texas–Houston Medical School. The dermatologist will also examine your scalp to ensure that there is not another cause for the excessive scaling.

If the flaking extends from the scalp to the eyebrows, the sides of the nose, or behind the ears: You may have a related skin condition called seborrheic dermatitis, which requires medical attention.

sometimes that medicated shampoos can't get into the scalp," says Dr. Mays. "Applying oil will soften and remove scaly buildups."

After applying the oil, cover your hair with a shower cap, then wash out the oil in the morning, using a regular or medicated shampoo.

For Long-Term Relief

home remedies

Alternate shampoos. Skin cells on the scalp quickly become resistant to the active ingredients in medicated shampoos. "People should probably buy shampoos with three different active ingredients and alternate them daily," says Dr. Mays.

Test tar-based shampoos. They're very effective, but they often leave a brown stain in light-colored hair. Try other products first, Dr. Mays advises. If your hair is brown or black, a tar shampoo is probably a good choice to include in your hair care routine.

mind-body techniques

Deal with the stress in your life. Dandruff tends to flare up during stressful times, says Dr. Mays. You may be able to keep it from getting worse by relaxing a little more—by going for long walks, leaving work at the office on weekends, and generally allowing yourself to unwind a little more.

depression

We all feel sad or discouraged from time to time, and usually we know why. It might be a troubled relationship, problems at work, or simply the winter blahs. As time passes, we work through the problems, and our moods begin to brighten.

Depression is an entirely different matter. "It's more than just a down mood," says Jack G. Modell, M.D., professor of psychiatry at the University of Alabama in Birmingham. "With depression, your feelings are controlling you, and you feel as though you just can't get past them."

It's not clear why, but women are twice as likely as men to suffer from depression. Signs of depression include losing pleasure in daily activi-

ties, diminished appetite, difficulty concentrating, changes in your usual sleep patterns, and feelings of guilt or worthlessness.

"If you start having three, four, or five symptoms every day for most of the day, and the feelings persist for more than 2 weeks, it's time for concern," says Kelly Conforti, Ph.D., a clinical psychologist and manager of psychotherapy services at the Mental Health Center at the University of New Mexico Health Sciences Center in Albuquerque.

The treatments for depression—everything from medications and "talk therapy" to changes in lifestyle—are surprisingly effective: Up to 80 percent of those who seek treatment will notice rapid improvement, usually within a few weeks.

For Immediate Relief

home remedies

Put pleasure on your schedule. Every day, jot down a few enjoyable activities—going for a walk, enjoying a long bath, or simply perusing a magazine that you haven't had time to read—that you're going to do. Give them the same priority that you would a serious business appointment.

"We have too many *should*s in our lives and not enough things that are enjoyable. That can lead to depression," says Dr. Conforti.

Limit coffee to a cup or two a day. Caffeine boosts mood temporarily, but some women feel a letdown when the caffeine wears off, says Neil Benowitz, M.D., professor of medicine at the University of California, San Francisco.

Get enough calcium. Research suggests that women who experience premenstrual depression may feel better when they consume calcium. One study found that women who took 1,200 milligrams of elemental calcium daily in the form of calcium carbonate experienced more than a 50 percent reduction in their premenstrual syndrome symptoms.

The best sources of calcium are low-fat milk and cheese. Many juices and breakfast cereals are fortified with calcium, says Mary Lake Polan, M.D., Ph.D., professor and chairperson of the department of gynecology and obstetrics at Stanford University School of Medicine.

alternative therapies

Try St. John's wort. This herb appears to help maintain healthful levels of mood-regulating brain chemicals. Varro Tyler, Ph.D., Sc.D., dean emeritus of the Purdue University School of Pharmacy and Pharmacal Sciences in West Lafayette, Indiana, and author of *Tyler's Honest Herbal*, advises taking 300 milligrams of St. John's wort extract three times daily.

THREE THINGS I TELL EVERY FEMALE PATIENT

JACK G. MODELL, M.D., professor of psychiatry at the University of Alabama in Birmingham, offers the following advice for coping with depression.

1

EXERCISE DAILY. It boosts levels of chemicals in the brain that regulate mood. "If all you can do at first is 5 minutes, that's fine," he says. Research has shown that people who exercise regularly are less likely to stay depressed. They'll also recover more quickly when their moods head south.

2

GET SOME SUN. Exposure to sunlight triggers the release of melatonin in the brain. Melatonin regulates your sleep and wake cycles, and it can have a powerful effect on energy and mood.

3

SHARE YOUR PROBLEMS WITH FAMILY AND FRIENDS. Chances are, others have experienced the same feelings. Their understanding and emotional support will go a long way toward helping you feel better. ■

It may interact with other medications, including some antidepressants. Don't combine St. John's wort with other drugs without checking with your doctor first.

For Long-Term Relief

home remedies

Stay in touch with your friends. It might be the best medicine for depression. A British study found that 65 percent of women with depression

when to see a doctor

If you're feeling "blue" and are also experiencing physical problems, such as fatigue or unexplained changes in your weight, see your family doctor. Many symptoms of depression mimic those caused by underlying medical problems, says Kelly Conforti, Ph.D., a clinical psychologist and manager of psychotherapy services at the Mental Health Center at the University of New Mexico Health Sciences Center in Albuquerque.

If your depressive feelings last longer than 2 weeks, or if you're thinking about suicide or death: These are symptoms of clinical depression, and you'll need professional help right away.

If you've had depression in the past, and you suspect that it's coming back: It is estimated that 50 to 60 percent of people who have had one episode of major depression will have another episode during their lives.

who met for 1 hour weekly with a volunteer "befriender" experienced a remission, compared with 39 percent of those who didn't get the extra support. That's about the same success rate that's seen in conventional therapy or from taking drugs, says study author Tirril Harris, Ph.D., a researcher with the Socio-Medical Research Center in London.

mind-body techniques

Manage negative thoughts. You have a surprising amount of control over the ideas and beliefs that flit through your mind. People are more likely to suffer from depression when they embrace negative thoughts, such as "I've wasted my life" or "This is the worst thing that's ever happened."

Turn the thoughts around, Dr. Conforti advises. "When you tell yourself things like 'Things are getting better' or 'I've made mistakes, but I think I can improve things,' you'll decrease your feelings of sadness or depression."

Stay in touch with your spirituality. "Studies have shown that people who are active in their churches or synagogues and feel a connection with God or some higher power have less depression," says Dr. Modell.

medical options

See a professional. Full-fledged depression is unlikely to disappear on its own. If your symptoms are mild, regular visits with a therapist are probably all you need. For more severe depression, antidepressant medications may be added.

"The best treatment is often a combination of therapy and medications," says Dr. Modell.

"Therapy will help you understand why you were having problems in the first place, and the medications will give you the energy and strength to make the most of the therapy."

Ask your doctor about hormone replacement. Postmenopausal fluctuations in estrogen and other hormones often contribute to insomnia and fatigue, which can increase the risk of depression.

"Trying estrogen replacement for a month or two will often solve the problem of sleep deprivation and restore a sense of well-being," says Neill Epperson, M.D., assistant professor of psychiatry at Yale University School of Medicine.

For more information on depression: Visit the Web site of the National Institute of Mental Health at www.nimh.nih.gov.

diarrhea

Diarrhea. The runs. Montezuma's revenge. These are just a few of terms that are used to describe the loose, watery stools that men and women get, on average, about four times a year. Diarrhea is so common that it's second only to respiratory infections as the most commonly reported illness in the United States.

Doctors divide diarrhea into two categories: Acute diarrhea, which tends to clear up within a few days, is typically caused by minor intestinal infections—or by the hot peppers on your favorite, hold-nothing-back pizza. Chronic diarrhea, on the other hand, can last 3 weeks or more. It's also caused by infections or by more serious conditions, such as diabetes or inflammatory bowel disease, says Susan C. Stewart, M.D., clinical assistant professor of medicine at the State University of New York Health Science Center in Brooklyn and past president of the American Medical Women's Association.

Diarrhea rarely requires medical treatment, including the use of over-the-counter anti-diarrhea medications. The drugs are effective, but they can trap bacteria or parasites in the intestine and slow your recovery.

Here are some better ways to reduce discomfort and speed diarrhea on its way.

For Immediate Relief

home remedies

Try yogurt. A cup of yogurt may bring you relief if your diarrhea stems from an infection. "It helps restore the balance of good and bad bacteria in your digestive tract," says Barbara Harland, Ph.D., professor of the department of nutritional sciences at Howard University College of Pharmacy, Nursing, and Allied Health Sciences in Washington, D.C.

Follow the BRAT diet. The letters stand for bananas, rice, applesauce, and toast. Each of these foods is very easy for your body to digest. Following the diet for a few days will give your intestines a chance to recover.

Drink a lot of fluids. Diarrhea removes a tremendous amount of water from body. When you lose water, you also lose electrolytes, essential minerals that you need to be healthy. Plain water will replace fluids, but it won't replace electrolytes.

"You need liquid with some substance to it, such as chicken broth," says Christine L. Frissora, M.D., assistant professor of medicine in the division of gastroenterology and hepatology at the Weill Medical College of Cornell University in New York City. Or you can drink rehydration solutions (available at drugstores), such as Pedialyte, which can also be used by adults.

For Long-Term Prevention

home remedies

Consider switching gum. Sugar-free gum contains the artificial sweeteners mannitol and sorbitol, which cause diarrhea in some people.

Take some of the heat out of your diet. Hot peppers add a lot of zest to pizzas, enchiladas, and other delicious foods, but they contain a fiery compound called capsaicin, which may trigger watery stools.

Wash your hands often. Your risk of getting intestinal infections will drop dramatically if you wash your hands often, especially before meals or after using the bathroom.

Travel wisely. It's not a coincidence that millions of Americans get diarrhea during the travel season. Water quality and food sanitation aren't always optimal in foreign countries, and your intestines may pay the price. Important travelers' guidelines include:

- Always use bottled water for drinking or brushing your teeth. Don't drink ice water unless you're sure the ice was made from sterilized water.

- Only eat fruits that you peel yourself, such as papayas, pineapple, or mangoes.

- Avoid raw vegetables or salad greens.

- Eat your meals in restaurants. Street vendors often sell delicious foods, but the risk of contamination is high.

WHAT WORKS FOR ME

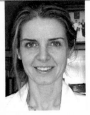

CHRISTINE L. FRISSORA, M.D., *assistant professor of medicine in the division of gastroenterology and hepatology at the Weill Medical College of Cornell University in New York City, occasionally travels overseas. Here's how she protects herself.*

I take Pepto-Bismol in tablet form to prevent diarrhea. I chew one tablet two times a day. It's so handy because you can just toss the package in your purse.

People who take Pepto-Bismol sometimes get alarmed when their tongues or the stools temporarily turn black. It's the body's normal response to the medicine—it's nothing to worry about. ■

diverticular disease

From the beginning of human history to the end of the 1800s, humans survived by eating whole grains, legumes, and other plant-based foods. They enjoyed meat, but it wasn't on the menu very often. And they certainly didn't eat the highly processed foods that we enjoy today.

Before thanking your lucky stars for progress, consider this: Diverticular disease, a condition in which portions of the intestinal wall weaken and bulge, used to be a rarity. Today, as many as half of older American adults (ages 60 to 80) have these intestinal pockets, and almost everyone over age 80 has diverticulosis. The disease is often "silent"; many people have it for decades without even knowing. But in some cases it results in cramps, diarrhea, bloating, or rectal bleeding.

What's the connection between the modern diet and diverticular disease? It all comes down to fiber, explains Susan C. Stewart, M.D., clinical assistant professor of medicine at the State of University of New York Health Science Center in Brooklyn and coeditor of *The Women's Complete Healthbook*. The fiber found in plant foods absorbs water in the intestine. It makes stools larger as well as softer, which decreases the amount of pressure that's required to push them out of the body.

Americans today, however, only get about half of *Prevention* magazine's recommended 25 to 35 grams of fiber a day. A low-fiber diet produces stools that are smaller and harder than they should be, which means that the intestine has to exert more pressure to push them along. The increase in pressure may cause the intestinal wall to bulge, much like a weak spot on a tire, explains J. Barry O'Connor, M.D., assistant professor of medicine at Duke University Medical Center in Durham, North Carolina.

In addition, a low-fiber diet often results in constipation. The harder it is to move your bowels, the more you strain—and straining increases pressure in the intestine.

Once the bulges, known as diverticula, form in the intestinal wall, you have them for good. However, there are a few ways to reduce the discomfort and also prevent them from forming.

For Immediate Relief

home remedies

Ease cramping with heat. One of the most common symptoms of diverticular disease is cramping, which often occurs after meals. A quick way to reduce the discomfort is to hold a hot-water bottle wrapped in a towel or a heating pad on your abdomen for 10 to 15 minutes. You can repeat the treatment as often as necessary to get relief.

Include more fiber in your diet. While the jury is still out on whether fiber can ease the painful effects of diverticular disease, the overall advantages of fiber make it worth your while to give it a try. "Studies evaluating the effect of fiber supplements on pain in diverticular disease are conflicting. Small studies suggest that fiber may alleviate pain, but larger studies show no effect. Although further research is needed to clarify this situation, the general health benefits of fiber justify increasing fiber intake nonetheless," says Dr. O'Connor.

For Long-Term Prevention

Eat more fruits and vegetables. Aim for eating five vegetables and four fruits a day. Along with legumes and whole grains, they're among the best sources of intestine-protecting fiber. In a study published in the *British Medical Journal*, researchers compared the stools of Africans, who primarily ate a very high fiber diet, with those of Euro-

when to see a doctor

If you're having severe abdominal cramps, or if the cramps are accompanied by fever, call your doctor immediately. People with diverticulosis sometimes develop an infection in one of the intestinal pockets, a potentially serious condition called diverticulitis, says J. Barry O'Connor, M.D., assistant professor of medicine at Duke University Medical Center in Durham, North Carolina. You'll probably need antibiotics to knock out the infection.

If you're having rectal bleeding: It's often caused by hemorrhoids, but it can also occur in those with diverticular disease. If the bleeding is severe, you could need surgery to correct the problem.

peans, who filled up mainly on a refined Western diet low in fiber. They found that the stools of the Africans were bigger and moved much more quickly through the intestine.

"It seems likely that the larger volume of stool associated with high fiber intake allows the colon to move the stool along with lower intestinal pressures," Dr. O'Connor explains.

Buy whole grain breads and flour. Even if you don't eat a lot of fruits or vegetables, you can get substantial amounts of fiber just by eating whole grain breads. Try to incorporate three to six servings of whole grains into your diet every day. "Two-thirds of the fiber in flour is lost in modern milling," says Karen Heitzman, M.D., associate professor of medicine at State University of New York Upstate Medical University in Syracuse. "Diverticular disease would be a disease none of us ever heard of if flour milling had not been invented."

Track fiber the easy way. Unless you walk around with a calculator in one hand and nutritional charts in the other, it's hard to tell when you're getting enough fiber to prevent diverticulosis. One way to make it easier is to follow these general rules.

"A serving of fruits or vegetables has at least 1 gram of fiber," says Dr. Stewart. If you have fruit at breakfast, lunch, and dinner, plus a couple of servings of vegetables at dinner and a high-fiber cereal—some of which provide more than 10 grams of fiber—in the morning, you'll almost automatically get all the fiber that you need.

Consider a fiber boost. If you find that you're not getting a lot of fiber in your diet—a common problem for those who travel or who eat away from home a lot—you may want to take a fiber supplement. Found in the "laxative" aisle in pharmacies, fiber supplements such as psyllium (found in Metamucil and Hydrocil) and methylcellulose (found in Citrucel) are an excellent way to supplement the fiber in your diet. Find one that is pleasant tasting, and take it one to three times a day for those times when you cannot get your usual food sources of fiber, says Dr. Stewart.

Drink plenty of water. It's absorbed by the fiber in the stools, which makes them larger as well as softer. This can help prevent constipation and the straining that accompanies it. Doctors advise drinking eight full glasses of water every day.

Follow a regular routine. The urge to have a bowel movement, called the gastrocolonic reflex, is usually strongest in the morning after breakfast. If you sometimes suffer from constipation, it's worth listening to the body's "gotta go" signals. The longer you wait, the harder it may be to move your bowels later.

medical options

Talk to your doctor if you overuse painkillers. "One study suggests that there is an increased risk of bleeding from diverticuli in patients who regularly and consistently use common over-the-counter pain medicines. However, despite this apparent increased risk of bleeding, it is important to remember that overall most patients with diverticuli will not develop bleeding," says Dr. O'Connor.

For more information on diverticular disease: Go online to visit the Web site of the National Institute of Diabetes and Digestive and Kidney Diseases at www.niddk.nih.gov.

dizziness and vertigo

Dancing in circles is fun. Ferris wheels and merry-go-rounds are fun. What isn't fun is feeling as though the world is whirling even when you're sitting still.

Dizziness that comes from out of the blue is surprisingly common, especially among older adults. Approximately 90 million Americans suffer from occasional dizziness, and about one in five adults ages 60 and older says that it interferes with their daily lives.

One common form of dizziness is called vertigo. Caused by damage in the inner ear, vertigo can make you feel as though the world is spinning around you, says Gordon B. Hughes, M.D., professor in the department of otolaryngology and communicative disorders at the Cleveland Clinic Foundation in Cleveland.

Other forms of dizziness or light-headedness may be caused by poor circulation, side effects from medications, or a condition called orthostatic hypotension, in which blood pressure temporarily drops when you're changing position—while bending over to tie your shoes, for example, or getting out of bed in the morning.

"Time alone cures most inner ear problems," Dr. Hughes adds. "But dizziness and vertigo can be disabling because they often occur without warning and can cause people to become reclusive or avoid their normal activities."

However, with a combination of medical care and home treatments, most people can reduce or even eliminate the discomfort.

For Immediate Relief

home remedies

Steady yourself. If you feel an attack of dizziness or vertigo coming on and you must walk, lightly rest your fingers on a table or another familiar piece of furniture. "The brain senses the touch and tells the legs what posture to maintain," says Dr. Hughes. Sit down or lie down, if possible.

Flex your legs. If you have orthostatic hypotension, the blood tends to pool in the legs and feet. Flexing your leg muscles before you stand up—by crossing and uncrossing your legs, for example—will help push blood back into circulation.

One study found that when men and women with orthostatic hypotension flexed their thigh and buttock muscles, their blood pressure upon standing rose by 30 percent, according to study coauthor Phillips Low, M.D., director of the Autonomic Disorders Center at the Mayo Clinic.

Hold your head still. Dizziness is often triggered by movement. Lying still for a few minutes will allow blood pressure to stabilize, and it also may reduce "confusion" in the inner ear.

Be careful after hot baths or showers. "When you're in a hot bath, the blood vessels dilate in order to dissipate the heat," says Robert Peterka, Ph.D., an associate scientist at the Neurological Sciences Institute at Oregon Health Sciences University in Portland. "If you get up too quickly, your brain may not get enough blood, which will make you temporarily feel lightheaded."

THREE THINGS I TELL EVERY FEMALE PATIENT

GORDON B. HUGHES, M.D., professor in the department of otolaryngology and communicative disorders at the Cleveland Clinic Foundation, offers this advice for people with dizziness or vertigo.

1 DON'T WALK IN DARKNESS. "If you're having trouble with your inner ear or the balance in your legs, keeping a light on and using your vision will help keep you properly oriented."

2 WEAR FLAT SHOES. They allow your feet to maintain a firm "platform" on the ground, which sends posture information signals to the brain.

3 AVOID RISKY ACTIVITIES. Forget ladders: If you're having trouble with dizziness or vertigo, getting on a ladder or other unstable surface is an accident waiting to happen. ∎

Get out of bed slowly. It allows your blood pressure to adjust to the change in position, which can prevent dizziness in some cases, says Dr. Hughes. When you're ready to get up, swing your legs over the side of the bed and rise to a sitting position. Wait for a minute or two, then slowly stand up.

alternative therapies

Try ginger capsules. They can help prevent the nausea that sometimes accompanies dizziness or vertigo. "If you use herbal medicines, be sure to follow the directions on the label," Dr. Hughes says.

medical options

Review your regular medications with your doctor. Many prescription and even some over-the-counter drugs, such as medications for treating high blood pressure, may cause dizziness. Make a list of all the drugs you're taking and show it to your doctor. In some cases, switching drugs is all that's necessary to eliminate the symptoms, says Dr. Hughes.

Consider anti-dizziness drugs. A number of prescription and over-the-counter drugs sedate the central nervous system and shorten the duration and severity of vertigo and dizziness attacks.

"You can take them around the clock if dizziness is frequent or severe," says Dr. Hughes. For quick relief, he recommends a prescription drug called lorazepam (Ativan), which is placed under the tongue. It works much more quickly than oral drugs.

Ask your doctor about head position therapy. Vertigo sometimes occurs when calcium

when to see a doctor

A yearly general checkup is always a good idea, says Gordon B. Hughes, M.D., of the department of otolaryngology and communicative disorders at the Cleveland Clinic.

If you're having chest pain, shortness of breath, loss of consciousness, or another new neurological symptom, call 911 or visit your emergency department at the hospital right away. These may be signs of potentially serious problems, such as a blocked coronary artery or a brain disorder.

If you've had a recent cold or flu: Dizziness is sometimes caused by inner ear viral infections, which commonly occur after these and other respiratory infections. If symptoms do not clear within several days, see your doctor for an examination and treatment.

mineral particles in the inner ear break free from their proper resting spots and stimulate the hairlike sensors that sense movement and changes in the position of the head. A technique called the canalith repositioning procedure, which should be done by a trained therapist, involves moving the head into different positions until the particles return to their proper locations.

Many patients who undergo this procedure once will remain symptom-free.

Long-Term Solutions

home remedies

Reduce your salt intake. Vertigo is sometimes caused by a condition called Ménière's disease, which occurs when fluid accumulates in the inner ear. One way to reduce the fluid buildup is to follow a low-salt diet, getting no more than 2,000 milligrams of sodium daily. "People need to read food labels to keep track of how much salt they're getting," says Dr. Hughes.

Stay physically active. People with vertigo or dizziness often lose their physical confidence and become increasingly sedentary. This can reduce the ability of the brain to monitor and fine-tune your sense of balance. "The idea is to keep moving, either with physical therapy or by getting regular exercises," says Dr. Peterka.

mind-body techniques

Reduce the stress in your life. "Emotional stress aggravates inner ear disorders, although the mechanisms aren't known," says Dr. Hughes. Your symptoms may be a sign that you need to unwind—by taking long walks, meditating, or participating in counseling or a support group.

dry eyes

Until fairly recently, it was unusual for women to suffer from dry eyes. It sometimes occurred after menopause, when declines in female hormones caused a drop in tear production. Eye dryness could also be a problem for those with autoimmune conditions or for women taking birth control pills or other medications.

Today, however, ophthalmologists see a lot of patients with dry eyes, including those who are otherwise in perfect health.

"Dry eyes are almost an epidemic because of our energy-efficient environment," says Stephanie Marioneaux, M.D., assistant professor of ophthalmology at Eastern Virginia Medical School in Norfolk. Modern homes, buildings, and cars are so airtight that people are exposed to filtered air that contains little or no moisture, she explains. The ultradry air pulls moisture from the skin, hair, and nasal passages—and, of course, from the eyes.

Dry air isn't the only reason that so many people are suffering from scratchy, irritated, desert-dry eyes. Staring at computer screens doesn't help. Neither does the use of contact lenses or hair dryers, or the never-ending exposure to air pollution and chemical vapors.

To moisturize your eyes and ease the irritation fast, here are a few things to try.

For Immediate Relief

home remedies

Use artificial tears. Available in pharmacies, artificial tears have a similar composition to your natural tears. You can use them six or eight times a day to supplement your own tear production and to soothe and moisturize the surfaces of the eyes, says Dr. Marioneaux.

It's a good idea to avoid artificial tears made with preservatives because they can trigger allergic reactions in some people, Dr. Marioneaux adds. Eyedrops that are preservative-free usually carry the label "PF."

Humidify the air. Indoor humidifiers can be inexpensive, and they fill the air with eye-protecting moisture.

Take a break from contact lenses. No matter what kind you wear, contact lenses dry the eyes and can make them sore and irritated. When your eyes are bothering you, switch to your regular glasses for a few days. Even a short break from contacts may be enough to eliminate the irritating dryness.

medical options

Save the tears. Normally, there are plenty of tears to coat the eyes and protect the delicate surfaces. After they've done their work, the tears leave the eye through a duct called the lacrimal punctum. If you're suffering from dry eyes, your doctor may recommend plugging the duct with silicone or collagen, which allows more of the tears to stay in the eyes, says Dr. Marioneaux.

For Long-Term Relief

home remedies

Remind yourself to blink. When you're engrossed in a movie or working on a computer, you probably keep your eyes open much longer than you normally would. The tears evaporate instead of lubricating the eye surface. Try to blink 12 to 15 times a minute, says Dr. Marioneaux. Blinking spreads tears over the surfaces of the eyes, which helps prevent dryness.

Adjust the car vents. The blast of air from the air conditioner or heater in the car might feel good on your face, but over time it will pull moisture from the surfaces of the eyes. Tilt the vents so that the airflow is below, above, or to the sides of your eyes.

Wear goggles. Women who are active often suffer from dry eyes because the rushing wind wicks away moisture. An easy, long-term solution is to wear protective goggles when you ski, cycle, or run.

when to see a doctor

If your eyes have been dry for more than 2 weeks, or if the dryness is causing considerable discomfort, make an appointment to see an ophthalmologist. There are a number of potentially serious conditions—such as Sjögren's syndrome, thyroid disease, or lupus—that can cause dry eyes, says Sandra Belmont, M.D., associate professor of ophthalmology at Cornell University in New York City.

If you have eye dryness and you're also taking medications: Ask your doctor to review your medications to see if any of them might be responsible. A number of drugs—including antihistamines, birth control pills, decongestants, and medications for depression and high blood pressure—can cause eye dryness.

If you're approaching menopause or are postmenopausal: You may need supplemental hormones to bring your natural hormones into balance. This is often enough to keep the eyes healthy.

earaches and ear infections

Ear pain and infections are often considered to be a childhood problem. In fact, ear infections are the most common reason children visit their doctor. As adults, women are less likely to get ear infections and the earaches that accompany them. But we're not immune.

Infections of the middle ear often follow on the heels of colds or allergies, which cause an increase in secretions that sometimes block the narrow passageway (the eustachian tube) that connects the back of the nose to the ear. The blockage prevents normal airflow, creating an environment that's ideal for infection.

Less common, but even more painful, is swimmer's ear, a condition that occurs when moisture in the external or outer ear canal causes breaks in the skin that allow harmful germs to move in. Despite the name, it isn't caused only by swimming. "It can occur when you get water in your ears when you shower, bathe, or wash your hair," says Gregory Bergman, M.D., assistant clinical professor at the Wright State University School of Medicine in Dayton and a family practice physician in Minster, Ohio.

Some ear infections, especially those involving the external ear canal, need to be treated promptly. Apart from the fact that ear infections can be extremely painful, they can potentially cause permanent hearing loss. Here are a few ways to get them under control.

when to see a doctor

If the pain is so bad that you're thinking about taking an analgesic, call your doctor. There's a good chance that an infection is developing in the outer or middle ear, and you'll probably need antibiotics, says Gregory Bergman, M.D., assistant clinical professor at the Wright State University School of Medicine in Dayton and a family practice physician.

If you have ear pain and there's also blood or pus coming from the ear: Your eardrum may have ruptured, and you'll need immediate medical attention.

If you've been feeling dizzy and can't figure out why: Dizziness is a common symptom of ear infections, even in the absence of pain, says Dr. Bergman.

For Immediate Relief

home remedies

Soothe the pain with heat. Applying heat to the ear improves circulation and quickly reduces the painful throbbing in the outer ear. The easiest approach is to rest your head on a heating pad or hot-water bottle wrapped in a towel, says Dr. Bergman.

Make the ears less hospitable with vinegar. There's no such thing as an "ear towel" for those prone to swimmer's ear, but the next best thing is to put in a few drops made from equal amounts of white vinegar and warm water. After putting in the drops, raise your head for 3 to 5 minutes and then tilt it so the excess runs out of your ears. The solution will change the acid level in the outer ear, inhibiting the growth of bacteria and fungi, says Dr. Bergman.

Take antibiotics. Most ear infections are caused by bacteria, and a course of antibiotics will usually stop the pain of a middle ear infection within 3 days. If you do need antibiotics, be sure to finish the prescription, adds Dr. Bergman. It's the only way to ensure that all of the harmful germs are eliminated.

For Long-Term Prevention

Blow away moisture. If you sometimes get earaches because of swimmer's ear, an easy solution is to dry the inside of the ear with a hair dryer, says Dr. Bergman. After swimming or showering, hold the hair dryer 8 to 12 inches away from your ear. Set the heat on low, pull your ear back with one hand, and let the dryer run for a few minutes to thoroughly dry the ear.

Keep cotton swabs out of your ears. Women often use them for removing earwax, but they irritate the ear canal and increase the risk of earaches, says Dr. Bergman.

Blow gently. Aggressive nose blowing increases pressure in the middle ear, which can damage delicate tissues and make you more vulnerable to infections, says Dr. Bergman.

Prepare for takeoff. Every year, millions of travelers experience ear pain while flying, usually during takeoffs and, more likely, landings, when the changes in air pressure are greatest. The only way to prevent the pain is to equalize the pressure in the ears. One way to do this is to repeatedly say words with a *k* sound, like koala, says Dr. Bergman. Chewing gum or swallowing repeatedly will also help.

eczema

The worst part about eczema isn't necessarily the painful sores or shedding skin flakes. It may not even be the itching, which people often describe as severe. The worst part about this persistent, inflammatory skin condition is that it often appears on the face, elbows, wrists, or other visible areas. Some people are so self-conscious during flare-ups that they're reluctant to leave the house.

Doctors aren't sure what causes eczema, although it's probably linked to defects in the immune system. It runs in families, and attacks can be triggered by changes in temperature, rising or falling humidity, or even the changes of seasons, says Thomas Helm, M.D., clinical associate professor of dermatology and pathology at State University of New York at Buffalo.

Eczema often makes its appearance during

childhood, and children with asthma have a higher risk of getting it. Many children outgrow eczema by the time they are teenagers, but it does persist beyond puberty in 30 to 50 percent of those who suffer from it as children. It's not uncommon for remissions to last for months or even years. Even though there isn't a cure for eczema, most people can control it with medications and simple home care.

For Immediate Relief

home remedies

Use steroid creams. The quickest way to reduce skin inflammation and itching is to apply an over-the-counter cream that contains hydrocortisone or other steroids, says Amy S. Paller, M.D., professor of pediatrics and dermatology at Northwestern University Medical School and head of the division of dermatology at Children's Memo-

when to see a doctor

If you have eczema and your usual treatments don't "clear" the rash, call your doctor for advice. It's common for medications and other treatments to lose their effectiveness over time, says Thomas Helm, M.D., clinical associate professor of dermatology and pathology at State University of New York at Buffalo.

If your skin develops moist patches or blisters: There's a good chance that you've developed an infection, probably due to scratching. You may need antibiotics or other medications to stop the infection and speed healing.

rial Hospital, both in Chicago. You can apply the creams up to two times daily to get relief.

Keep your hands busy. Doctors advise people with eczema not to scratch—and nearly everyone ignores the advice because the itching is so intense. But it's still good advice because scratching irritates the skin and can make the itching worse. One solution is to keep your hands busy with enjoyable activities, such as knitting, quilting, or painting.

Use moisturizers daily. They keep the skin moist and pliable, which helps stop irritation and itching. The best time to apply a moisturizer is right after you bathe or shower because it will seal in water and give it a chance to be absorbed.

For Long-Term Relief

home remedies

Take quick baths and showers. The water should be warm, not hot. Extra-long baths in hot water may trigger flare-ups in some people.

Pat yourself dry. After bathing, don't rub the skin vigorously with a towel. Air drying is best, but if you can't take that much time, pat your skin with a towel for gentle drying.

Spend some time in the sun. Exposure to the ultraviolet light in sunshine sometimes prevents flare-ups. Your doctor may "prescribe" spending 10 to 15 minutes in the sun each day.

Of course, too much sun can be just as harmful as too little. Ask your doctor whether sunshine will be helpful for you and whether or not you'll need to use a sunscreen to prevent skin damage.

Calm the immune system. When eczema doesn't respond to home treatments or over-the-counter creams, your doctor may recommend a stronger steroid cream or ointment, or new medications called immunomodulators. A study of more than 1,000 children and adults showed that an immunomodulating ointment called tacrolimus improved or completely eliminated eczema in more than 80 percent of the people who used it. "They have all of the benefits of topical or oral steroids, with few of the risks," Dr. Helm says.

Ask about phototherapy. A fancy word for "light exposure," phototherapy involves exposing the skin to precise amounts of ultraviolet light from specialized lamps. It's a very effective way to prevent flare-ups—or to help skin rashes and inflammation heal more quickly.

fatigue

t's early afternoon, and lunch is followed by one big yawn after another. Ready for a snooze? Join the club: Millions of Americans barely have enough energy to get through the day, and the problem is getting worse all the time.

Americans are spending more time working and less time sleeping or simply having fun. According to a survey conducted by the National Sleep Foundation, 60 percent of women don't get the 8 hours of sleep that they need to feel refreshed and energized.

"Most women need about 8 hours of sleep in order to wake up feeling rested and to have energy throughout the day," says Lynn Mack-Shipman, M.D., an endocrinologist and assistant professor of internal medicine at the University of Nebraska Medical Center in Omaha. "Sleep deprivation is a common cause of fatigue."

It's not the only one, however. Many women are low in iron. That's the mineral essential for creating hemoglobin, the iron-based protein in blood that ferries the oxygen that the body needs for energy. Thyroid conditions can also lead to fatigue, says Dr. Mack-Shipman. So can stress, which is almost at epidemic proportions these days.

"The average woman today has many responsibilities, such as a full-time job, child rearing, housework, and taking care of aging parents," says Dr. Mack-Shipman. The stress from personal and professional responsibilities, along with the physical burden of trying to do too much, leaves many women feeling exhausted all the time.

Because fatigue is a common symptom of medical problems, it's essential to see your doctor as soon as you notice that your energy isn't what it should be. In most cases, however, it's possible to recharge your batteries with a variety of at-home techniques.

For Immediate Relief

Adjust your sleep schedule. Many women get into the habit of keeping late hours—but the alarm clock still goes off at the same time every morning. If you aren't getting enough sleep at night, there's no way you're going to feel energetic during the day.

The solution is simple: Try to go to bed a little earlier. You can't shift your body's internal clock all at once, so you have to work in increments. Go to bed about 15 minutes earlier than usual. Do

Dealing with Altitude Sickness

every year, millions of Americans take their vacations at high altitudes, where they hike, camp, climb rocks, or ski. It can be both exhilarating and relaxing to leave the confines of an office and spend time trekking up a mountain trail. But women who are planning vacations in areas where the altitude is above 8,000 feet need to be on the lookout for altitude sickness.

As you ascend to high altitudes, the amount of oxygen in the air declines. Because less oxygen reaches the body's cells, you start breathing faster to compensate. This brings more oxygen to the blood, but not enough to provide all that your body needs. About one in four people who hike to elevations above 8,000 feet will experience altitude sickness, which is potentially life threatening, says Benjamin Honigman, M.D., chief of emergency medicine at the University of Colorado School of Medicine in Denver. "The higher you climb, the greater your chances are of getting sick," he adds.

The early symptoms of altitude sickness include fatigue, headache, light-headedness, weakness, nausea, or difficulty sleeping. "If you're beginning to feel any of these symptoms, climb back down to a lower elevation immediately," says Dr. Honigman. "Stay there until you feel better. Once your body's adjusted, you can continue climbing."

Here are a few additional ways to combat altitude sickness.

Pace yourself. "Even if you're an active, fit individual, don't hike as far on day 1 as you would on day 2 or 3," says Dr. Honigman. "This gives your body time to adjust to the lower oxygen level. If you hike up to a level of 12,000 feet, limit yourself to hiking no more than 1,500 feet per day."

Sleep low. Respiration slows at night, which makes it even harder for the body to get enough oxygen. If you're hiking to high altitudes, it's a good idea to descend every night when it's time to sleep. "For example, if you're at 10,000 feet, hike down to 8,000 feet to sleep," says Dr. Honigman.

Drink plenty of fluids. The body loses a lot of water when you climb to high altitudes, so it's essential to take in plenty of fluids. "I recommend doubling your usual intake of water or a nutritious beverage," says Dr. Honigman. "If you normally drink 2 quarts of fluid each day, drink 4 quarts."

Take ginkgo. "We don't really know why it helps, but recent studies indicate it may help prevent altitude sickness," says Dr. Honigman. Ask your physician about this in advance of your next hike.

Ask your doctor about preventive medicine. "Some people are more prone to altitude sickness than others," says Dr. Honigman. "If you've experienced it before, talk to your doctor about taking the prescription medicine acetazolamide (Diamox). It increases respiratory rate and helps your body adjust to the higher elevations better." ■

this for a few weeks until it feels like the "right" time. Then move your bedtime back another 15 minutes. Keep doing this until you're getting a full 8 hours' sleep. Most women can make the transition easily, and you'll find that your energy levels will be higher throughout the day.

Get your body moving. Exercise doesn't produce energy directly; as a matter of fact, it consumes energy. But women who walk, jog, work in the yard, or are otherwise physically active generally notice that fatigue is much less of a problem.

"Physical activity stimulates the release of beta-endorphins, hormones that make you feel alive, refreshed, and energized," explains Dr. Mack-Shipman. Exercise is also beneficial because it tires the muscles, which in turn will make it easier to sleep at night.

Vary your routine. Women who are new to exercise often complain that doing the same things every day is too boring to stay motivated. That's why many people who start exercise plans drop out within a few weeks or months. The solution is to identify a dozen or more physical activities that you enjoy—it could be swimming, working in the garden, bicycling, or even walking through the mall—and swap them around so that you never get bored.

"Try running one day and lifting weights the next. Or do something entirely different, like tai chi or ballroom dancing," Dr. Mack-Shipman suggests.

THREE THINGS I TELL EVERY FEMALE PATIENT

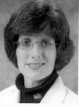

LYNN MACK-SHIPMAN, M.D., an endocrinologist and assistant professor of internal medicine at the University of Nebraska Medical Center in Omaha, sees a lot of women whose main symptom is fatigue. Here's what she advises.

DO EVERYTHING YOU CAN TO RELAX. "Stress can zap anyone of their energy," says Dr. Mack-Shipman. "Practice relaxation techniques. I've actually written a prescription for one of my patients to enroll in a yoga class."

Yoga isn't the only way to relax, of course. Some women cut back on their work hours. Others practice relaxation techniques such as meditation or visualization. Exercise is a great stress-reducing technique because it stimulates the releases of "calming" chemicals in the brain.

FOCUS ON COMPLEX CARBOHYDRATES. Whole grains, legumes, and other plant foods are rich in complex carbohydrates, which are broken down slowly during digestion. This allows glucose (blood sugar) to be produced at a steady pace, which helps maintain energy.

AVOID SIMPLE CARBOHYDRATES. There's nothing wrong with having a sweet snack on occasion, but the sugars in snacks and sodas, known as simple carbohydrates, cause blood sugar levels to spike. The body responds by releasing large amounts of insulin, which can make you feel tired. ■

Energize with essential oils. "Smelling certain scents can invigorate your body and mind and help you feel more energetic," says Alan Hirsch, M.D., neurologic director of the Smell and Taste

when to see a doctor

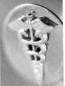

If you feel as though you sleep well at night, but you're still exhausted during the day, make an appointment to see your doctor. You could have a sleep problem that's preventing you from getting all the rest you need, says Lynn Mack-Shipman, M.D., an endocrinologist and assistant professor of internal medicine at the University of Nebraska Medical Center in Omaha.

Insomnia is probably the most common sleep disorder, but it's not the only one. Your doctor might advise you to have a sleep test, which will measure brain waves, respiration, and other factors that can affect the quality of your sleep, Dr. Mack-Shipman explains.

If you've been fatigued for months, and nothing you try seems to help: You should ask your doctor about getting tested for iron deficiency anemia. If you are anemic, getting adequate amounts of iron will reverse the symptoms within weeks or even days.

If the fatigue is accompanied by weight gain, intolerance to cold, and constipation: These are classic symptoms of an underactive thyroid, says Dr. Mack-Shipman.

If you have increased thirst and you're also urinating frequently: You could have diabetes, which is often accompanied by severe fatigue.

Treatment and Research Foundation in Chicago. The scents of peppermint and jasmine essential oils are especially energizing, he says.

The easiest way to use "scent therapy" is to put a few drops of essential oil on a handkerchief, then take a few minutes to enjoy the aroma. Another option is to use an aromatherapy diffuser, available from mail-order catalogs and some health food stores. It will fill the air with the special scents.

For Long-Term Prevention

Get enough iron. Millions of American women don't get enough iron in the diet. This is especially common during the childbearing years because women lose a little blood each month during menstruation. Even when a woman doesn't have full-fledged iron deficiency anemia, low levels of this mineral can result in fatigue.

"Some women don't consume enough iron-rich foods, such as red meats, because they are concerned about gaining weight," says Dr. Mack-Shipman. Without sufficient amounts of iron, the red blood cells can't carry as much oxygen, which results in fatigue.

The best sources of iron are lean red meats, poultry, eggs, and fish, says Dr. Mack-Shipman. Other options include fortified breakfast cereals, potatoes, and beans. The Daily Value for iron is 18 milligrams, she says.

Drink plenty of water. "Dehydration, even in its earliest stages, can make you feel tired and weak," says Dr. Mack-Shipman. Try to drink eight full glasses of water daily, she advises.

Lose weight sensibly. Women who are trying to lose weight often depend upon restrictive diets such as those high in protein and low in carbohydrates, and others that are very low in calories. These diets aren't very effective for weight loss, and they're even worse for maintaining healthful energy levels, says Cindy Polich, R.D., a medical nutritionist at the University of Nebraska Medical Center in Omaha.

"Following one of these 'starvation' diets can lead to fatigue and weakness," she says. "When you don't get enough carbohydrates, you deplete your short-term energy supplies."

Whether or not you're trying to lose weight, you want to choose a variety of foods from the food guide pyramid, focusing on carbohydrates such as whole grains, legumes, and fruits and vegetables. "The body converts carbohydrates into glucose, which is used for energy," Polich explains.

Maintain a healthful weight. Women who are above a healthy weight are more likely to experience fatigue. Extra weight can also increase your risk for a sleep disorder, called apnea, in which breathing is reduced at night. Your body responds by waking up momentarily in order to take a deep breath. You might not be aware of the disturbance in your sleep, but your energy levels are sure to suffer the next day.

A "Hidden" Cause of Fatigue

The thyroid is a small gland at the base of the front of the neck. It uses iodine from the blood to produce and store thyroid hormone, which plays a major role in the body's metabolism. Women who produce too little thyroid hormone, a condition called hypothyroidism, will feel tired, weak, or depressed.

Doctors estimate that 17 percent of women will have thyroid problems by the time they reach their 60th birthdays. "The condition often comes on gradually, over months or years, so it's not always diagnosed right away," says Gay Canaris, M.D., assistant professor of internal medicine at the University of Nebraska College of Medicine in Omaha. As a result, the symptoms often go unnoticed by either the patient or her doctor and are easily attributed to other medical problems, overwork, or stress, Dr. Canaris adds. Hypothyroidism is diagnosed by a blood test that measures thyroid gland function.

Women with a family history of thyroid disorders, or those with autoimmune conditions such as lupus, have a higher risk of developing hypothyroidism. Women who have recently given birth are also at risk, Dr. Canaris says.

Hypothyroidism is easy to treat with medications. Once your hormone levels are back to normal, most thyroid symptoms will improve. "You just have to take one small pill a day of synthetic thyroid hormone," says Dr. Canaris. "It's really very simple." ■

fever

t seems ironic, but trying to lower a mild fever may be counterproductive: The rise in temperature that occurs when you're ill may enhance the body's defense mechanisms against viruses and bacteria—when it does, you recover more quickly.

On the other hand, even a slight fever can make you feel a lot worse, and doctors agree that it makes more sense to reduce the discomfort than to wait for nature to takes it course, says Steven Mostow,

when to see a doctor

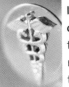 **If your temperature climbs to 102°F or higher:** It's common for children to develop high fevers, but adults rarely do unless they have something more serious than a simple cold or flu, says Anne L. Davis, M.D., a pulmonologist and associate professor of medicine at New York University School of Medicine and an attending physician at Bellevue Hospital, both in New York City.

If you have underlying medical problems, such as heart or lung disease: "Any fever, even a low-grade one, should be taken seriously, especially in older people, because fever increases the body's oxygen demands, which can put a strain on the heart and other already damaged organs," says Dr. Davis.

If the fever is accompanied by teeth-chattering chills that last more than 10 minutes at a time: This is a sign that bacteria may have entered the bloodstream, which can result in a serious infection. Call your doctor immediately.

M.D., professor of medicine and infectious diseases and associate dean at the University of Colorado Health Sciences Center in Denver. And there's no evidence that lowering a fever for comfort interferes with recovery, he adds.

Fevers can be caused by dozens of conditions, from ear or urinary tract infections to simple colds and flu as well as certain inflammatory, immunologic, or malignant disorders, and some medications. As long as fever is your main symptom, and your temperature doesn't spike above 102°F, it's fine to treat it at home, says Anne L. Davis, M.D., a pulmonologist and associate professor of medicine at New York University School of Medicine and an attending physician at Bellevue Hospital, both in New York City. Here are a few helpful strategies.

For Immediate Relief

home remedies

Drink enough water. Your body loses a lot of water when you have a fever, which can dehydrate the brain and other tissues and leave you feeling weak and tired. Try to drink a sufficient amount of water so that you will need to urinate once every 1 to 2 hours—that's about eight glasses of water a day—until the fever is gone. Caffeine-free, nonalcoholic beverages and 100 percent fruit juices diluted by half with water are also helpful.

Take an over-the-counter painkiller. In addition to their pain-relieving properties, aspirin, ibuprofen, and acetaminophen are very effective at lowering fever, says William J. Hall, M.D., president of the American College of Physicians–American Society of Internal Medicine in Philadelphia and chief of general medicine of the geriatrics unit, professor of medicine, pediatrics, and oncology at the University of Rochester School of Medicine in New York.

Some people need to be careful about which of these drugs they choose. For example, acetaminophen is less likely to cause stomach upset than aspirin or ibuprofen. And doctors warn that children with the flu or other respiratory infections should never be given aspirin because it can increase the risk for Reye's syndrome, a potentially serious neurological disorder. If you have a chronic disease or are taking other medications, consult with your doctor before using any over-the-counter drug.

alternative therapies

Try willow bark. Available in a dried form for making tea, willow bark contains salicin, which is very similar to the active ingredient in aspirin. To make a tea, steep 2 teaspoons of dried bark in 1 cup of boiling water for 20 minutes. Willow bark has a bitter taste, so you'll probably want to flavor the tea with cinnamon, ginger, or other sweet-tasting herbs.

Sip cinnamon tea. Herbalists have used it for centuries for reducing inflammation and lowering fever, and modern science shows that it works. Cinnamon contains a compound called cinnamaldehyde, which fights bacteria and helps reduce infections.

To make a tea, pour 1 cup of boiling water over two or three sticks of cinnamon; add a few whole cloves for flavor. Let the tea steep, covered, for 20 minutes, then drink it down. You can repeat the treatment several times a day.

Brew some ginger tea. It has a pleasant flavor, and it contains a variety of chemical compounds that can reduce fever. You can make teas with powdered ginger, but the fresh root may be more effective. It also tastes better. Grate 1 tablespoon of ginger, cover it with 1 cup of boiling water, and let it steep 10 minutes.

fibromyalgia

Women who develop fibromyalgia often confuse it with the flu, at least at first. It typically causes muscle stiffness, headaches, poor sleep, and an overwhelming sense of fatigue. People with fibromyalgia hurt all over, and they are often too tired to perform even the simplest daily activities. Unlike the flu, however, fibromyalgia doesn't go away in a week or two. It's a chronic condition, which means it can last months, years, or even decades.

Estimates show that 3.4 percent of American women suffer from fibromyalgia. It's most common in women of childbearing age, but children, the elderly, and men can also be affected.

Tender Spots Signal
Fibromyalgia

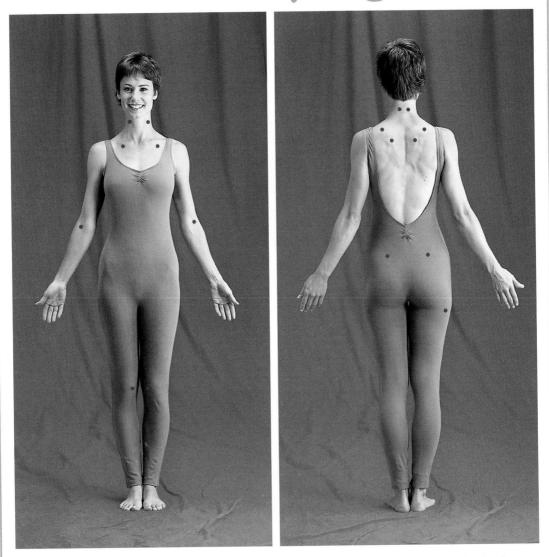

According to the American College of Rheumatology, people with fibromyalgia have widespread pain, along with tenderness in at least 11 of 18 "tender point" locations, shown here.

How can you tell if your symptoms are caused by fibromyalgia? The telltale sign is "tender points"—extremely sensitive areas that generally appear in the neck, spine, shoulders, and hips, says Lenore Buckley, M.D., a rheumatologist and professor of internal medicine and pediatrics at Virginia Commonwealth University School of Medicine in Richmond. Depression is another common symptom. Research has shown that between 18 and 36 percent of people with fibromyalgia suffer from depression at any given time.

Another characteristic of fibromyalgia is poor sleep. It's not that people with this condition sleep too little; in fact, many people with fibromyalgia sleep 10 (or more) hours a night. The problem is that they fail to achieve the deeper levels of sleep that they need to feel refreshed. The lack of deep sleep can interfere with the ability to focus and concentrate during the day. It can also make people feel groggy and "out of it" when they wake up in the morning.

Scientists still aren't sure what causes fibromyalgia. One theory is that injuries affecting the central nervous system play a role—which may explain why a large percentage of whiplash victims develop it. Some scientists have linked fibromyalgia to changes in muscle metabolism, which may result in diminished bloodflow and, in turn, fatigue.

Some evidence indicates that fibromyalgia is triggered by bacterial or viral infections. Research has shown, for example, that 10 to 25 percent of people with Lyme disease, a bacterial infection transmitted by ticks, will develop fibromyalgia.

Fibromyalgia is a challenge to diagnose because many of the symptoms are similar to those caused by other disorders. If you have tender points and widespread pain that has lasted more than 3 months, and tests show that you don't have lupus, arthritis, or Lyme disease, you could have fibromyalgia.

So far, there isn't a cure for fibromyalgia. That doesn't mean you have to live with it forever. The severity of the symptoms tends to come and go, and it's not uncommon for fibromyalgia to spontaneously disappear. In the meantime, here are a few ways to reduce the pain and discomfort.

For Immediate Relief

home remedies

Get a massage. "I have found in my patients with fibromyalgia that a massage stops the pain," says Denise Borrelli, Ph.D., a nationally certified massage therapist and clinical director of A Healing Touch Holistic Healing Center in Medford, Massachusetts.

Massage is relaxing, which makes it much easier for people with fibromyalgia to get the sleep they need. "Some of my patients have been able to cut back on their sleep medications after they started getting massages regularly," says Dr. Borrelli.

There are a bewildering variety of massage techniques to choose from. "I recommend Swedish massage because the long, gentle strokes are very soothing," Dr. Borrelli says. "I advise against deep muscle tissue massage because it can irritate nerve endings and cause more pain," she adds.

Depending on where you live, massage can cost anywhere from $30 to $100 per hour. To find a massage therapist in your area, contact the American Massage Therapy Association at 820 Davis Street, Suite 100, Evanston, IL 60201, or call the association's toll-free number, (888) 843-2682. Or go to the association's Web site at www.amtamassage.org.

Enjoy pool therapy. Warm-water pool therapy is a great way to relax the muscles and reduce the pain, says Dr. Buckley.

Exercise as much as you can. Walking, biking, water exercise, and other forms of aerobic exercise have been shown to reduce muscle pain and tenderness. Regular exercise also stimulates the production of endorphins, chemical messengers in the brain that promote feelings of relaxation and well-being.

If you have fibromyalgia, it probably won't be easy to start an exercise program because your muscles will be sore and achy. But it's worth pushing through the initial discomfort. As your muscles get stronger, you'll find you have more energy and endurance, and the intensity and frequency of the pain will gradually diminish.

If you haven't been physically active, you'll want to start out with stretching exercises before launching into full-fledged workouts. "Walking is more of an intermediate exercise for women to work up to," says Dr. Buckley. "Take a brisk 5-minute walk, then gradually increase the time and

THREE THINGS I TELL EVERY FEMALE PATIENT

LENORE BUCKLEY, M.D., a rheumatologist and professor of internal medicine and pediatrics at Virginia Commonwealth University School of Medicine in Richmond, offers this special advice for women with fibromyalgia.

FOCUS ON SLEEP. "It's hard for doctors to help people with fibromyalgia until we take care of the sleep problem," Dr. Buckley says. "Many people don't get the 7 or 8 hours of deep, uninterrupted sleep that they need, which leaves them feeling tired and unable to concentrate."

DO EVERYTHING POSSIBLE TO RELAX. The more stress you have in your life, the more anxiety and pain you'll experience. "Stress re-

duction helps people feel better overall, and it also helps them sleep better at night," says Dr. Buckley. Everyone relaxes in different ways, and you'll have to experiment to find what works best for you. "I advise people to do whatever appeals to them, whether it's walking, water exercise, deep breathing, meditation, or yoga."

EXERCISE IS CRITICAL. "It's very difficult for fibromyalgia patients to get better who are not part of an exercise program," says Dr. Buckley. "Regular, gentle exercise, such as walking or warm-water exercises, can help loosen up stiff muscles and get the blood flowing again—all of which will help ease pain." ▪

intensity until you're walking briskly for 40 minutes three times a week."

Avoid caffeine. Coffee, tea, and other caffeine-containing beverages are America's favorite pick-me-ups, but people often forget just how stimulating they can be. If you have fibromyalgia, consuming caffeine close to bedtime can make it difficult to get the deep, restorative sleep that you need.

Your doctor may advise you to limit your consumption of caffeine-containing beverages to one or two servings daily—and to avoid them altogether in the afternoon and evening.

For Long-Term Relief

home remedies

Take a yoga class. Even though regular exercise is among the best ways to ease the discomfort of fibromyalgia, people are often too tired or sore to get started. One way to get the muscles primed for action is to practice yoga. "If yoga is the exercise you choose, start with a beginning class," says Dr. Buckley.

Sign up for aquacise. "Warm-water exercises are very beneficial for fibromyalgia patients because they relax the muscles and decrease pain," says Dr. Buckley. "The water supports the muscles, so you're not working against gravity," she adds.

Some people head straight to a local pool, but it's better to sign up for an aquacise program tailored for those with fibromyalgia. "It's important to make sure that you're doing the moves correctly so you don't hurt yourself," says Dr.

when to see a doctor

If you've had widespread pain for 3 months or more, see your doctor right away. It's one of the classic signs of fibromyalgia, says Lenore Buckley, M.D., a rheumatologist and professor of internal medicine and pediatrics at Virginia Commonwealth University School of Medicine in Richmond.

If you feel pain at specific "tender points": People with fibromyalgia typically have tender areas on the shoulders, elbows, hips, or buttocks.

If you're always fatigued, and you can't figure out why: Fibromyalgia isn't the only condition that can result in low energy or lethargy. If you're exhausted all the time and there doesn't seem to be a good reason for it, see your doctor.

Buckley. Your doctor can refer you to a physical therapy program that includes water exercises. Many health clubs and YMCAs and YWCAs also offer aquacise classes in cooperation with the Arthritis Foundation.

Try to think positively. It's hard to be upbeat and positive when you're hurting, but it's worth making the effort. Studies have shown that people who dwell on their pain and unhappiness experience a lot more stress—which in turn increases pain.

In one large study, researchers at the University of Missouri in Columbia compared drug and nondrug treatments for fibromyalgia. They found that people who exercised or practiced cognitive-behavioral therapy—in which they learned to substitute positive thoughts for negative ones—

experienced less pain and fatigue. They also performed daily tasks more easily than those who only took drugs.

A good place to start is to make an appointment with a psychological therapist. In the meantime, do everything you can to relax. Set aside time each day to meditate, listen to music, or simply unwind.

medical options

Consider antidepressants. Even if you aren't suffering from depression, medications such as amitriptyline (such as Elavil or Endep) and fluoxetine (Prozac) can be extremely helpful for fibromyalgia. Apart from reducing muscle pain, these medications also make it easier to sleep, which can significantly boost energy and help you to stay active.

Today's antidepressants are safe and effective, but they may cause side effects, such as a dry mouth or grogginess.

Ask your doctor about drug combinations. In a study at Newton-Wellesley Hospital in Newton, Massachusetts, people with fibromyalgia were treated with Elavil, Prozac, or a combination of the two drugs. Those who took both drugs experienced twice the improvement of those taking the drugs separately. In fact, 12 of the 19 participants in the study reported improvements of at least 25 percent.

Researchers suspect that the combination of Elavil and Prozac may change pain perception in people with fibromyalgia. The medications also affect bloodflow to pain-receptive regions of the brain, and they enhance the body's production of "feel-good" chemicals such as serotonin.

Take a sleep aid. "The main goal in the pharmaceutical treatment of fibromyalgia is to help people get some sleep," says Dr. Buckley. "The pain often keeps people up at night, and even when they do fall asleep, the pain often wakes them up."

For more information on fibromyalgia: See the Web site of the National Institute of Arthritis and Musculoskeletal and Skin Diseases at www.nih.gov/niams. Other helpful Web sites include the Fibromyalgia Network at www.fmnetnews.com and the Arthritis Foundation at www.arthritis.org.

flu

Nothing ruins a woman's plans for the day—or the week—like coming down with a cold. Colds are annoying, uncomfortable, and messy. But they can't compete with the discomfort—and danger—of the flu. Short for "influenza," the flu is a highly contagious illness that's responsible for more than 20,000 deaths in the United States every year.

Women cross their fingers every fall and winter, hoping they won't get the flu. The problem with the flu virus is that it's constantly changing, or mutating, in order to outfox the body's immune system. The virus changes so rapidly that vaccine manufacturers have to design new formulas every year in order to combat the newest strains.

A mild case of the flu bears some resemblance to a serious cold, causing coughs, achy muscles, and a sore throat. More often, the flu feels like no cold you've ever had. "With the flu, you feel like you have been hit with a giant pile driver," says Steven Mostow, M.D., professor of medicine and infectious diseases and associate dean at the University of Colorado Health Sciences Center in Denver.

Utter exhaustion is usually the first symptom. After that, you may have intense head and muscle aches, a high fever, chest congestion, and a severe cough.

Kay A. Bauman, M.D., professor of medicine and associate dean at the John A. Burns School of Medicine at the University of Hawaii in Honolulu, says she has no trouble keeping up with her work and exercise routines when she has a cold—but a recent bout of the flu wiped her out. "I was flat on my back," Dr. Bauman explains. "A cold makes your head feel miserable. The flu is allover misery."

There isn't a miracle cure for flu. Medications can help, but mainly what you have to do is take it easy until the infection passes. In addition, it's important to boost your body's defenses and take a few steps to ease the worst of the discomfort.

For Immediate Relief

home remedies

Eat immune-boosting foods. When you're sick, more than ever it's important to choose foods that

---

THREE THINGS I TELL EVERY FEMALE PATIENT

STEVEN MOSTOW, M.D., professor of medicine and infectious diseases and associate dean at the University of Colorado Health Sciences Center in Denver, gives his patients the following important advice.

CALL YOUR DOCTOR INSTEAD OF COMING TO THE OFFICE. The flu is highly contagious, and the last thing you want is to spread the virus to other patients in the waiting room. When people call Dr. Mostow and describe classic flu symptoms, he simply phones in a prescription for an antiviral drug. Women with the flu usually feel so lousy that they welcome the chance to stay home in bed

rather than make the trip to the office, he adds.

DON'T ASK FOR AN ANTIBIOTIC. The flu is caused by viruses, which aren't affected by antibiotics, Dr. Mostow explains. Too many people (including doctors) use antibiotics unnecessarily, which make the germs stronger and the drugs less effective.

GET VACCINATED. No remedy or immune-boosting strategy can compare with the preventive power of the flu vaccine. Everyone, including women, should get the vaccine annually, Dr. Mostow says. ■

shore up the immune system, such as green leafy vegetables (which are rich in vitamins A and C), citrus fruits, tomatoes, strawberries, carrots, and pumpkin. Even small amounts of produce can make a big difference: One study found that eating about one medium carrot or two small carrots significantly boosted immune cell activity.

Remember that old rule. An apple a day just might keep the doctor away! When invading viruses go chomping and chewing their way through your healthy cells, they leave behind a trail of free radicals, tiny land mines that can blow up your immune system's defenses. Quercetin, a natural plant chemical found in apples as well as in onions, berries, and tomatoes, is one of the top technicians on the bomb-defusing squad.

"Quercetin disarms free radicals, disrupting the tricks those pathogens use to sabotage us," says David L. Katz, M.D., director of the Yale D. Griffin Prevention Research Center in Derby, Connecticut. Try to get nine servings of quercetin-containing fruits and vegetables every day.

Make an antiviral soup. To stimulate your body's defenses, chop up fresh vegetables, add plenty of onions and garlic, and cook them in 8 ounces of steaming chicken broth per serving. Both onions and garlic contain compounds that have antiviral properties.

Cut back on fat and sugar. Until the virus is gone, try to eat as little fat as possible, no more than 25 percent of daily calories, because it reduces the ability of the immune system to work efficiently. It's also important to avoid sweet foods because sugar undermines phagocytosis, the process by which viruses are destroyed by white blood cells.

Drink hot tea. It's an old folk remedy for the flu, and there's good evidence that it works. Drinking several cups of steaming tea daily will thin mucus and help relieve congestion.

Breathe moist air. Take a long, hot shower or plug in a humidifier. Moisture in the air soothes irritated tissues in the throat and airways, says Dr. Mostow.

when to see a doctor

 If you suspect that you have the flu, call your doctor right away. There are a number of prescription drugs that can dramatically reduce discomfort as long as you take them a day or two after symptoms appear, says Steven Mostow, M.D., professor of medicine and infectious diseases and associate dean at the University of Colorado Health Sciences Center in Denver.

If your symptoms seem unusually severe: High fever, difficulty breathing, and other common flu symptoms can also be caused by other conditions, including pneumonia and heart disease. In addition, some strains of flu can make people so ill that they require hospitalization, so call your doctor right away if you're suffering from any severe symptoms.

If you start feeling better, then take a turn for the worse: The original flu infection could have set the stage for a secondary bacterial infection—which means you'll need to take antibiotics as soon as possible. Call your doctor immediately if you suspect an infection.

Enjoy herbal teas. A number of herbal teas contain compounds that soothe sore throats and also break up congestion in the airways. Some of the best include slippery elm bark and marshmallow root, which relieve sore throats; and thyme and eucalyptus leaf, which help loosen congestion. Teas made from boneset or yarrow are especially good because they have immune-boosting properties.

To make a tea, pour 1 cup of boiling water over crushed, dried herbs as indicated for each: slippery elm bark (powdered only) or marshmallow root, steep 2 teaspoons for 10 minutes; thyme, eucalyptus leaf, or yarrow, steep 1 teaspoon for 10 minutes; or boneset, steep $1/2$ teaspoon for 30 minutes. Strain the leaves, and drink the tea while it's hot. You can drink several cups of herbal tea a day—except drink only 3 cups daily of thyme or eucalyptus leaf.

Gargle with an echinacea tonic. Mix about $1/2$ teaspoon of echinacea tincture in 8 ounces of warm water. Gargling with the mixture will help numb a sore throat. When you're done gargling, swallow the liquid, which will fortify your body with an immune-boosting blast of echinacea. You may do this several times a day.

Allow yourself some downtime. No one enjoys taking time away from work or family responsibilities when they're sick, but it's a mistake to ignore your pounding head and rattling cough. You have to listen to what your body's telling you, says Dr. Bauman. "If it's saying, 'Go to bed,' well, you should go to bed," she says.

food allergy

In the past few years, a number of airlines have eliminated the customary practice of handing out bags of peanuts to hungry passengers. The reason: Many people—male and female alike—are allergic to peanuts, and for those whose allergy is severe, even the scent molecules that waft from a newly opened bag can trigger life-threatening reactions.

Fortunately, most food allergies aren't this serious. People who eat the "wrong" foods may break out in hives or welts. Or they may have nausea, diarrhea, or other digestive problems. Once the offending foods clear the system, the symptoms rapidly disappear.

But whether your allergies are minor or severe, there's only one long-term solution: to avoid the foods that make you sick. This isn't always easy because people with food allergies are rarely allergic to just one food. They usually react to whole groups of foods, such as shellfish or certain grains. Identifying the culprit—and avoiding it—can take some work. As little as $1/5,000$ teaspoon of an offending food can potentially cause a reaction. Women who are allergic to peanuts, for example, could have problems if a cook merely used the same spatula when baking different types of cookies, one of which contained peanuts. If you're allergic to a certain food or foods, you have to avoid them entirely—probably for the rest of your life.

Food allergies occur when the immune system mistakes an entirely innocent protein for a harmful intruder. It overreacts and launches a full array of immune cells to counteract the "attack," which is what causes the symptoms, says Clifton T. Furukawa, M.D., the Seattle-based vice president of the American Academy of Allergy, Asthma, and Immunology.

While most food allergies cause only minor symptoms, people with extreme sensitivities may experience a life-threatening reaction called anaphylaxis, which can literally shut down the airways and cause blood pressure to plummet. Anaphylaxis is more common in people with food allergies than in those who are allergic to insect stings or medications.

Food allergies often begin in childhood, although adults, too, can develop them. Children with food allergies tend to be sensitive to eggs and milk, while adults are more likely to be allergic to shellfish or nuts. Children sometimes outgrow food allergies, but if you developed the problem as a grown woman, it's unlikely to go away, says Dr. Furukawa.

Researchers are investigating ways to reverse the body's sensitivity to potential allergens in foods, but for now there isn't a cure for food allergies. All you can do is make sure to avoid the "wrong" foods, and know what to do should an emergency strike.

For Immediate Relief

home remedies

Act quickly. If you have a minor food allergy and you accidentally eat what you shouldn't, most reactions can be treated with an antihistamine, and

WHAT WORKS FOR ME

ANNE MUÑOZ-FURLONG *is chief executive officer of the Virginia-based Food Allergy and Anaphylaxis Network—and the parent of a daughter, now 17, who once suffered from severe food allergies. She quickly learned to be especially vigilant when they enjoyed meals away from home.*

We never went to restaurants during their busiest times. We usually ate at 5:00 P.M., not 7:00 P.M., because that's when restaurant staffs are fresh and we could get their attention.

When I ordered, I would carefully explain to the waiter what would happen if we were accidentally served the wrong food. Once they understood the consequences, they were much more willing to work with us.

Sometimes the waiter would accidentally bring the wrong dish. I would order a new serving—but I would keep the old serving on the table. Otherwise, the chef might merely remove the offending item—for example, the cheese on a hamburger. He would think he'd done the right thing, but the food would still be contaminated with the offending protein. ■

you can simply wait for the symptoms to pass. But for those with severe allergies, waiting can cost them their lives. You have to be prepared to take immediate action—by giving yourself an anti-anaphylaxis injection and getting to an emergency room immediately.

Always carry a self-injector. Women with severe food allergies are advised to keep a self-injector handy. Products such as the EpiPen or AnaKit contain a medication called epinephrine. It helps reverse anaphylaxis by stimulating the heart, opening the airways, and reducing swelling of the throat.

If you have a history of food allergies but haven't had a serious reaction for years, it's easy to get complacent and leave the injector at home—either because you forgot it at the last minute or because you figured you wouldn't need it. Don't take that chance. When researchers looked at 32 people who had died from food allergy reactions, they found that only three of them were carrying their injectors.

"I tell patients they should always carry three doses of epinephrine," says Sandra M. Gawchick, D.O., codirector of the division of allergy and clinical immunology at Crozer-Chester Medical Center and clinical associate professor of pediatrics at Thomas Jefferson University Medical Center in Philadelphia. "They have one extra in case they drop one, another to buy them time until they get medical help, and a third in case they need another dose."

Use the medicine at the first sign of symptoms. Even if you're not completely sure if you're having an allergic reaction, give yourself the injection anyway. "I advise patients to inject the epinephrine first and ask questions later," says Dr. Furukawa. The sooner you get the injection, the better your chances of making a full recovery.

The advantage of the EpiPen is that it's fully automatic: Just remove the safety cap, push the tip against the outer thigh to release the medicine, and hold it in place for several seconds. Then get to an emergency room right away.

Practice. It takes time to learn to use self-injectors properly, so it's important to practice ahead of time. "You need about 30 pounds of pressure to trigger the EpiPen, so if you just tap it lightly, it won't work," says Ira M. Finegold, M.D., assistant clinical professor of medicine at Columbia University and chief of the division of allergy and clinical immunology and director of the R. A. Cooke Institute of Allergy at St. Luke's–Roosevelt Hospital Center, both in New York City. "That's why it's important to practice using it."

If you experience an allergic reaction and need to give yourself a shot, it's fine to raise your skirt slightly and put the shot into your thigh through panty hose, Dr. Finegold adds. If at all possible, avoid injecting yourself through thick fabric because you could get an infection when the needle goes through dirty clothing.

Avoid alcohol when eating out. Alcoholic beverages can increase the body's absorption of allergy-causing proteins, says Marianne Frieri, M.D., Ph.D., director of allergy and immunology at Nassau University Medical Center in East Meadow, New York, and professor of medicine at the State University of New York at Stony Brook.

At home, where it's easier to control your exposure to potential allergens, it's fine to enjoy a beer or a glass of wine. But when you're eating away from home, avoiding alcohol will give you an extra measure of protection.

Never take chances. Many people with food allergies don't take their condition seriously. They may assume that "just a tiny taste" won't hurt. Or they may depend on medication to get them out of a tight spot. This is a dangerous mindset, says Dr. Frieri. "Food allergies can be life threatening. People need to take their symptoms seriously."

For Long-Term Prevention

home remedies

Keep a food diary. It can be tricky to know what food or foods you're allergic to. The only way to find out which foods are friends and which are foes is to keep a comprehensive food diary. Every day, jot down everything you eat. Be specific: Don't write "salad" when you really ate lettuce, onions, tomatoes, and grated cheese. At the same time, note any physical symptoms that occur. If you keep the diary for several months, you'll start to narrow down the possible suspects.

Talk to your doctor about an elimination diet. This involves giving up, one at a time, the foods that you suspect are causing symptoms. If you felt that you had a reaction after eating shrimp, for example, you would give up shrimp for a few weeks. If you don't have additional symptoms, you may have discovered the culprit.

Of course, you might be allergic to more than one food, so you might have to repeat the process several times. Once you have a good idea what's causing the problems, the solution is obvious: You'll have to give up the foods completely.

Because there are so many ingredients in packaged foods, and because people with food allergies may react to similar proteins that are found in different foods, you'll need to work with your doctor to ensure that you're eliminating the proper foods—and to make sure that you're getting adequate nutrition while the elimination diet is under way.

Read food labels carefully. Packaged foods can contain dozens of ingredients—and sometimes you'll find ingredients where you least expect them. Surprising numbers of packaged foods contain soybeans, for example. Milk proteins are commonly used in packaged foods, even some that you wouldn't suspect of containing dairy.

The terms on food labels can be confusing, so you'll need to work with your doctor to identify possible offenders. For example, many products contain "casein" or "caseinates." These include milk protein, and foods that contain them can cause allergic reactions.

Check labels frequently. Food manufacturers often change the ingredients in their recipes. A food that was "safe" in the past might contain allergy-causing ingredients in the future. The only way to be safe is to read the labels every time you shop.

Keep foods and utensils separate. Some people with food allergies are so sensitive that the merest brush with an offending food can trigger anaphylaxis, says Dr. Gawchick. If you are at risk, you have to be careful that you don't inadvertently breathe, taste, or touch the foods that you're allergic to.

If you're allergic to peanuts, for example, make sure that family members don't use "your" cutting board when making peanut butter sandwiches. If you're allergic to shrimp, eating foods that were fried in the same oil could be just as harmful as eating the shrimp itself, says Dr. Finegold.

Call restaurants ahead of time. Eating away from home can be risky for people with food al-lergies. Asian restaurants, for example, typically use the same woks to cook all the dishes. Even if the chef assures you that your dish doesn't contain a certain ingredient, traces of it might remain on the utensils. Doctors refer to this as cross-contamination.

Rather than trusting a waiter to communicate your concerns to the chef, it's worth calling the restaurant ahead of time to express your concerns—and to find out if they're willing to accommodate you, says Anne Muñoz-Furlong, chief executive officer of the

Stay on Guard for Hidden Allergens

Women with life-threatening food allergies need to look for harmful ingredients in some unexpected places. Food is the main offender, of course, but food allergens can also be found in cosmetics, shampoos, and other items that you'd never think of eating.

It's possible, for example, for a woman who's allergic to nuts to develop a severe reaction if she uses a shampoo made with almond oil, says Hugh A. Sampson, M.D., director of the Elliot and Roslyn Jaffe Food Allergy Institute at Mount Sinai School of Medicine in New York City.

"One of my patients was allergic to nuts—and he developed wheezing and hives when the shampoo, which contained nut oils, got near the lips and eyes," he says.

Shaving creams, moisturizers, and lipsticks are often made with oils made from peanuts, al-monds, or soybeans, adds Clifford W. Bassett, M.D., assistant clinical professor of medicine at the State University of New York Health Science Center in Brooklyn and an attending physician and faculty member of New York University School of Medicine.

Even chewing gum is a potential problem for some people because it may contain cow's milk proteins, Dr. Bassett says.

Reading the labels may not always help because nonfood items rarely list all the ingredients—and those that are listed may be in scientific terms that are difficult to interpret. While nothing is completely foolproof, in some cases it may be helpful to call the manufacturer—use the Internet to find the number—to inquire about ingredients before using any product that can potentially get into the nose, mouth, or eyes. ■

Food Allergy and Anaphylaxis Network, based in Virginia.

Even if you call ahead, be sure to explain the issues to the waiter. If you're allergic to shellfish, for example, let the waiter know that the steak you've ordered can't be cooked in the same pan or section of the grill that's used to prepare shellfish, explains Dr. Gawchick.

Order simple foods. When you're eating out, it's a good idea to order foods that undergo minimal preparation. A baked potato, for example, is unlikely to be cross-contaminated with other foods, whereas french fries are prepared in oil that may be used to fry other foods.

Wear a medical alert bracelet or necklace. Anaphylaxis and other food allergy symptoms can come on very quickly—too quickly, in some cases, for people to care for themselves. Teach your friends and family about your self-injector so that they can help during a time of crisis. It's also helpful to carry a personalized card that lists your name, your doctor's name and phone number, and a list of foods that you're allergic to.

For more information about food allergies: Visit the Web site of the Food Allergy and Anaphylaxis Network at www.foodallergy.org.

gallstone attacks

The gallbladder is a small pouch that's connected to the liver at one end and the small intestine at the other. It's like a squeeze bottle; every time you eat, the gallbladder contracts and pushes out bile, a digestive fluid that breaks down fats, into the small intestine.

Bile consists of cholesterol, minerals, and other substances. Trouble begins when some of these substances form hard little deposits, or stones. The stones themselves don't cause problems unless they lodge in the tiny openings, or ducts, that lead to the small intestine. The bile flow is interrupted and tension builds up, causing fierce abdominal pain.

Gallstones are potentially serious because the blockages can cause an infection in the gallbladder. The gallbladder could even burst open, causing even more problems, some life threatening. Most gallstones are "silent," however: About 60 percent of those who have them never get sick.

But any woman who's had one gallstone attack will know that she doesn't want another one. Here are a few ways to reduce the discomfort and prevent future problems.

For Immediate Relief

home remedies

Avoid dietary triggers. One way to prevent gallstone attacks is to avoid foods that are high in fat. Fat in the diet signals the gallbladder to contract more than usual, which can trigger attacks in some cases. "The things that usually give people the most trouble are fried foods," says Thomas R. Gadacz, M.D., professor and chairman of the department of surgery at Medical College of Georgia in Augusta.

medical options

Consider surgery. If you're having frequent attacks of gallstone pain, your doctor may recommend that you have your gallbladder removed, a procedure called cholecystectomy. More than 500,000 Americans have gallbladder surgery every year, for good reason: We can function just fine without it.

Consider nonsurgical options. If the gallstones are small and consist mainly of cholesterol, your doctor may be able to eliminate them with medications. Prescription drugs such as ursodiol (Actigall) contain bile acids, which literally dissolve the stones. The drawback to this approach is that the drugs often cause side effects, and you may need to take them for months or even years.

Another nonsurgical approach is extracorporeal shock wave lithotripsy (ESWL), a procedure in which shock waves are transmitted through the abdomen to crush the stones. Once the stones are small enough, they will pass through the bile ducts without causing blockages.

For Long-Term Prevention

home remedies

Maintain a healthy weight. Research has shown that middle-aged women who are overweight or obese may be twice as likely to develop gallstones as those who are leaner. Maintaining a

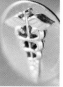

when to see a doctor

If you have unexplained abdominal pain or nausea, especially after meals, call your doctor right away. There's a good chance that you have gallstones, says Thomas R. Gadacz, M.D., professor and chairman of the department of surgery at Medical College of Georgia in Augusta.

If you have a history of gallstones and the attacks have become more frequent or severe: Gallstones are often "silent," but frequent or severe attacks mean that you're probably going to need medical treatment, says Dr. Gadacz.

healthful weight is among the best ways to prevent gallstones from forming, says Dr. Gadacz.

Lose weight slowly. Dropping a few pounds can prevent gallstone attacks, but losing weight too quickly can make the problem worse. Crash diets typically call for restricting fat intake to fewer than 10 grams daily. With so little fat in the diet, the activity of the gallbladder slows too much, which can make stonelike deposits more likely to form, says Dr. Gadacz. So-called yo-yo dieting, in which women repeatedly lose weight and gain it back, increases the risk for gallstones even more. (For a complete guide to healthy weight loss, see chapter 6.)

Get regular exercise. A study of more than 3,000 women found that those who walked briskly for 20 minutes 5 to 7 days a week were 20 percent less likely to get gallstones than those who were sedentary. (To start an exercise program, see chapter 5.)

gas

Passing gas elicits giggles from 9-year-olds, but for millions of American adults, it's not a laughing matter.

Every day, our bodies produce 1 to 3 pints of intestinal gas—and people pass it, on average, about 14 times a day.

There are three main sources of intestinal gas, says Henry C. Lin, M.D., director of the gastrointestinal motility program and section of nutrition at Cedars-Sinai Medical Center in Los Angeles. The first is the air we swallow when we eat, drink, chew gum, or talk. The second is stubborn carbohydrates, including beans, that are difficult for the body to digest. The third is bacteria that move from their normal abode in the colon into the small intestine.

It isn't possible to eliminate gas completely, but there are ways to reduce the volume. Here's what experts advise.

For Immediate Relief

home remedies

Identify gas-producing carbohydrates. The worst offenders include beans, cabbage, Brussels sprouts, broccoli, and asparagus. They contain a sugar called raffinose, a major trigger of gas. You don't want to give up these foods completely because they are very good for your health, but it may be worth eating them a little less often.

Switch to regular gum. Sugar-free chewing gums contain a sugar called sorbitol, which can trigger gas in some people.

Eat more rice. Most starch-containing foods—such as wheat, corn, and potatoes—produce gas during digestion. Rice, however, doesn't have this effect.

Drink from a glass. All carbonated beverages, including beer and sodas, contain gas—and gas that goes into the body will eventually come out. One solution is to pour carbonated drinks into a glass, which allows some of the gas to escape.

For Long-Term Relief

medical options

Talk to your doctor. If gas is making you uncomfortable and nothing you do seems to help, ask your doctor if you should be tested for bacterial overgrowths, Dr. Lin advises. It's possible that eliminating the troublesome bacteria will eliminate much of the gas as well.

You should also see your doctor if you're belching a lot or if you have heartburn or stomach pain. Along with gas, these are common symptoms of gastritis (inflammation of the stomach), ulcers, and a condition called gastroesophageal reflux disease, says Dr. Lin.

gastroesophageal reflux disease

Women who have heartburn after meals find it embarrassing, especially when they're dinner guests.

Nearly everyone suffers from heartburn sometimes. As long as it doesn't happen often, it's more of an annoyance than a serious medical problem.

Also called gastroesophageal reflux disease (GERD), heartburn occurs when a muscular ring of muscle at the base of the esophagus (the tube that carries food to the stomach) weakens or opens at the wrong times. This allows harsh stomach acids to splash upward into the esophagus, causing the characteristic burning.

There's no reason to suffer from the discomfort of GERD, says Joshua Ofman, M.D., assistant professor of medicine in the division of gastroenterology at Cedars-Sinai Medical Center in Los Angeles. It's usually easy to control with simple measures, including avoidance of certain foods, and medication if needed.

For Immediate Relief

home remedies

Chew gum. It stimulates the flow of saliva, washing digestive juices back down to the stomach. It also helps neutralize the burning acid, says Tim McCashland, M.D., associate professor of medicine in the department of gastroenterology at the University of Nebraska Medical Center in Omaha.

Take over-the-counter relief. Antacids containing magnesium or aluminum compounds provide quick relief from heartburn. Other helpful medications include famotidine (Pepcid-AC) and cimetidine (Tagamet), which reduce stomach acid.

For Long-Term Relief

home remedies

Take small servings. They put less pressure on the stomach than eating large amounts all at once, says Dr. Ofman. It's also helpful to loosen your belt or clothing: Tight clothes increase pressure on the stomach and can force the acid upward, he explains.

Raise the head of your bed. It's harder for stomach acid to flow upward when your torso is slightly elevated. Elevate the head of your bed 6 to 8 inches with blocks.

Maintain a healthful weight. It's one of the best ways to prevent GERD, says Dr. Ofman. "For most women, even a loss of 10 to 15 pounds can relieve the symptoms."

Cut back on chocolate. And on coffee, alcohol, and fatty foods. They weaken the esophageal muscle, causing painful symptoms for hours later.

alternative therapies

Add turmeric to recipes. This flavorful kitchen herb stimulates the flow of saliva and can help neutralize acid buildups.

gout

Once known as the "rich man's disease," gout is rare in women.

Gout is a form of arthritis, and perhaps the most painful. It occurs when there are high levels of uric acid in the blood. Uric acid is a waste product formed by the breakdown of proteins, especially proteins called purines. When uric acid reaches high concentrations, it may begin to form sharp little crystals, which literally stab into joints, often in the big toe, causing intense inflammation.

People who eat a lot of purine-rich foods, such as shellfish and organ meats, have a high risk of getting gout. Some people have a genetic tendency to produce abnormally high amounts of uric acid, or their bodies are unable to eliminate it efficiently. Other risk factors for gout include a history of kidney disease, high blood pressure, heavy drinking, or the use of blood pressure medications. It can be triggered by drinking large amounts of alcohol or eating too much rich food.

"Gout is often inherited," says Elizabeth Tindall, M.D., associate clinical professor of medicine at Oregon Health Sciences University in Portland. If someone in your family had it, you're at a higher risk of getting it, too, she adds.

Gout is known as a male disease, and for good reason: Men are at a significantly higher risk of getting it than are women.

But that doesn't mean you're safe. "Women can be slowly building up high amounts of uric acid in their bodies for 20 years. They'll have no symptoms—until they wake up in the middle of the night with severe pain in their large toe," says Dr. Tindall. "The pain can make a grown woman cry."

During an acute attack, the joint will be red, hot, and painful, Dr. Tindall adds. "Some of my patients say they couldn't walk—they couldn't even stand to have the bed sheet touching their foot."

Although gout usually affects the big toe, it can also strike the elbow, ankles, or other joints in the body. The pain only lasts a day or two, but it can feel like forever. Here are some tips for stopping gout fast—and making sure that it doesn't come back.

For Immediate Relief

home remedies

Take ibuprofen. When gout first strikes, take ibuprofen or another over-the-counter pain reliever right away, advises Dr. Tindall. The drugs curtail the body's production of prostaglandins, chemicals that cause pain and inflammation.

But stay away from aspirin. It can block the excretion of uric acid from the kidneys, thereby worsening a gout attack.

Pamper your foot. "Lie on the bed and make sure the foot doesn't have any weight on it—remove your shoes and socks as well as a sheet or blanket," says Dr. Tindall. "All those things can cause pain just by touching the area."

Apply ice—or heat. Different things work for different people, says Dr. Tindall. Cold is often helpful because it reduces swelling. Wrap some ice cubes in a washcloth and hold it on your toe for 10 to 15 minutes. If you don't like the sensation of cold, it's fine to apply a heating pad or hot-water bottle wrapped in a towel.

medical options

Ask your doctor about colchicine. Available by prescription, it will stop the pain of gout within an hour or two. However, it works best if you take it within 12 hours after an attack begins. If you wait much longer, it won't be as effective.

Consider corticosteroids. Given orally or by injection, corticosteroids are powerful drugs that are considered the "gold standard" for stopping inflammation. Because of the risk of side effects, however, they're usually used only when other treatments don't work.

For Long-Term Prevention

home remedies

Stop drinking alcohol. "Alcohol is the number-one dietary-related cause of gout because it interferes with the ability of the kidneys to excrete uric acid," says Dr. Tindall. Some women can get away with drinking small amounts of alcohol, but others may have to give it up altogether.

Get purines out of your diet. Foods that are high in purines include anchovies, shellfish, gravies made with organ meats, and red meats.

Women do need some red meat in the diet in order to get enough iron, Dr. Tindall adds. "I

recommend keeping the serving to about the size of a deck of playing cards. It's fine to have that much twice a week."

Drink a lot of water. Six to eight glasses daily is ideal. Water increases the amount of uric acid excreted by the kidneys, Dr. Tindall explains. It's especially important to drink water when you're exercising or working hard. "You don't want to get dehydrated because that can trigger a gout attack," she says.

Exercise regularly. It will keep your weight down, which reduces the amount of uric acid that the body produces. Dr. Tindall advises her pa-

when to see a doctor

 If the joint in one of your big toes is red, swollen, and warm to the touch, call your doctor. There's a good chance you're suffering a gout attack, says Elizabeth Tindall, M.D., associate clinical professor of medicine at Oregon Health Sciences University in Portland.

If symptoms similar to those caused by gout are affecting joints besides the big toe: It could be gout, or it could be a different form of arthritis or even an infection, says Dr. Tindall.

If the attacks are happening frequently: There are a number of prescription drugs that will help prevent attacks of gout. It's important, however, to use the drugs exactly as they're prescribed. "People will take the drugs in the beginning, but as the pain goes away, they'll tend to forget," says Dr. Tindall. "If you're taking prescription drugs for gout, you must take them every day in order to prevent future attacks."

tients to get aerobic exercise—jogging, swimming, riding a bike, or aerobic dancing, for example—most days of the week.

In addition to regular exercise, women with a history of gout should think about controlling their weight by following a plant-based diet, one that includes only a small amount of meat and is rich in fruits, vegetables, whole grains, and legumes. "If you limit red meat, you'll automatically consume less fat and fewer calories, along with cutting down on the purines," she says.

For more information about gout: Visit the Web site of the Arthritis Foundation at www.arthritis.org. Or go to the Web site for the National Institute of Arthritis and Musculoskeletal and Skin Diseases at www.nih.gov/niams.

gum problems

Bacteria are among the leading causes of illness worldwide, which is why people do everything possible to keep them in check. Despite this wise vigilance, one bacterial hot zone often gets overlooked.

Hundreds of species of bacteria live in the human mouth. Some bacteria are harmless; others cause gum disease and tooth decay. Gum disease affects about 75 percent of adults over age 35 to some degree.

Every time you eat, bacteria in the mouth feed on food particles and form a sticky gel called plaque, which adheres to the teeth and wedges beneath the gum line. The bacteria in plaque release toxins that irritate and break down gum tissues, causing gum disease. This condition (also called periodontal disease) is an infection of the tissues surrounding and supporting teeth and a major cause of tooth loss in adults.

The mildest form of gum disease is gingivitis, which causes bleeding and swelling around the gums. This is a signal that your immune system is kicking in, trying to fight the infection with inflammation. "If you catch it early, gingivitis is a fully reversible condition," says Jonathan Korostoff, D.M.D., Ph.D., assistant professor in the department of periodontics at the University of Pennsylvania School of Dental Medicine in Philadelphia. But if gum disease advances to periodontitis, the gums and bone that support the teeth can become seriously damaged.

Here's what you need to do.

For Immediate Relief

home remedies

Brush at least twice daily. Brushing your teeth removes plaque and takes away the nourishment that bacteria need to thrive. It's especially important to brush before bedtime because the cleansing flow of saliva is reduced at night.

Use soft-bristled brushes. They're less likely to damage the gums than hard brushes. "Brush with more of a gentle circular motion rather than an aggressive up-and-down motion," says Dr. Korostoff. "Studies have shown that to effectively brush, it takes 4 to 5 minutes to do your entire mouth," he adds.

Switch on an electric brush. This kind requires less strength and coordination than manual brushes, so people tend to brush their teeth longer, says Dr. Korostoff.

Rinse in a pinch. Between regular brushings, rinse your mouth with an antimicrobial over-the-counter mouthwash. "I'm not sure they have a dramatic effect on plaque buildup, but the physical action of rinsing does remove particles and plaque," says Dr. Korostoff.

Floss daily. It's the only way to remove plaque and bacteria that hide between the teeth. Don't use a lot of force—it can damage the gums. "You want to do it in a nice, controlled fashion," says Dr. Korostoff. Guide the floss along both sides of each tooth. "You want to go up and down about six times on each tooth surface," he adds.

Use an oral irrigator. People don't always have enough manual dexterity (or patience) to floss correctly. Oral irrigation devices such as WaterPik or Hydro Floss direct a strong jet of water between the teeth and around the gums, which removes food particles as well as plaque and bacteria, says Dr. Korostoff.

medical options

Have your teeth professionally cleaned. Your dentist (or a dental hygienist) will remove plaque and tartar from the teeth and beneath the gums. If this doesn't eliminate the infection, you may need antibiotics. They're usually taken orally, although your dentist may insert an antibiotic gel directly into parts of the gums.

"People rarely need medications for gum problems," Dr. Korostoff adds. "I usually clean the teeth, and that's enough."

Ask about periodontal pockets. If you have gum disease, these pockets form where tooth meets gum. Ask your dentist how your gums are

One More Reason to Keep Flossing

eft unchecked, gum disease is more than a mouth problem—it can boost the risk of other health conditions, including heart disease, stroke, diabetes, respiratory infections, and premature birth.

"Women with gum disease are three to eight times more likely to go into premature labor than those with healthy gums," according to Marjorie Jeffcoat, D.M.D., chairperson of the department of periodontics at the University of Alabama School of Dentistry in Birmingham, who is heading a study of 2,500 women. "The more severe the disease is, the greater your odds are of premature labor."

Meanwhile, experts are discovering that some health woes can make gum disease worse. "Diabetes inhibits immune response, leaving you more vulnerable to infection," explains Jack Caton, D.D.S., professor of periodontology at the University of Rochester in New York and president of the American Academy of Periodontology.

And as osteoporosis thins your bones, it can leave your jawbone more vulnerable to erosion due to gum disease, explains Dr. Jeffcoat.

So what is the best gum protection plan? Brush twice a day, floss once a day, and have a dental checkup and cleaning twice a year, Dr. Jeffcoat says. ∎

when to see a doctor

If your gums are swollen, red, or bleeding, you need to see your dentist right away. These are early signs of gum disease, says Jonathan Korostoff, D.M.D., Ph.D., assistant professor in the department of periodontics at the University of Pennsylvania School of Dental Medicine in Philadelphia.

If your gums are inflamed and you also have diabetes: Diabetes increases the risk of gum disease. Research also suggests that people with oral infections may have difficulty controlling their glucose (blood sugar) levels.

doing. The earlier that gum disease is diagnosed and treated, the better.

Long-Term Solutions

home remedies

Quit smoking. The American Academy of Periodontology has found that smokers are almost three times as likely to suffer gum damage as nonsmokers. Giving up cigarettes is the best solution, but if you're not ready to quit, at least cut back. Research suggests that people who smoke fewer than 10 cigarettes daily have half the risk of developing serious gum disease of those who smoke more than 30 cigarettes daily.

medical options

Talk to your doctor about supplemental hormones. A small study of 70 postmenopausal women found that those who were on hormone replacement therapy had less gum inflammation and bone loss than those who weren't taking hormones. The supplemental estrogen appeared to reduce tissue-damaging inflammation in the gums, according to researchers at the University of Nebraska Medical Center College of Dentistry in Lincoln.

For more information on preventing and treating gum problems: Visit the Web site of the American Dental Association at www.ada.org.

hay fever

For women with allergies, hay fever is an annual rite of spring. Your eyes well up, your nose springs a leak, and your ears and throat start itching.

"There's a reason they call it hay fever, even though it doesn't cause a fever and it isn't triggered by hay," says Harold S. Nelson, M.D., an immunologist and codirector of clinical research at the National Jewish Medical and Research Center in Denver. "The term was coined in the 19th century because people with hay fever have fatigue and difficulty thinking, as if they had a feverish illness."

People can be allergic to potentially anything, but those with hay fever are usually sensitive to pollen—and it's everywhere. Ragweed plants, for example, can release up to 1 million pollen granules a day.

Other common causes of hay fever are grasses, which release their eye-watering payload in summer; a variety of weeds, which cause problems in summer and early fall; and trees, which come into bloom in the spring.

Hay fever may also be due to dust mites, molds, and pet dander, adds Sandra M. Gawchick, D.O., codirector of the division of allergy and clinical immunology at Crozer-Chester Medical Center and clinical associate professor of pediatrics at Thomas Jefferson University Medical Center in Philadelphia.

It's impossible to avoid all of the allergens that nature throws at you, but reducing the amount that you breathe will help keep your symptoms at manageable levels. In addition, there are a variety of medications that can dramatically reduce the discomfort.

For Immediate Relief

home remedies

Take an antihistamine. Available over the counter, antihistamines that contain chlorpheniramine (like Chlor-Trimeton) or diphenhydramine (like Benadryl) are very effective at relieving allergy symptoms. The problem with these drugs is that they often cause side effects, including drowsiness or a dry mouth. The newer, nonsedating antihistamines, such as loratadine (Claritin) and fexofenadine (Allegra), are as effective, and they're much less likely to cause side effects.

Time your antihistamines. If your allergies keep you up at night, your doctor may advise you to take one of the older antihistamines at night,

when drowsiness isn't a problem. Then, in the morning, you can take one of the nonsedating drugs. However, the drowsiness from the bedtime dose may continue into the next day, so this strategy may not work for everyone, says Dr. Nelson.

Wash your hair before going to bed. Pollen particles that cling to your hair will coat the pillows at night, giving you an extra 8 hours to breathe them in. Washing your hair at night will remove the pollen before it has a chance to get into your airways.

Close the windows and use the air conditioner. It will trap pollen before it has a chance to get inside. It's also a good idea to use the clothes dryer instead of hanging your laundry outside. Fabrics are natural traps for pollen, especially when they're damp.

Substitute washable throw rugs for wall-to-wall carpets. Carpets trap a tremendous amount of pollen, which can leave you sneezing and rubbing your eyes long after the allergy season is gone. Washing carpets will remove pollen as well as pet dander and other potential allergens.

Use the hot cycle. Cool water will remove pollen, but it won't kill allergy-causing dust mites, which accumulate on rugs, shower curtains, sheets, and bedspreads. Water hotter than 130°F will kill the mites, along with their eggs.

Stay inside in the morning. "Pollen counts are highest between the hours of 6:00 A.M. and 10:00 A.M.," says Dr. Gawchick.

Keep the grass cut short. Mowing the lawn every few days, especially in the spring, will prevent the grass from sprouting pollen-producing flowers.

Keep your work clothes outside. Then, when it's time to come back inside, change into clean clothes—and leave your pollen-laden jeans on the porch. Washing your "outside" clothes after every wearing will help keep their pollen loads low.

Wear a microfiber mask when working outside. Available at hardware stores, the masks slip over the nose and mouth and are held in place with a rubber band. They'll prevent large amounts of mold or pollen from getting into your airways.

alternative therapies

Take stinging nettle. A natural antihistamine, stinging nettle has been used around the world to combat allergies. Start off by taking 20 drops of a 1:1 tincture or 1 teaspoon of a 1:5 tincture once a day for the first few days. Then begin taking this dose three times a day. Stinging nettle is available in health food stores and some pharmacies.

Add onions to recipes. And eat plenty of apples. They're among the richest sources of quercetin, a natural plant nutrient that appears to inhibit allergic reactions. You can also buy quercetin supplements in health food stores. The recommended dose is 600 milligrams, taken two or three times daily.

For Long-Term Relief

home remedies

Track pollen counts. When pollen counts are high—usually between 20 and 100 grains per cubic meter—you may want to stay indoors. You can get the latest information on pollen and spore counts in your area on the Web site of the National Allergy Bureau at www.aaaai.org/nab.

Use a nose spray. One of the most effective over-the-counter sprays contains cromolyn sodium (Nasalcrom). If you start taking it a few weeks before allergy season begins and continue using it four times daily during the spring and summer, you'll have a dramatic reduction in sneezing and other allergic nasal symptoms.

If nothing seems to help, keep a food diary. The allergy-causing particles in pollen may be similar to proteins found in common foods. If your symptoms include itching in the mouth or swollen lips, it's possible that allergens in carrots, celery, cantaloupe, or other foods are partly re-

when to see a doctor

If your hay fever symptoms are accompanied by a fever or a bad headache, call your doctor. Persistent nasal congestion sometimes results in sinusitis, a bacterial infection in the sinuses that may require antibiotics, says Sandra M. Gawchick, D.O., codirector of the division of allergy and clinical immunology at Crozer-Chester Medical Center and clinical associate professor of pediatrics at Thomas Jefferson University Medical Center in Philadelphia.

If the nasal discharge is greenish or yellowish instead of clear: This can be a sign of a bacterial infection, which may require medical care.

sponsible. Unfortunately, there isn't a cure for this condition, called "oral allergy syndrome," but avoiding the "wrong" foods will eliminate the problems, says Dr. Gawchick.

Ask your doctor about steroid nasal sprays. Available by prescription, nasal sprays that con-

tain steroids will lessen nasal itching and reduce nasal swelling that increases congestion. Some people will see an improvement in as little as 12 hours, but others may need 3 to 10 days of use before they see relief of these allergy symptoms, adds Dr. Gawchick. The drugs are usually used in combination with antihistamines.

headaches

More than 45 million Americans suffer from headaches, with pain that ranges from a mild twinge to the skull-pounding agony of migraines. For reasons that still aren't clear, women are more likely to suffer from headaches than men.

The two most common types of headaches are tension headaches and migraines. Even though they share the name "headache," they're as different as night and day.

With tension headaches, the pain is felt all over the head, including in the small muscles around the eyes and behind the ears. As the name suggests, tension headaches are often but not always associated with muscle tightness in the back of the neck or on the scalp. The pain is usually mild or moderate, and it tends to be triggered by emotional factors, such as stress, anxiety, fear, or anger.

Migraines are much more disabling. They cause moderate to severe throbbing or pulsing pain, usually on one side of the head. The pain of migraines, which can last as long as 3 days, is

often accompanied by nausea and sensitivity to light or sound. About 20 percent of migraines are preceded (or accompanied) by visual disturbances that include wavy lines, dots, flashing lights, or blind spots. Some people experience changes in their usual sense of touch, taste, or smell prior to the attacks.

Doctors still aren't sure what causes migraines. They have discovered that people who get migraines have overactive areas in the brain stem. It's thought that changing levels of hormones affect this part of the brain, which may be why women get migraines more frequently than men.

"Some women get migraines due to the falling estrogen levels that are associated with their menstrual cycles," says Stephen D. Silberstein, M.D., director of the Jefferson Headache Center at Thomas Jefferson University Hospital in Philadelphia.

Another hormonal factor that contributes to migraines is pregnancy. "Some women find that they get more migraines during the first trimester, when their levels of estrogen and progesterone change," Dr. Silberstein explains. "The migraines usually go away during the second and third trimesters, when hormones level off. Then, after women give birth, they often return within the first week because of falling estrogen levels."

Hormonal fluctuations are just one explanation for migraines. Doctors have identified dozens of things that can set them off, including stress, bright lights, food preservatives (such as nitrites and nitrates), or even changes in the weather. Migraines also tend to run in families. If your parents got these head bangers, there's a higher risk that you'll get them, too.

Tension headaches are easier to treat than mi-

graines, but nearly all headaches, regardless of the type, can be managed with a combination of medications and self-care strategies.

For Immediate Relief

home remedies

Use over-the-counter painkillers. They're very effective at stopping tension headaches, says Dr. Silberstein. Aspirin, ibuprofen, naproxen, and acetaminophen are all equally effective.

"The FDA has approved three over-the-counter products for treating migraines," he adds. A product called Excedrin Migraine, for example, contains aspirin, acetaminophen, and caffeine.

THREE THINGS I TELL EVERY FEMALE PATIENT

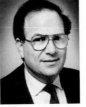

STEPHEN D. SILBERSTEIN, M.D., director of the Jefferson Headache Center at Thomas Jefferson University Hospital in Philadelphia, offers the following advice for women coping with headaches.

1

DON'T WAIT TO GET HELP. Women often assume that headaches are "normal"—and they suffer for years or decades without getting help. "Most women with tension or migraine headaches can get successful treatment that will keep them under control," Dr. Silberstein says. Before your doctor's appointment, keep a journal noting the dates, severity, and duration of the headaches; any possible triggers; and the headache's impact on your life, such as missed workdays, suggests Dr. Silberstein.

2

THEY'RE NOT "ALL IN YOUR HEAD." In the past, doctors sometimes dismissed headaches as being a sign of emotional problems. Nothing could be further from the truth. "Headaches are a biological disorder of the brain, and we can usually control them," says Dr. Silberstein.

3

TAKE TIME FOR YOURSELF. "Write a prescription for yourself to relax," Dr. Silberstein advises. "Schedule time to do anything you want, whether it's listening to relaxing music, meditating, or reading a book. Everyone needs this special time to relax—and it may prevent headaches." ∎

Other migraine medications contain ibuprofen. All of the products work for a nondisabling migraine, so you can take these if your pain is not so severe that you are unable to function. Everyone responds differently, so you may have to try several medications to find the one that works best.

Take a hot shower. "It may relieve tension headaches because the warm water loosens and relaxes muscles in the back of the neck and head," says Dr. Silberstein.

Ice it down. Cold compresses are helpful for all types of headaches because they numb the area and also constrict blood vessels, which can reduce the painful pounding. Apply either an ice pack or a plastic bag filled with ice cubes and wrapped in a towel to the painful area for about 10 to 15 minutes. Or wrap a bag of frozen peas in a towel and place it on your forehead, Dr. Silberstein suggests.

alternative therapies

Try feverfew. It's been used for thousands of years to treat headaches, and there's some evidence that it's effective. A common herb, feverfew contains compounds called sesquiterpene lactones, which reduce spasms in blood vessels in the brain. The research isn't conclusive, but feverfew appears to be more effective at preventing migraines than at stopping them once they begin. The recommended doses vary, depending on the form. If you're using fresh feverfew, take one leaf once daily; for freeze-dried feverfew tablets or capsules, take 300 milligrams daily; for fresh plant tinctures, take 40 drops daily; and for standardized extracts in tablet form, take a daily dose that provides the equivalent of 0.25 to 0.50 milligram of parthenolide.

One more point about feverfew: Many herbs are dried with traditional methods, but this destroys the active compounds in feverfew. It's best to use tinctures made from fresh leaf, or tablets or capsules that contain freeze-dried herb.

Reach for rosemary. This fragrant kitchen spice does more than perk up roasts and poultry—it also appears to prevent some stress-related headaches by keeping the blood vessels dilated. The easiest way to use rosemary is to enjoy it in a tea. Pour 1 cup of boiling water over 1 teaspoon of dried rosemary leaves. Cover and let it steep 10 minutes, strain the leaves, and drink.

For Long-Term Prevention

home remedies

Drink more fluids if you're active. Some people get migraines mainly when they exercise, possibly because they allow themselves to get dehydrated, says Dr. Silberstein. "To prevent dehydration, be sure to drink eight 8-ounce glasses of water each day," he advises. "If you're working out and perspiring, you're losing water, and it needs to be replaced."

Take riboflavin. Researchers have found that brain cells in some people with migraines produce insufficient amounts of energy. One way to boost energy production and prevent headaches might be to flood the cells with vitamin B_2, also known as riboflavin.

when to see a doctor

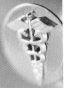

If you're experiencing headaches more than usual, or if the pain seems to be getting worse, see your doctor right away. Headaches can be caused by a variety of potentially serious neurological problems, including tumors, says Stephen D. Silberstein, M.D., director of the Jefferson Headache Center at Thomas Jefferson University Hospital in Philadelphia.

If the pain mainly occurs on one side of the head: You're probably suffering from migraines, which are a lot more serious (and painful) than garden-variety tension headaches.

If the headaches that you experience are accompanied by nausea or vomiting or if you're experiencing auras—visual disturbances that may include waving lines, flashing lights, or blind spots in your vision that precede or accompany (or both) the headache: You may be experiencing the classic form of migraines, and you'll probably need medications to get them under control.

In a study in Belgium, 55 migraine sufferers were given either 400 milligrams of riboflavin or a placebo. At the end of the 3-month study, 56 percent of the riboflavin group reported a decrease in the frequency of their migraine attacks. In the placebo group, only 19 percent had a similar benefit.

The amount of riboflavin used in the study was much higher than the amounts that most people get—235 times the Daily Value of 1.7 milligrams, to be exact. "It's difficult to get that much riboflavin from foods, and the study wasn't recommending that all migraine sufferers take the study amount in supplement form," Dr. Silberstein says. "But women with migraines might consider asking their doctors for advice on whether to try a supplement and the dosage that's right for them," he adds.

Keep a food journal. There's little scientific evidence that eating certain foods causes migraines, but many people believe that when they quit eating the "wrong" foods, their migraines disappear. For some migraine sufferers, the desire to eat particular foods, however, can be a warning sign of an impending migraine attack, adds Dr. Silberstein.

The next time you get a migraine, take a few minutes to jot down everything you ate in the past 48 hours, Dr. Silberstein suggests. If you keep the journal consistently, you may discover that the headaches are consistently preceded by a craving for certain foods.

Some of the foods that are commonly associated with migraines include:

- Ripened cheeses such as Cheddar, Stilton, Brie, and Camembert

- Fermented, marinated, or pickled foods

- Chocolate

- Sour cream

- Nuts or peanut butter

- Sourdough breads or crackers

- Broad beans, lima beans, fava beans, or snow peas

- Foods with monosodium glutamate (MSG), such as soy sauce, seasoned salt, or meat tenderizer
- Papayas, figs, raisins, or avocados
- Citrus fruits
- Processed meats, such as bologna and pepperoni
- Alcoholic beverages

Cut back on caffeine. "Some people get 'Saturday migraines' because they drink a few cups of coffee every day during the week, then don't drink any on the weekends," says Dr. Silberstein. "Caffeine withdrawal is what causes their migraines."

The solution isn't to drink coffee or tea 7 days a week but to cut back on caffeine overall—or to switch to decaf. This gives the brain a chance to become less sensitive, which in turn can reduce the frequency of headaches.

Keep a regular sleep schedule. Women who keep irregular hours—by staying up late on weekends, for example, then sleeping until noon the next day—are more likely to suffer from headaches than those who keep regular hours. "Make sure that the bedroom is dark, peaceful, and quiet," Dr. Silberstein adds. "When your body is resting, your brain is resting."

mind-body techniques

Take up yoga or meditation. Stress probably doesn't cause headaches, but it does act as a trigger in those who are susceptible to migraines or tension headaches. Some of the best ways to relax and reduce stress include yoga, deep breathing, and meditation, says Dr. Silberstein.

Try progressive relaxation. This relaxation technique calls for tensing and then relaxing every muscle in your body, starting with your toes and working upward to your skull. It can take 20 minutes or more to complete a session, but it's worth it. People who practice progressive relaxation say it helps them feel rested and relaxed—and less likely to suffer from headaches.

medical options

Ask about prescription relief. Medications for migraines are divided into two main groups: those that prevent migraines and those that can quickly reduce the pain of attacks.

Doctors have found that medications—such as divalproex sodium (Depakote) and topiramate (Topamax)—used to control some types of seizures can also prevent migraines. To stop migraines that are already under way, doctors usu-

WHAT WORKS FOR ME

STEPHEN D. SILBERSTEIN, M.D., *director of the Jefferson Headache Center at Thomas Jefferson University Hospital in Philadelphia, says,* "When I get a bad headache, I take an over-the-counter analgesic or migraine-specific medication."

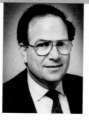

"If I'm at work, I take a break by closing the door to my office, shutting off the lights, and unwinding," he adds. "I go into a mild trance, a very calm, relaxing state." ■

ally prescribe a class of drugs known as "triptans," which include sumatriptan (Imitrex), rizatriptan (Maxalt), naratriptan (Amerge), and zolmitriptan (Zomig). The medications work by attaching to a receptor for serotonin, a neurotransmitter in the brain.

For the fastest relief possible, doctors often advise people with migraines to use sumatriptan in an injectable form, Dr. Silberstein adds.

Consider biofeedback. It's a technique that teaches people to control muscle tension, lower blood pressure, and even divert blood away from the head at the first signs of headaches. Biofeedback is simple to learn, but it requires the use of sophisticated equipment that allows patients to monitor changes in their physical signs. Ask your doctor if a referral to a biofeedback specialist would be helpful.

For more information about headaches: Visit the Web site for the National Headache Foundation at www.headaches.org. The telephone number is (888) NHF-5552. Or go to the Web site for the American Council for Headache Education at www.achenet.org.

hemorrhoids

Hemorrhoids are one of those intimate conditions that no woman feels comfortable talking about. But there's nothing mysterious about them. Hemorrhoids occur when veins in the rectum become stretched, swollen, and inflamed. Basically, they're like the varicose veins that you see on people's legs, except they are in a much more sensitive area.

Most hemorrhoids occur inside the anus, where there aren't many nerve endings. These internal hemorrhoids aren't painful, but if they protrude outside the anus, they can become sensitive and sometimes cause bleeding. Hemorrhoids that start on the outside of the anus, on the other hand, can swell or form a hard lump caused by a blood clot. This type of hemorrhoid, called a thrombosed external hemorrhoid, causes acute pain.

Constipation is the main cause of hemorrhoids. When you strain to have a bowel move-

ment, the increase in internal pressure damages the walls of the veins. If you're pregnant, you're especially vulnerable because the growing uterus also causes an increase in vein-damaging pressure.

Hemorrhoids usually go away in a few days to a week, but they can make your life miserable in the meantime. Here are some quick ways to reduce the discomfort and prevent hemorrhoids from coming back.

For Immediate Relief

home remedies

Use baby wipes for a few days. Toilet paper can feel like sandpaper when you have hemorrhoids. "The best thing people can use is alcohol-free baby wipes," says Bruce A. Orkin, M.D., director of the division of colon and rectal cancer and associate professor of surgery at George Washington University in Washington, D.C.

Take baths instead of showers. Soaking the area in warm water two or three times a day will shrink swollen tissues and reduce the discomfort.

Soften the stools. When you have hemorrhoids, having a hard bowel movement can be agony. To soften stools in a hurry, use an over-the-counter stool softener or a fiber supplement that contains psyllium (like Metamucil) or methylcellulose (like Citrucel), following the directions on the label. Stool softeners may be taken twice a day. Fiber supplements with psyllium, such as Metamucil and Fibercon, should be taken one or two times per day with plenty of fluids, adds Dr. Orkin.

For Long-Term Prevention

home remedies

Increase the fiber in your diet. Found in fruits, vegetables, whole grains, and other plant foods, fiber helps prevent hemorrhoids—and reduces discomfort if you already have them. Gradually increase your fiber intake to avoid bloating.

"Fiber acts like a sponge and soaks up water," Dr. Orkin says. The water makes stools softer, which reduces straining during bowel movements.

According to *Prevention* magazine, everyone should eat 25 to 35 grams of fiber daily. "I tell patients to choose cereals with 5 to 7 grams of fiber per serving," Dr. Orkin says. Add to that a few servings of fresh fruits, raw or lightly steamed vegetables, and fiber-rich foods such as whole grains and legumes, and you'll automatically get all the fiber that you need.

Drink a lot of water. It's absorbed by stools in the intestine, which makes them softer. Plan on drinking eight full glasses of water daily. If you drink coffee, tea, or a caffeinated soft drink, only count that as two-thirds of a serving toward your fluid intake for the day, recommends *Prevention* magazine. These drinks can pull water out of your stool.

Use the bathroom right after breakfast. That's when the body's urge to go is strongest. If you wait until later in the day, you'll probably have to strain more, which increases the risk of hemorrhoids.

Don't dawdle. The more time you spend on the toilet, the more likely you are to suffer from hemorrhoids. "You shouldn't need to sit there for more than a few minutes to have a bowel movement," says Dr. Orkin.

when to see a doctor

If you're having rectal bleeding, even if it's just a few drops on the toilet paper, see your doctor right away. Most bleeding is caused by hemorrhoids, but it can also be caused by colon cancer, says Heidi Nelson, M.D., chairperson of the division of colorectal surgery at the Mayo Clinic.

If the discomfort is accompanied by changes in bowel habits or unusually thin stools: These are other common symptoms of colon cancer.

If a hemorrhoid is causing excruciating (not just annoying) pain: The hemorrhoid could have a blood clot inside that may need to be removed by your doctor.

hepatitis

Hepatitis has been called a "silent" illness because many people don't even know they have it until it's discovered during a routine blood test, sometimes years after they were first infected. If symptoms are present, they are likely to be mild and intermittent. They may include fever, dark urine, light-colored stools, loss of appetite, nausea, vomiting, abdominal pain, and jaundice (yellowing of the skin and whites of the eyes).

Even when it doesn't cause symptoms, hepatitis can result in serious and sometimes permanent damage. An inflammation of the liver, hepatitis is usually caused by a virus. The severity of the disease depends on the type of virus that's involved.

The main types of hepatitis are labeled A, B, and C. Hepatitis A, the mildest form of the disease, is often caused by exposure to something contaminated with the stool of someone who's infected. Typically it is spread by household members or food handlers who fail to wash their hands after using the bathroom. Hepatitis B is often spread by sexual contact or the transfer of contaminated blood—by an accidental needle stick, for example. Hepatitis C, the most serious form of the disease, is spread mainly by tainted blood; it's common among drug addicts who share hypodermic needles.

Hepatitis A almost always clears up on its own, says Samuel Meyers, M.D., a gastroenterologist and clinical professor of medicine at Mount Sinai School of Medicine in New York City. Types B and C, however, may become chronic and may require a combination of medications and lifestyle adjustments to keep the infection and symptoms under control.

For Immediate Relief

home remedies

Drink plenty of water. Vomiting is a common symptom of hepatitis in the early stages, says Dr. Meyers. Drinking a lot of fluids—doctors usually recommend drinking at least 64 ounces daily—will help prevent dehydration.

Rest—and keep resting. "The classic symptom of hepatitis is fatigue and weakness," says Dr. Meyers. "You don't have to stay in bed, but it's important to rest or take naps whenever you feel tired."

Avoid ibuprofen or other painkillers. They're processed by the liver, so taking them can slow your recovery time or lead to further damage.

"If you're feverish, you can put a cold compress on your head," says Dr. Meyers. "The less medication you use, the better off you'll be."

Don't drink alcohol. When you have hepatitis, the effects of alcohol on the liver are magnified: A single beer or glass of wine is the equivalent of having four or five drinks when you're healthy, Dr. Meyers explains. Even small amounts of alcohol are likely to increase damage to the liver.

Take milk thistle. It contains a chemical compound called silymarin, which is thought to reduce damage to liver cells and also help the cells regenerate.

Look for supplements that contain 150 milligrams of milk thistle extract that's been standardized to contain 70 percent silymarin. Take one capsule three times daily as long as the infection lasts. It can be used for both acute and chronic hepatitis.

Boost immunity with maitake. A type of mushroom, maitake stimulates the body's defensive white blood cells and may reduce symptoms of hepatitis, according to Douglas Schar, Dip.Phyt., an herbalist in London and Washington, D.C. He recommends taking 4 to 6 grams of tableted powdered maitake daily as long as you're having symptoms.

Take immune globulin immediately. If you suspect you've been exposed to hepatitis B—because your spouse is infected, for example—a prescription medication called immune globulin may eliminate the virus and prevent infection.

"You have to take it very early," Dr. Meyers adds. "If symptoms have already appeared, immune globulin won't help."

Treat chronic hepatitis with interferon. About 6 percent of those infected with hepatitis B, and nearly everyone who gets hepatitis C, are unable to eliminate the virus from their bodies, says Dr. Meyers. Your doctor may recommend taking interferon, which may eradicate the virus in some

when to see a doctor

If you have flulike symptoms— such as fatigue, fever, loss of appetite, and nausea—that linger more than 2 weeks, see your doctor. Hepatitis is often confused with the flu in the early stages, says Samuel Meyers, M.D., a gastroenterologist and clinical professor of medicine at Mount Sinai School of Medicine in New York City.

If you have dark urine or pale stools: These are classic signs of hepatitis. They indicate that the liver isn't working properly and may be inflamed.

If you develop symptoms about 2 weeks after having unprotected sex: Hepatitis B is commonly spread by sexual contact.

cases. Interferon, a synthetic version of a substance that is naturally produced by the body's cells that stimulates immunity, may cause depression, hypothyroidism, loss of appetite, and flulike symptoms.

Long-Term Solution

Exercise if you can. Walking, biking, and other forms of exercise can help restore some of the energy that hepatitis takes away. But don't overdo it, Dr. Meyers advises. "If you get tired, rest. You have to use common sense."

For more information about hepatitis: Visit the Web site of the American Liver Foundation at www.liverfoundation.org.

hives

Stress. Food. Heat. Cold. Whatever the cause, hives grace your skin with a mass of inflamed, itchy bumps.

One out of five women will get hives at least once. If you've had them before, chances are you'll have them again, especially if you have a family history of hives or suffer from hay fever, food allergies, eczema, or asthma, says Gillian Shepherd, M.D., an allergist/immunologist and associate professor of medicine at Weill Medical College of Cornell University in New York City.

Hives usually come and go within a few hours; they're intensely itchy, but relatively brief. In rare cases, though, they become chronic, lasting for months and even years.

"Hives can be caused by everything under the sun—and even the sun itself," notes dermatologist Wilma F. Bergfeld, M.D., head of clinical research in the department of dermatology at the Cleveland Clinic Foundation in Cleveland. "Your body is visibly reacting to *something*."

The most common triggers are things you ingest: foods such as nuts, chocolate, shellfish, berries, and tomatoes; and medications like antibiotics, pain relievers, and sedatives. A trigger prompts mast cells in the skin to release chemicals, called histamines, that cause swelling and itching, notes Mary Ruth Buchness, M.D., clinical associate professor of dermatology and medicine at New York Medical College in Valhalla.

"Some people also get them from stress or chronic infections, like hepatitis B," adds Dr. Buchness. "Others react to something physical, like heat, exercise, air conditioning, and even pressure from a tight belt or the elastic on their underwear."

If you've got hives, the first order of business is to relieve the itching and inflammation, then take steps to avoiding what gets under your skin. Here's what doctors recommend.

when to see a doctor

If hives last longer than 24 hours, cover approximately 10 percent of your skin (one whole arm, a thigh, or your entire stomach, for example) or don't blanch (turn white) when you press them: Contact your doctor, advises allergist-immunologist Gillian Shepherd, M.D., associate professor of medicine at Weill Medical College of Cornell University in New York City.

If hives worsen rapidly or if you have difficulty breathing, feel light-headed, or grow nauseated, you may be suffering from anaphylactic shock, an extreme drop in blood pressure and other problems, which is a sign of a severe, bodywide allergic reaction. Go to the nearest emergency room. You may need a shot of epinephrine (a drug similar to the natural adrenaline in our bodies) to open your breathing passages and keep your blood pressure from dropping dangerously low.

For Immediate Relief

Cool the itch. To reduce swelling, constrict blood vessels, and slow the release of histamines, place a few ice cubes inside a wet towel or paper towel and apply to the affected area. Let it melt there 1 or 2 minutes, then take it off. Reapply within minutes or as needed until the itching subsides, says Dr. Bergfeld. Cold baths and showers lasting 15 to 30 minutes will also provide relief from itching.

Choose your anti-itch lotion carefully. Try over-the counter anti-itch treatments, like Sarna Anti-itch Lotion or Aveeno Anti-itch Concentrated Lotion, available at your local drugstore, says Dr. Buchness. Avoid creams containing antihistamines or those ending in "caine," such as benzocaine, which may cause an allergic reaction when applied to the skin.

Bathe in oatmeal. For additional relief, Dr. Buchness recommends natural colloidal oatmeal powder, available over the counter in various brands, added to a lukewarm bath.

Take an antihistamine. If needed, try 25 milligrams of diphenhydramine (Benadryl) every 4 hours, advises Dr. Buchness. If this makes you too drowsy, ask your doctor for a nonsedating prescription alternative, such as fexofenadine (Allegra) or loratadine (Claritin), Dr. Bergfeld suggests.

Try herbal antihistamines. If drugstore antihistamines bother you, consider antihistamine alternatives, such as stinging nettle. Take one or two capsules of freeze-dried nettle leaf extract every 2 to 4 hours until symptoms disappear. This remedy may come as a surprise to you since rubbing against stinging nettle plants in the

---

THREE THINGS I TELL EVERY FEMALE PATIENT

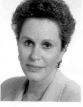

WILMA F. BERGFELD, M.D., a dermatologist and the head of clinical research in the department of dermatology at the Cleveland Clinic Foundation in Cleveland, offers this special advice.

1 **LIQUID ANTIHISTAMINES BRING FASTER RELIEF.** They're absorbed into the blood in only 15 to 20 minutes, compared with 30 to 45 minutes for pills, but they also contain more sugar. If you're obese or have diabetes, you'll need to remember to factor in the additional sugar to your diet.

2 **HIVES AND HEAT DON'T MIX.** Avoid hot showers or intense workouts. Heat increases bloodflow to the skin, encouraging the release of more histamines.

3 **CONSIDER ALL CAUSES.** Not only can you have multiple allergies at once, but the source of your hives may change over time. ■

wild irritates the skin and causes hivelike welts. When taken orally, however, it contains substances that heal hives, says David Edelberg, M.D., founder of the American Whole Health Centers in Chicago.

Quercetin, a bioflavonoid from citrus fruits and buckwheat, is another effective antihistamine. Take 400 milligrams of quercetin tablets twice daily until symptoms disappear, suggests Andrew Weil, M.D., director of the program in integrative medicine and clinical professor of medicine at the University of Arizona College of Medicine in Tucson and author of *Eight Weeks to Optimum Health*. Both are available at health food stores.

mind-body techniques

Calm yourself. Not only does stress sometimes cause hives, but it can aggravate an outbreak you already have, notes Dr. Buchness. She recommends stress-busting activities, such as biofeedback, acupuncture, meditation, or anything that calms you. (For additional steps you can take to handle stress, read chapter 7.)

Long-Term Solutions

home remedies

Avoid known triggers. "Hives usually show up within a couple of hours after contact with a stimulus," says Dr. Buchness. So once you discover the cause, it makes sense to avoid it in the future.

Play detective. For chronic hives, keeping a food diary may help scout out the source. But if you're not having luck, your doctor may order some tests. "With chronic cases, we seldom find the cause," Dr. Buchness admits. "But most hives eventually go away as mysteriously as they came."

For more information on hives: Visit Allergy, Asthma, and Immunology Online (sponsored by the American College of Allergy, Asthma, and Immunology) at http://allergy.mcg.edu/advice/urtic.html.

inflammatory bowel disease

Unpredictability is one of the biggest challenges of inflammatory bowel disease. It can cause no symptoms for months or even years—and then it flares up with a vengeance, causing abdominal cramps, diarrhea, weight loss, and other painful (and frightening) symptoms.

Though it sounds like a single condition, there are two main types of inflammatory bowel disease, or IBD: Crohn's disease, which can damage any part of the digestive tract, and ulcerative colitis, which affects only the colon, explains Theodore M. Bayless, M.D., clinical director of the Meyerhoff Inflammatory Bowel Disease Center at Johns Hopkins Hospital in Baltimore and coeditor of *Advanced Therapy of Inflammatory Bowel Disease*.

Despite these differences, the conditions have many things in common. During flare-ups, patches of the intestine become raw and irritated. The inflammation is usually limited to the intestinal surface, but sometimes the damage extends all the way through the intestinal wall.

No one's sure what causes IBD, but it appears to be an immune disorder—a condition that occurs when the immune system "mistakenly" attacks the body's tissues.

There isn't a cure for IBD, but most people can manage it successfully with medications, lifestyle changes, surgery, or a combination of these treatments.

For Immediate Relief

home remedies

Keep track of what you eat. For some people, eating fatty foods can result in cramping or diarrhea; for others, spicy foods or caffeine is a problem. When the disease is "active," try to figure out which foods make your symptoms worse. Many physicians recommend avoiding dairy products. However, these are excellent sources of calcium, so don't eliminate them from your diet if you can tolerate them.

Eat smaller meals. It's usually easier for the intestines to handle small, frequent meals than single large servings.

Ease discomfort with a hot-water bottle. Place it on your abdomen when you're experiencing cramps to reduce some of your pain, suggests Sunanda V. Kane, M.D., a specialist in IBD in the section of gastroenterology and nutrition at the University of Chicago Hospitals and Health System.

Take extra calcium. Evidence suggests that it reduces the severity and frequency of abdominal cramps, says Dr. Kane. She advises taking 1,200 to 1,500 milligrams of calcium daily, based on the amounts used in studies.

alternative therapies

Drink chamomile or peppermint tea. The herbs contain compounds that reduce spasms in

---

THREE THINGS I TELL EVERY FEMALE PATIENT

WILLIAM TREMAINE, M.D., professor of medicine and director of the Inflammatory Bowel Disease Clinic at the Mayo Clinic, has some special advice for patients with inflammatory bowel disease.

1 TALK TO YOUR FAMILY AND FRIENDS. People with intestinal disorders are often too embarrassed to discuss their conditions with others—but the support you get from family will help you cope with this difficult condition.

2 JOIN A SUPPORT GROUP. It's a great place to get emotional support as well as practical tips for controlling IBD. The Crohn's and Colitis Foundation of America Web site (www.ccfa.org) will steer you to a support group in your area.

3 DO YOUR HOMEWORK. The more you learn about the disease, the better you'll be able to manage it, says Dr. Tremaine. ∎

the intestine, which can help ease gas and painful cramps. To make a tea, pour 1 cup of boiling water over 1 to 2 teaspoons of dried herb, cover, and let it steep for 10 to 15 minutes. Keep in mind that peppermint taken close to bedtime may cause heartburn by relaxing the esophagus.

For Long-Term Relief

home remedies

Avoid aspirin or ibuprofen. They're a very common cause of IBD relapses because they weaken the mucosa, the protective coating that lines the intestine.

If you smoke, try to quit. "For people with Crohn's disease, smoking increases relapses," Dr. Bayless says.

Exercise—and relax. Emotional stress doesn't cause IBD, but it can make the symptoms worse. An excellent way to reduce stress is to get regular exercise. As a bonus, exercise helps prevent weight gain in those taking steroids to control their symptoms, says Dr. Kane. (For step-by-step details on starting an exercise program, see chapter 5.)

medical options

Control IBD with medications. Not so long ago, the main treatment for IBD was corticosteroids—drugs that are rife with side effects. There are many more options today, including drugs that modify the immune system and get the inflammation under control, says Stephan R. Targan, M.D., director of the Inflammatory Bowel Disease Center at Cedars-Sinai Medical Center in Los Angeles.

For more information about IBD: Visit the Web site of the Crohn's and Colitis Foundation of America at www.ccfa.org. Or look up "digestive diseases" at the Web site of the National Institute of Diabetes and Digestive and Kidney Diseases at www.niddk.nih.gov.

irritable bowel syndrome

Women who live with irritable bowel syndrome (IBS) soon develop a sixth sense about the locations of public restrooms. They have to because the symptoms of IBS—usually abdominal pain, cramping, and diarrhea—can come on with very little warning.

Before leaving the house, women with IBS invariably ask themselves, "Is my bowel going to act up today?" says Nancy Norton of Milwaukee, founder of the International Foundation for Functional Gastrointestinal Disorders.

IBS is very unpredictable. Some women will have sudden attacks of diarrhea, sometimes several times a day. For others, diarrhea may alternate with constipation, painful gas buildups, or other digestive upsets.

There's still a lot of mystery surrounding IBS. Normally, the muscular walls of the intestine contract and relax in a predictable and rhythmic way.

Research has shown that in people with IBS, the contractions are stronger and last longer—although it's not yet clear if this is the underlying cause of the condition, says Marie Borum, M.D., associate professor in the division of gastroenterology at George Washington University in Washington, D.C.

Since doctors haven't discovered what causes IBS, there still isn't a cure. However, there are a number of medications that can control the symptoms. In addition, there are a number of home care strategies that will go a long way toward reducing the discomfort.

For Immediate Relief

home remedies

Cut back on coffee and tea. Caffeine may irritate the digestive tract, so it's a good idea to avoid anything containing caffeine.

Take fatty foods off the menu. They're difficult for the body to digest, which can result in more gas and indigestion.

Choose soluble fiber supplements over bran. Some IBS sufferers find that bran and other foods rich in insoluble fiber worsen their condition. If you're one of them, switch to a soluble fiber supplement, such as psyllium.

Be prepared. There will be times when you simply can't afford to be incapacitated with intestinal woes—when you're overwhelmed at work, for example, or you're planning an overseas flight. For short-term control of diarrhea, it's fine to take over-the-counter diarrhea remedies such as loperamide (Imodium), says Eugene Bozymski,

M.D., professor of medicine at the University of North Carolina at Chapel Hill.

Reduce gas. Bloating or distention due to intestinal gas is one of the most common symptoms of IBS and can also lead to cramping and abdominal pain. Over-the-counter products that contain simethicone (such as Maalox or Gas-X) may help relieve intestinal gas. Or you may want to try an over-the-counter product called Beano. It contains an enzyme that assists in the digestion of some sugars and may help prevent gas from forming.

Eat less dairy. Millions of Americans have a condition called lactose intolerance: They don't produce enough of the enzyme (lactase) that's needed to digest a sugar (lactose) found in dairy foods. If you're lactose intolerant and also have IBS, even small amounts of milk, cheese, or other dairy foods may cause symptoms.

If you're lactose intolerant, you might be able

when to see a doctor

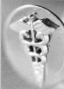

If diarrhea or other common symptoms of IBS are accompanied by weight loss, see a doctor right away. You could have a more serious digestive condition, called Crohn's disease, says Marie Borum, M.D., associate professor in the division of gastroenterology at George Washington University in Washington, D.C.

If you notice rectal bleeding or if you've had recent changes in your symptoms: Some of the same signs of IBS can also be caused by colon cancer. You'll want to get a checkup right away.

to enjoy small servings of dairy foods, especially if you have them with other foods. You can try adding lactase enzyme (Lactaid) to dairy products. Or you may have to avoid dairy products altogether. You may have to experiment a bit to find out which approach works for you.

alternative therapies

Relax the intestine with herbs. Chamomile and valerian relax intestinal contractions. Valerian may be especially helpful because it also reduces stress, a common trigger of IBS. Pour 1 cup of boiling water over 1 to 2 teaspoons of dried chamomile flowers. Cover and let it steep for 10 to 15 minutes. For valerian, take two 500-milligram root tablets 30 minutes before bed.

You can buy herbal teas and supplements at pharmacies and health food stores.

Try peppermint. Another herb that relaxes the intestinal muscles, it appears to be very helpful for those with IBS, says Mark Stengler, N.D., a naturopathic physician at La Jolla Whole Health Medical Clinic in California.

In one study, out of 52 people with IBS who took one peppermint capsule before meals for 1 month, most reported having less abdominal pain, bloating, and diarrhea.

If you decide to try peppermint capsules, look for products that are enteric-coated: They dissolve in the intestine instead of in the stomach, thereby reducing stomach upset. Look for capsules with 0.2 to 0.4 milliliter of oil.

Try cognitive therapy. Studies have shown that using a type of "talk therapy" can help you feel better by changing the way you view your problems. Cognitive therapy involves keeping a

THREE THINGS I TELL EVERY FEMALE PATIENT

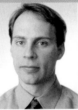

MARK STENGLER, N.D., a naturopathic physician at La Jolla Whole Health Medical Clinic in California, suffered from IBS for years. Here are his strategies for getting the symptoms under control.

1

EXERCISE REGULARLY. There's no scientific evidence that it controls IBS, but many patients report that it helps. "Choose an exercise that you really like, such as taking walks with a friend," Dr. Stengler advises.

TAKE CONTROL OF STRESS. "When you're under stress, the sympathetic nervous system gets stimulated and the normal contractions of the intestines are altered," he explains. Some of the best ways to reduce stress include yoga, prayer, and meditation. "You'll have to experiment to find what works best for you," he says.

2

TRY PASSIONFLOWER. An herb, it reduces digestive discomfort, Dr. Stengler explains. If you're using a 1:1 tincture, take 20 drops three times daily. If you're using capsules, take two 500-milligram tablets three times daily. ■

3

diary of your symptoms and your feelings about them. A therapist can help you reframe your feelings so you gain control over your IBS symptoms.

For Long-Term Relief

Include more fiber in your diet. It's among the best strategies for controlling IBS, says Dr. Borum.

Prevention magazine recommends getting 25 to 35 grams of fiber daily. If you start the day with a high-fiber cereal, snack on fruit throughout the day, and include several servings of vegetables with meals, you'll almost automatically get all the fiber you need.

There are several types of fiber, and they aren't quite interchangeable. If your main symptom is diarrhea, try to increase your intake of soluble fiber, found in fruits, oatmeal, rice, barley, and psyllium, says Elaine Magee, R.D., author of *Tell Me What to Eat If I Have Irritable Bowel Syndrome.* If constipation is the problem, you'll do better focusing on the insoluble fiber found in legumes, whole wheat, and vegetables.

Keep a regular meal schedule. Having breakfast, lunch, and dinner at the same times every day will help regulate digestion and prevent "sneak" attacks of IBS.

Eat cooked vegetables. They're easier to digest than raw vegetables, says Dr. Stengler.

Pay attention to your diet. Everyone with IBS reacts to different foods. If you find that you spend 30 minutes in the bathroom every time you eat oatmeal, for example, you'll probably want to try another hot cereal. It will take some trial and error to find out which foods make your symptoms worse—and which make them better.

Talk to your doctor about antidepressants. Patients with more severe symptoms may benefit from antidepressants. They have been shown to relieve some of the symptoms of IBS, especially when people are also suffering from pain and depression.

Your doctor may recommend one of the tricyclic antidepressants, such as imipramine (Tofranil) or amitriptyline (Elavil). Apart from reducing stress and depression, these drugs may decrease stool frequency, which is helpful for some people with IBS.

Other medications that may be helpful to some people include fluoxetine (Prozac) or paroxetine (Paxil). These drugs tend to be used when people with IBS are suffering from constipation as well as depression.

Ask about new treatment options. A new drug shows great promise for easing IBS. In a study of 800 people with IBS, those who took a medication called tegaserod daily for 12 weeks had 20 percent less abdominal pain and 25 percent less constipation.

Look into hypnosis. Performed by doctors or other trained professionals, hypnosis and behavior modification techniques may be useful in reducing stress and relaxing the intestinal muscles. Studies show that they may be helpful in reducing abdominal pain and bloating associated with IBS.

kidney infections

Even women who get frequent urinary tract infections are surprised—and dismayed—by how sick they feel when the infection moves upward from the bladder to the kidneys.

The kidneys are the body's main filters. They remove waste products from the blood and ship them to the bladder for disposal. An infection in the kidneys, called pyelonephritis, can result in excruciating pain. There's also a risk that the infection will spread to other parts of the body.

"Women get kidney infections more than men because they tend to ignore bladder infections, instead of getting them treated right away," says Larrian Gillespie, M.D., president of Healthy Life Publications in Beverly Hills, California, and author of *You Don't Have to Live with Cystitis.*

Kidney infections tend to occur when bacteria that have multiplied in the bladder travel upstream through the ureters, the tubes that connect the kidneys to the bladder. It's common, in fact, for women to have infections in the kidneys and bladder at the same time.

Once you have a kidney infection, you're going to need antibiotics. While you're waiting for the drugs to work, there are a number of ways to reduce the discomfort. You can also take steps to prevent future infections.

For Immediate Relief

home remedies

Drink as much as you can hold. Water helps flush the infection from the kidneys, and it also dilutes the concentration of bacteria in the bladder, which can prevent kidney infections from getting started, says Dr. Gillespie. For long-term protection, *Prevention* magazine recommends drinking at least eight 8-ounce glasses of water daily.

Use pain relievers as needed. While you're waiting for antibiotics to work, taking aspirin or ibuprofen will help reduce fever and muscle aches, says Dr. Gillespie. Just follow the directions on the label.

Apply heat. Women with kidney infections often feel better when they apply a hot-water bottle to the abdomen or below the ribs, says Dr. Gillespie.

when to see a doctor

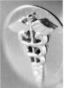

If you have pain in the flank (below the ribs toward the back), fever, or nausea and vomiting, see a doctor right away. These are classic symptoms of kidney infections, says Larrian Gillespie, M.D., president of Healthy Life Publications in Beverly Hills, California, and author of *You Don't Have to Live with Cystitis.*

If the urine is cloudy or tinged with blood or if it has an unpleasant smell: You probably have an infection somewhere in the urinary tract—either in the bladder or the kidneys.

Get a prescription. Kidney infections always require antibiotics and cannot be treated with herbs, says Dr. Gillespie. Some women get so sick that they're given the drugs intravenously, but oral medications are usually effective. The antibiotics—such as trimethoprim with sulfamethoxazole, ciprofloxacin, or ofloxacin—are usually taken for 7 to 14 days to eliminate every trace of infection.

Reduce bladder irritation. Women with kidney infections often experience intense urges to urinate, even after they've just used the bathroom. An over-the-counter medication called phenazopyridine (such as Pyridium) reduces the "gotta go" symptoms, says Dr. Gillespie.

For Long-Term Relief

Inhibit bacteria with baking soda. If you have a bladder infection and want to ensure that it doesn't spread to the kidneys, mix $1/4$ teaspoon baking soda in a glass of water and drink it once a day. It makes the urine more alkaline, which helps prevent bacteria from thriving, says Dr. Gillespie.

Keep bacteria away from the urethra. Women often get kidney or bladder infections when germs from the anal area get inside the urethra, the tube that carries urine from the body. When you use the bathroom, always wipe from front to back, which pushes bacteria out of harm's way, says Mary Jane Minkin, M.D., clinical professor of obstetrics and gynecology at Yale University School of Medicine.

Wash before sex. Washing the genital area—with soap and water, or simply warm water—removes bacteria that might otherwise slip into the urethra, says Dr. Minkin. Urinating after sex is also helpful because it flushes away bacteria that were lucky enough to get inside.

Drink cranberry juice daily. Research has shown that cranberry juice contains chemical compounds that make it more difficult for bacteria to stick to cells in the urinary tract. Women who get a lot of infections will often drink one or two glasses of cranberry juice daily as a preventive measure. Dried cranberries, which contain the same infection-fighting chemicals, are also a good bet.

Eat active, live-culture yogurt. The "good" bacteria in live-culture yogurt help to maintain a healthy balance of bacteria in the body, which translates into fewer bladder infections, says Dr. Minkin.

kidney stones

If you haven't checked the color of your urine lately, it might be a good time to start: The darker it is, the more concentrated it is—and the greater your risk for developing kidney stones.

When minerals and other substances in urine become too concentrated, they may form hard little crystals on the kidney walls. You won't have a problem as long as the rough little stones stay in place. But sometimes a stone breaks free and squeezes through one of the ureters, the tubes that connect the kidneys to the bladder, or the urethra, which carries urine from the bladder out of the body.

Kidney stones can often cause extreme pain. "I've known people who were involved in car accidents because they were so distracted by the severe pain of their kidney stones," says Howard Heller, M.D., assistant professor in the department of internal medicine at the University of Texas Southwestern Medical Center in Dallas. Conversely, some people may experience little or no pain—but this is fairly rare.

Large kidney stones can cause bleeding, infection, and severe kidney damage. And passing one stone doesn't guarantee it won't happen again. Quite the opposite: People who have passed a stone once have a 50 to 70 percent chance of a repeat performance.

For Immediate Relief

home remedies

Dilute the urine. You can help kidney stones pass more quickly—and prevent them from coming back—by drinking nine to ten 8-ounce glasses of water daily. To accomplish this, Dr. Heller recommends drinking two glasses with meals, one between meals, one at bedtime, and, for people who frequently get stones, one more during the night. "Increasing fluid intake can significantly reduce the risk of stones," says Dr. Heller. "It's the cheapest medicine we have."

Enjoy lemonade. It counts toward your water total, and it also contains citrate, a chemical that inhibits the formation of kidney stones.

Take something for pain. Kidney stones can be excruciatingly painful until they pass—which can take anywhere from a few minutes to hours or even days. To reduce the pain, take acetaminophen, or, if that doesn't work, try ibuprofen or another over-the-counter analgesic, Dr. Heller advises. Just follow the dosage directions on the label. For severe pain, your doctor may prescribe stronger medications.

medical options

Crush the stones. When a kidney stone is too large to pass by itself, your doctor may crush the stone with a procedure called extracorporeal shock wave lithotripsy (ESWL). Sound waves pass through the abdomen and are absorbed by the stone, which often crumbles. The smaller fragments then pass out of the body in the urine.

See a surgeon. Stones that don't respond to sound waves may need to be surgically removed. With a recently developed procedure called percutaneous nephrolithotomy, a surgeon can remove stones with a tiny tube that's inserted through the back into the kidney. "This has been a major advance in removing kidney stones," says Dr. Heller.

Long-Term Solutions

As always, drinking plenty of water is an important factor in the prevention of kidney stones. For some people, the following changes in diet may also be helpful—but be sure to first consult your doctor to make sure that these changes are right for you.

Reduce the oxalates in your diet. Meats (especially organ meats), spinach, rhubarb, beets, chocolate, and many other foods contain substances called oxalates, which are an important cause of kidney stones.

"Brewed tea is also high in oxalates," says Dr. Heller. "The darker the tea, the more oxalates it contains."

Talk to your doctor about calcium. You need calcium for strong bones, but some people absorb it a little too well and wind up with large amounts in the urine.

"For someone who forms a lot of stones, I would initially advise them to restrict their calcium intake by having no more than one-half to one serving of dairy foods daily," says Dr. Heller. "Then I would increase their dietary calcium each visit as long as the urine calcium is reasonably controlled."

If you're on a low-calcium diet, your doctor should perform regular urine tests to determine the optimal level of calcium for preserving bone strength while reducing the risk of kidney stones.

Enjoy beer on occasion. According to the research of Pirjo Pietinen, D.Sc., professor at the National Public Health Institute in Helsinki, Finland, beer increases the amount of water in urine, which reduces the concentration of stone-forming calcium. In his 3-year study, Dr. Pietinen found that the risk of kidney stones dropped 40 percent with each beer drunk daily. However, excessive alcohol consumption can lead to health problems, so limit your drinks—men can have one or two 12-ounce glasses, while women should stick to one glass a day.

when to see a doctor

If you have pain that began around the flank (the area under the ribs toward the back) and then moved toward the groin, call your doctor. You're probably passing a kidney stone, says Howard Heller, M.D., assistant professor in the department of internal medicine at the University of Texas Southwestern Medical Center in Dallas. This pain can be severe and may be accompanied by fever, nausea, burning with urination, blood in the urine, or the inability to urinate.

If you've had kidney stones along with a rapid heartbeat, insomnia, or increasing irritability: You could be producing too much thyroid hormone, which increases calcium levels in the urine.

If you get frequent urinary tract infections: They're a common cause of a class of kidney stones called struvite stones.

Give up antacids. Both calcium- and aluminum-based antacids increase the concentration of stone-forming calcium in the urine. People with a history of kidney stones should switch to H_2 blockers (such as Tagamet), medications that control stomach acid without increasing the risk of stones, says Dr. Heller.

Eat less meat. The protein in beef, chicken, and pork breaks down in the body to form uric acid, a common cause of kidney stones. For patients with high uric acid or with high urine calcium, Dr. Heller advises eating no more than 8 ounces of meat daily.

Eat more citrus fruits. Like lemonade, citrus fruits and juices such as oranges, grapefruit, and orange juice contain stone-inhibiting citrate.

Cut back on sodium. Salt in the diet increases the amount of stone-forming calcium in the urine. People who get kidney stones due to high urine calcium should reduce their salt intake to fewer than 2,500 milligrams daily. To do this, Dr. Heller recommends using fresh or frozen foods instead of canned or processed ones, eating at home rather than in restaurants, and avoiding the temptation to add salt to your food.

medical options

Prevent stones with medications. People at high risk for kidney stones often take medications to prevent them. If you tend to form calcium stones, your doctor may prescribe a thiazide diuretic (water pill).

For uric acid stones, you may need a medication called allopurinol (Zyloprim), which prevents stones from forming by lowering uric acid production. Potassium citrate (Urocit-K) has also been shown to prevent stones in patients with high uric acid, and, by raising pH levels, it may actually help to dissolve small stones.

For more information about kidney stones: Go online to visit the Web site of the National Institute of Diabetes and Digestive and Kidney Diseases at www.niddk.nih.gov.

laryngitis

The human voice produces sounds when air from the lungs causes folds in the larynx, or "voice box," to vibrate. When tissues in the larynx swell, usually due to inflammation or an infection, they don't vibrate the way they should. This causes the most melodious voice to get raspy—or even disappear for a few days.

If you develop laryngitis and you also have a sore throat or stuffy nose, you probably have a minor viral infection and will get your voice back in a week or two, says Gregory Grillone, M.D., an otolaryngologist and director of the Voice Center at Boston University Medical Center.

Anything that irritates the vocal cords—smoking, a talkative night with girlfriends, or cheering your kid's soccer team—can cause temporary inflammation and voice loss, Dr. Grillone adds. Long-term laryngitis, on the other hand, is more likely to be caused by underlying problems, such as heartburn (in which acids from the stomach irritate tissues in the throat) or polyps (growths on the vocal folds).

Persistent laryngitis should always be evaluated by a doctor. In most cases, however, you can soothe the larynx and regain your voice with some simple home remedies.

For Immediate Relief

home remedies

Rest your voice. It's the best way to help the vocal cords recover. Talk as little as possible—and don't whisper: It irritates the larynx even more than talking.

Drink hot liquids. Water is fine, or you can brew cups of decaffeinated tea. Warm liquids soothe irritated tissues in the throat and may help the irritation heal more quickly, says Dr. Grillone.

Take long showers. Or plug in a humidifier. Breathing humid air will soothe and moisturize the injured tissues, says Dr. Grillone.

Avoid alcohol and caffeine for a few days. They remove water from the body and will make the larynx even drier.

Take care of heartburn. You'll feel—and talk—a lot better if you get your stomach acid under control. There are many strategies for reducing heartburn. They include:

- Elevate the head of your bed a few inches. That will make it harder for acids in the stomach to travel upstream.

- Take antacids or acid-reducing drugs, such as Tagamet.

- Avoid fatty foods, including chocolate. They weaken the circular muscle that prevents acid in the stomach from getting into the esophagus.

alternative therapies

Drink cinnamon tea. It reduces inflammation as well as pain. To make a tea, pour a cup of boiling water over 1 teaspoon of powdered cinnamon. Let it steep, covered, for 20 minutes, and drink it down.

THREE THINGS I TELL EVERY FEMALE PATIENT

GREG GRILLONE, M.D., directs the Voice Center at Boston University Medical Center. He advises women with laryngitis to do the following:

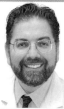

1 **DRINK AS MUCH WATER AS YOU CAN HOLD.** It hydrates the vocal cords, speeds healing, and reduces the raspy irritation.

2 **FOLLOW THE "ARM'S-LENGTH" RULE.** To preserve (or restore) your voice, don't talk to anyone who's more than an arm's length away.

3 **AVOID OVER-THE-COUNTER COLD REMEDIES.** The same active ingredients that ease congestion will remove moisture from the vocal cords. ■

when to see a doctor

When laryngitis lasts longer than 2 weeks, make an appointment to see your doctor. Persistent hoarseness may be a symptom of vocal cord damage or even cancer, says Gregory Grillone, M.D., an otolaryngologist and director of the Voice Center at Boston University Medical Center.

If the hoarseness is accompanied by trouble swallowing, or if there's a lump in the throat: These are also warning signs of cancer.

You may want to add honey to the tea, which will soothe the throat, and a squeeze of lemon, which stimulates saliva production and will help keep the tissues lubricated.

Long-Term Solutions

home remedies

If you smoke, try to quit. Cigarette smoke is irritating and a common cause of hoarseness.

Wear a protective mask. Pollen, mold, high office humidity, and even simple yard dust can irritate the larynx and lead to hoarseness or full-fledged laryngitis.

A paper "surgical" mask will filter out the coarsest particles. But a protective respirator, available in hardware stores, is a better choice when you're doing things like refinishing furniture, laying carpet, or adding a pressed wood door to a shed, where you're working with power tools or with paints or other chemicals like varnishes and adhesives.

lupus

Lupus has been called the "disease with a thousand faces" because it causes an incredible variety of symptoms, ranging from fatigue, achiness, and swollen joints to persistent fever, anemia, sensitivity to sunlight, and skin rashes. In severe cases it can damage the heart, lungs, kidneys, and other vital organs.

Lupus is an autoimmune condition, which means that the immune system "mistakenly" attacks healthy tissues throughout the body, resulting in inflammation. It's difficult to estimate how many Americans suffer from lupus because its symptoms vary widely, even in the same individual over time, and its onset is often hard to determine. Studies have shown, however, that lupus is much more common among women, affecting them about eight to 10 times as often as men. It usually strikes during the childbearing years, but older women, too, can get it.

"Researchers aren't sure why more women than men are diagnosed with lupus, but one possibility is that it's due to environmental exposure to toxins," says Michael Lockshin, M.D., director of the Barbara Volcker Rheumatology Center at the Hospital for Special Surgery in New York City. What these toxins are, however, and exactly what role they play in the development of lupus has yet to be determined.

It's also possible that lupus is triggered by bacteria or viruses. Because so many more women than men get the disease, researchers are also exploring a hormonal connection, specifically the role of estrogen.

There's no way to prevent lupus, nor is there a single test to diagnose it. If your doctor suspects that you have lupus, one of the tests you may be given is a blood test called an immunofluorescent antinuclear antibody (ANA) test. A positive result doesn't necessarily mean that you have lupus; other diseases and some drugs can cause false positives. In fact, only a minority of patients with positive ANA have lupus, but the test is almost always positive in lupus. Another test is the erythrocyte sedimentation rate. This is a blood test that examines how fast the red blood cells settle to the bottom of the test tube. If the red blood cells settle faster than normal, it could indicate a systemic disease, including lupus. Your doctor may also order a blood count test because people with lupus can have low numbers of white blood cells. Low platelets or red blood cells and low hemoglobin are also common signs of lupus.

Because lupus causes so many possible symptoms, and because the disease is so unpredictable—it's common for women to experience extended periods of remission, followed by sudden flare-ups of symptoms—there isn't a one-size-fits-all treatment plan. Here are some of the strategies that your doctor may recommend.

For Immediate Relief

home remedies

Take aspirin or ibuprofen as needed. Many women with lupus will experience joint pain or swelling, which can significantly reduce their ability to get around. Aspirin and ibuprofen can help because they reduce inflammation as well as pain, says Dr. Lockshin.

Always use sunscreen. "About one-third of lupus patients are very sensitive to the sun," says Dr. Lockshin. Even small amounts of sun exposure can trigger a flare-up of symptoms. "Use a sunscreen with an SPF of at least 15," he adds. Be sure to reapply it often, especially if you're swimming or perspiring, which will wash the sunscreen off the skin.

Avoid the sun's peak hours. "Stay out of the sun between 10:00 A.M. and 3:00 P.M.," Dr. Lockshin advises. That's when the sun's rays are strongest. "If you're doing outdoor activities, such as walking or gardening, do them first thing in the morning or later in the evening."

Exercise as much as you're able. Many women with lupus are so achy and fatigued that the very idea of exercise is enough to make them want to take a nap. But it's worth exercising anyway, even if you don't feel like it, since regular exercise can promote both physical and mental well-being.

Some of the best exercises are bicycling, swimming, and walking. You'll probably want to avoid pounding exercises such as running, which can put additional stress on joints that are already tender. But before you start an exercise program, ask your doctor to recommend a type and level of activity that's right for you.

Get the immune system under control. When lupus is "active," the immune system can destroy tissues throughout the body. Sooner or later, your doctor will probably give you prescription medications to suppress immunity and also reduce inflammation and pain. Some of the medications commonly used for lupus include corticosteroids, azathioprine (Imuran), and cyclophosphamide (Cytoxan).

The drugs can be very effective, but they're also rife with side effects. If your doctor prescribes corticosteroids, you will be given "tapering" doses, in which the amounts of medication are slowly reduced over time, which gives the body a

when to see a doctor

 If you have unexplained fatigue, muscle or joint pain, low-grade fever, hair loss, or a facial rash, such as spots about 1 to 2 inches in diameter on the cheeks or eyebrows, call your doctor right away. These are the classic symptoms of lupus, and you should get tested for it right away, says Michael Lockshin, M.D., director of the Barbara Volcker Rheumatology Center at the Hospital for Special Surgery in New York City. A butterfly-shaped rash across the nose or cheeks, while an important sign doctors use to diagnose lupus, is relatively uncommon, at least at the onset of the disease.

chance to adjust to the change. The other medications don't require tapering.

Long-Term Solutions

Eat as well as you can. There aren't specific dietary guidelines for people with lupus, but eating a well-balanced diet is essential to keep the immune system healthy. Doctors usually advise women to restrict their consumption of red meat and other fatty foods and to eat a variety of whole grains, legumes, and fruits and vegetables. This is a good plan for anyone, even if you don't have lupus, notes Dr. Lockshin.

Get plenty of rest. "Physical exhaustion tends to trigger flare-ups," says Dr. Lockshin. "Getting a good night's sleep, and doing that on a regular basis, is one of the things women can do to help manage the disease," he explains. "It's believed that sleep is also the time the body repairs cellular damage, so it may be helpful for the immune system."

Beware of colds or the flu. Even though lupus puts the immune system into overdrive, women with this condition are actually more susceptible to infections of all kinds, including colds and the flu, from the treatments and the disease itself. And when they do get sick, it may take them longer to recover.

It's impossible to avoid cold and flu viruses, of course, and certain treatments for lupus may reduce the effectiveness of the immune system, reducing your ability to fight any infection. If you do get infected, be sure to see your doctor. Even minor infections can be much more serious when you're also dealing with lupus.

Do everything you can to reduce stress. Women with lupus have been known to have flare-ups when they're going through difficult times, says Dr. Lockshin. "Everyone experiences stress, but people with lupus should try to avoid it," he says. "Professional counseling to help the woman and her family deal with this chronic illness may be helpful." Friends and family can also provide emotional and social support. Many organized groups for lupus also exist. To locate a support group in your area, check with your doctor or local hospitals.

Some women with lupus ask Dr. Lockshin whether they should practice stress reduction techniques, such as deep breathing, biofeedback, meditation, or yoga. Since these can sometimes be helpful, he usually advises anyone who wants to try them to go ahead.

For more information about lupus: Visit the Web site of the Lupus Foundation of America at www.lupus.org.

lyme disease

Ever since Lyme disease was first identified in the United States in 1975, millions of Americans have been nervous about hiking in woods, fields, and other areas occupied by deer ticks, which transmit this sometimes painful bacterial infection.

It's reasonable to be concerned about Lyme disease, especially if you live in a high-risk region, such as the northeastern, upper midwestern, and Pacific coast states. But there's no reason to limit your activities because of it.

"There's a lot of unwarranted anxiety in this country about Lyme disease," says Robert T. Schoen, M.D., a leading Lyme disease researcher and clinical professor of medicine at Yale University School of Medicine. The number of ticks infected with the bacterium varies by region. Fewer than 5 percent of adult ticks south of Maryland are infected while up to 50 percent are infected in some areas of the Northeast. Even if you do get bitten, it takes more than 24 hours for the tick to transmit the bacteria into a human. You can greatly reduce your chances of getting the disease by simply removing the tick as soon as you see it.

Unfortunately, removing ticks isn't always easy—they're not much larger than a sesame seed, so even when you're looking for one, you won't always spot it. The only way many people know they've been exposed to the Lyme bacterium is when they develop symptoms, such as fatigue, fever, joint pain, and a skin rash that looks like a bull's-eye.

For Immediate Relief

medical options

Take antibiotics. For all the worries about Lyme disease, it's usually easy to treat. If you are diagnosed with Lyme disease, your doctor will give you a course of antibiotics consisting of amoxicillin or doxycycline. In most cases, that will knock out the infection for good.

For Long-Term Prevention

Dress properly. If you live in an area that's known to harbor deer ticks, it's worth wearing a long-sleeved shirt and pants when you go outside. Tuck the pants into your socks or boots. You may want to wear light-colored clothing, which makes it easier to spot any ticks that happen to climb on board.

Avoid high-risk areas. There's no reason to stay inside during the spring and summer months, when tick season is at its height, but it's a good idea to steer clear of areas where ticks are likely to thrive, especially moist, shady areas that have a ground cover of leaves or low-lying vegetation.

Use repellent. Before going outside, spray insect repellent on your clothing and any exposed skin. Adults should use an insect repellent that contains 20 to 30 percent DEET. Don't use any DEET-containing products on children under age 2. If you want to use DEET on a child over 2, never use a product that contains more than 10 percent—and always consult a pediatrician first.

Keep up with yard maintenance. Even if you live in the suburbs, deer ticks probably aren't far away. To keep them from getting too cozy, keep your grass cut short and clear leaves or brush from around the house and yard. If you live in a heavily wooded area, thinning the trees to let more sunlight through will also cut down on ticks by reducing the amount of habitat available for the deer and mice that carry the pests.

Remove ticks promptly. Ticks that haven't started feeding can be flicked off the skin with a washcloth or towel. Once they're embedded in the skin, however, they really hang on—and your risk for developing Lyme disease begins to rise.

To remove a tick, grip it close to the skin with a pair of tweezers. Pull with steady pressure, and the tick will pop right out. Try not to squeeze the body, which could cause the bacteria that are in the tick to be injected into the skin. After removing the tick, disinfect your skin and wash your hands with soap and water.

Consider the vaccine. Researchers have developed a vaccine that can reduce, by about 78 percent, the risk of Lyme infection in people ages 15 to 70. People who live in tick-infested areas and engage in activities that may put them at risk

when to see a doctor

If you develop a persistent fever or joint pain during the warm months, or if you have an unexplained rash, see your doctor right away. Even if you never saw a tick, you could be infected with the Lyme bacterium, says Robert T. Schoen, M.D., clinical professor of medicine at Yale University School of Medicine.

should consider the vaccine, says Dr. Schoen. It isn't foolproof, but it will provide significant protection.

The vaccine is given as a series of three shots over a 12-month period. "Studies have shown that it's safe and effective," says Dr. Schoen. "Talk to

your doctor to determine your individual risk, and then decide if the vaccine is right for you."

For more information about Lyme disease: Visit the Web site of the Centers for Disease Control and Prevention at www.cdc.gov. Click on the banner "Health Topics A–Z," and scroll down to "Lyme disease."

macular degeneration

Sunlight, beautiful as it is, packs some hidden hazards for the eyes, which is a big part of the reason that millions of women may lose some of their ability to see.

As you get older, the macula, a thin membrane at the back of the eyes, sometimes breaks down, making your vision a little blurry. This condition, called macular degeneration, is the leading cause of vision loss in older women.

There are two main forms of macular degeneration. The "dry" form, known as age-related macular degeneration, is thought to be caused by free radicals in the body that are formed whenever you're exposed to sunlight, cigarette smoke, and air pollution; they're also a natural by-product of your body's metabolic processes. The less common, "wet" form of the disease occurs when there's leakage from abnormal blood vessels in the eyes. The risk for both forms increases with age.

"You can repair some of the damage by improving circulation to the eyes and getting the appropriate nutrients," says Robert Abel Jr., M.D., clinical professor of ophthalmology at Thomas

Jefferson University School of Medicine in Philadelphia and author of *The Eye Care Revolution*.

Just as important, there are steps you can take that will protect your eyes from both forms of this free radical free-for-all.

For Immediate Relief

home remedies

Fill up on spinach. Along with other leafy greens, such as kale and Swiss chard, it's rich in a plant pigment called lutein, which prevents eye-damaging blue light in sunshine from harming the eyes. It also "neutralizes" free radicals, says Dr. Abel.

One small study found that people who ate $\frac{1}{2}$ cup of cooked spinach four to seven times a week for a year had significant improvements in night vision. "One man told me that he was thrilled to be able to read a clock after years of struggling with blank spots in his vision," says study leader Stuart Richer, O.D., Ph.D., a vision researcher with the Veterans Administration in Chicago.

Add a little fat to your greens. Your body can't absorb much lutein unless you consume it with a little fat. Adding a teaspoon of olive oil to lutein-rich vegetables will boost blood levels of the nutrient by as much as 88 percent.

Give your vision a boost. Women with mild forms of macular degeneration will see clearly most of the time, but they may need a little help when they're reading or watching TV. "Aids for low vision in the later stages of the disease, such as magnifiers, telescopic lenses, and closed-circuit reading devices, can make a real difference," says Dr. Abel.

For reading, an inexpensive pair of reading glasses may be all you need. "If you wear glasses, make sure your prescription is up-to-date," Dr. Abel adds.

Be careful when driving at night. Some people with macular degeneration have perfectly good vision during the day but lose some of their ability to see after dark, says Dr. Abel.

alternative therapies

Have a daily cup of bilberry tea. It's rich in chemical compounds called anthocyanosides, which strengthen blood vessels in the eye and inhibit the effects of free radicals. "Bilberry is especially good for improving night vision," says Dr. Abel. "You'll notice the difference very quickly."

Use ginkgo supplements. Available in health food stores, ginkgo improves circulation in the eyes. Better circulation means that you'll get additional nutrients into the damaged areas, says Dr. Abel. He recommends taking 15 drops of ginkgo extract, dropped into a sip of water, once or twice daily for 1 month.

THREE THINGS I TELL EVERY FEMALE PATIENT

ROBERT ABEL JR., M.D., clinical professor of ophthalmology at Thomas Jefferson University School of Medicine in Philadelphia, offers the following advice for keeping the eyes healthy.

1 DRINK EIGHT GLASSES OF WATER DAILY. "The eye is basically a bag of water with two lenses," Dr. Abel says. "Most of us don't drink enough water to replenish the fluids and get an improved circulation of nutrients."

EAT LIVE-CULTURE YOGURT. Or take probiotic supplements. Levels of stomach acid de-

2 cline with aging, which reduces the absorption of important nutrients. Yogurt and digestion-friendly supplements will help the eyes stay nourished.

3 TAKE OMEGA-3 SUPPLEMENTS. They help repair damaged tissues in the eyes. Fish contains some omega-3s, but supplements—especially those containing a high concentration of an omega-3 called DHA—give a more concentrated dose. Take 400 to 500 milligrams daily, Dr. Abel advises. ■

For Long-Term Relief

Wear sunglasses. Wraparound shades are your best choice because they provide the most protection from ultraviolet (UV) light in sunshine. "Everyone should wear sunglasses when they go outside," says Dr. Abel.

Get extra vitamin C. It accumulates in the watery portions of the body, including in the eyes. It's extremely effective at blocking the effects of free radicals, says Dr. Abel. He recommends supplementing your diet with 1,000 milligrams of vitamin C daily.

Eat a variety of fruits and vegetables. They contain a variety of antioxidant compounds, including lycopene and zeaxanthin, which have been shown to "mop up" free radicals in the eyes.

Put fish on the menu. A study of 2,900 people found that those who ate fish once or more a month had half the risk of developing macular degeneration as those who ate fish less often.

Limit your consumption of fat. Studies have shown that people who get a lot of fat in the diet, especially the saturated fat that's found in meats and full-fat dairy foods, have a much higher risk of macular degeneration. "Saturated fat contributes to blocked arteries, which reduces circulation in the eyes," Dr. Abel explains.

To protect your eyes as well as your heart and arteries, doctors advise limiting fat consumption to 25 percent (or less) of total calories.

when to see a doctor

If your vision is a little blurry, or if you're seeing a small blind spot in the middle of your field of vision, or if you notice that straight lines appear to be distorted, see an ophthalmologist. These are classic symptoms of macular degeneration, says John D. Hunkeler, M.D., clinical professor of ophthalmology at the University of Kansas School of Medicine in Kansas City.

If the change in vision occurred suddenly: You could have a leakage of blood in the brain that's affecting the optic nerve.

If your vision is blurry and you also have diabetes: You could have a potentially serious condition called diabetic retinopathy—which, without prompt treatment, can lead to blindness.

Talk to an ophthalmologist. The "wet" form of macular degeneration can sometimes be treated with a technique called photodynamic therapy. The damaged blood vessels are coated with a light-sensitive dye, then exposed to light from a laser.

"It's often possible to seal off the blood vessels without damaging other parts of the eye," says John D. Hunkeler, M.D., clinical professor of ophthalmology at the University of Kansas School of Medicine in Kansas City.

For more information on macular degeneration: Visit the Web site of the National Eye Institute at www.nei.nih.gov.

memory problems

Don't be too hard on yourself the next time you lose the car keys. Many women begin experiencing memory lapses around their 50th birthdays, and in adults 70 years and older, declines in memory are nearly universal. Blanking out occasionally is exasperating, but no big deal.

Occasional forgetfulness isn't a sign of Alzheimer's disease. It doesn't mean that you're destined to spend the rest of your life forgetting names or wondering why you put the mail in the freezer. What it probably means is that cells in your brain aren't getting all the nourishment or stimulation that they need to withstand the normal wear and tear of aging.

"Some people, whether because of their behavior or their genetic makeup, are able to avoid or slow the usual declines in memory function," says Stanley Birge, M.D., director of the Older Adult Health Center at Washington University School of Medicine in St. Louis.

Health problems such as high blood pressure and high cholesterol may contribute to memory lapses and other mental declines, so it's important to talk to your doctor if you find you're forgetting things more than you used to.

But in most cases occasional forgetfulness doesn't mean you're losing your mental faculties. There's a good chance you can significantly improve your memory—and reduce the risk of further declines—with a variety of mental tactics and simple lifestyle changes.

For Immediate Relief

home remedies

Exercise your mind. "People who remain active socially and are engaged in demanding cognitive activities may be able to reduce the usual aging of the brain," says Dr. Birge. Crossword puzzles and games of Scrabble will keep the brain challenged. Volunteer work is helpful. So are hobbies, or simply reading magazines and newspapers.

"You don't want to do just one thing," Dr. Birge adds. "You want to keep the brain operating at a multitude of activities."

Review important information. The brain has more trouble taking in new information as you get older. You can overcome this by mentally reviewing information that you want to retain.

The next time you meet someone new, for example, repeat the name in your mind several times. If you tend to lose the car keys, keep them in the same place and mentally visualize where they are.

"The better the preparation, the stronger the memory," says James McGaugh, Ph.D., director of the Center for the Neurobiology of Learning and Memory and professor of neurobiology and behavior at the University of California, Irvine.

Reinforce your memory with a cup of coffee or tea. Laboratory studies suggest that the caffeine in coffee, tea, and sodas may enhance long-term memory when it's consumed shortly after learning new things.

Take a nutritional supplement. As you get older, the small intestine loses some of its ability to absorb vitamin B_{12}, which plays a role in memory and other mental functions. Lean meats, eggs, and low-fat dairy foods provide abundant amounts of B_{12}. Vegetarians, however, may need to take a supplement. The Daily Value for vitamin B_{12} is 6 micrograms.

Drink more water. People who don't drink enough can get dehydrated, which affects bloodflow to the brain, leading to fatigue and making it harder to remember things. Try to drink at least eight 8-ounce glasses of water daily.

alternative therapies

Give ginkgo a try. Available in pharmacies and health food stores, this herb improves circulation and helps brain cells get all the nutrients they need to stay healthy. Researchers at the Medical Research Centre at the University of Surrey in Guildford, England, found that people ages 50 to 59 who took 120 milligrams of ginkgo three times daily had improvements in memory, concentration, and alertness.

"Now we have proof positive that ginkgo can boost memory in healthy young people," says Douglas Schar, Dip.Phyt., an herbalist in London and Washington, D.C.

Drink sage tea. Folk healers have traditionally recommended sage for improving memory, and new research suggests it could work. Sage contains two chemical compounds—1,8-cineole and alpha-pinene—which block an enzyme that may be linked to Alzheimer's disease.

THREE THINGS I TELL EVERY FEMALE PATIENT

STANLEY BIRGE, M.D., director of the Older Adult Health Center at Washington University School of Medicine in St. Louis, gives this important advice.

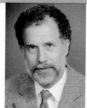

BE SURE TO EXERCISE REGULARLY.
Walking, biking, and other forms of exercise increase bloodflow to the brain. In addition, exercise stimulates different parts of the brain. When people engage in physical activity, their risk of cognitive impairment is dramatically reduced.

TALK TO YOUR DOCTOR ABOUT HORMONE REPLACEMENT THERAPY. The hormone estrogen protects memory in several ways. It reduces free radical damage, increases bloodflow, and stimulates growth factors that are involved in the repair of damaged neurons. Supplemental estrogen may help after menopause, when a woman's natural supply of the hormone declines.

TAKE CONTROL OF STRESS. Sustained high levels of cortisol and other stress hormones may block the ability to remember important information, such as names or telephone numbers. People who reduce their levels of cortisol—with exercise, meditation, or other pleasurable activities—are less likely to experience degenerative damage in the brain. ■

The problem with sage is that is also contains a compound called thujone, which may be toxic in large doses. It's fine to enjoy sage tea on occasion, but you don't want to drink it every day.

Boost cell communication with huperzine A. A supplement based on a Chinese herbal remedy, huperzine A (HupA) is thought to protect the brain's supply of acetylcholine, a chemical messenger that may break down over time. Studies of people with Alzheimer's disease have shown that 60 percent of those who took HupA had significant improvements in mental function, says Alan Kozikowski, Ph.D., director for the drug discovery program at the Institute for Cognitive and Computational Sciences at Georgetown University Medical Center in Washington, D.C.

Improve your memory with PS. Short for phosphatidylserine, PS is a component of brain cells that regulates chemical messengers, or neu-rotransmitters. One study showed that people who took PS found it easier to recall the names of people they'd recently been introduced to.

Long-Term Solutions

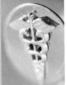

home remedies

Eat brightly colored fruits and vegetables. They contain chemical compounds called flavonoids, antioxidant compounds that blunt the effects of free radicals, unstable oxygen molecules in the body that may damage blood vessels in the brain and increase the risk of memory declines. In one study, animals that were given flavonoid-rich blueberries or spinach daily were able to reverse memory impairments.

"If you want to slow down the free radical aging process, blueberries are the leader of the pack," adds Ronald Prior, Ph.D., head of the USDA Phytochemical Laboratory at Tufts University in Boston. "With ½ cup of blueberries, you can just about double the amount of antioxidants that most Americans get in one day."

Take extra vitamin E. Scientists have found that vitamin E reduces levels of memory-clouding free radicals in the brain. Vitamin E is found mainly in nuts, wheat germ, and cooking oils, as well as in supplement form. The optimal dose hasn't been determined, but Dr. Birge advises patients to take 800 IU of vitamin E daily.

Enjoy citrus fruits. They're among the best sources of vitamin C, an antioxidant nutrient that promotes healthy bloodflow by preventing cholesterol and other fatty substances from accumulating in blood vessels in the brain. Vitamin C also makes vitamin E work more effectively and

when to see a doctor

If your memory is progressively getting worse, see your doctor immediately. Memory declines may be caused by potentially serious—and treatable—conditions, such as depression, thyroid disorders, or nutritional deficiencies, says Stanley Birge, M.D., director of the Older Adult Health Center at Washington University School of Medicine in St. Louis.

If your memory gets worse and you're taking a new medication: Many prescription drugs, including those used to control high blood pressure, may cause impairments in memory. Changing to a new drug will often resolve the problem.

improves its ability to block cell-damaging free radicals, says Dr. Birge.

Add some folate. In new research, older people with lower levels of the B vitamin folate in their blood found it harder to hold on to new information that was coming at them quickly.

"Folate is one of the most valuable nutrients you can take for healthy memory function throughout life," says Jay Lombard, M.D., director of the Brain Behavior Center in Nyack, New York. Dr. Lombard thinks that folate helps memory by "recycling" chemicals that brain cells need to communicate and fighting artery plaque, which can reduce bloodflow to the brain.

Pick the right pain reliever. If you take over-the-counter nonsteroidal anti-inflammatory medications, such as ibuprofen, for the treatment of arthritis, it may delay the effects of memory loss. Although these drugs are readily available over the counter, they should not be taken without medical supervision. Older people are particularly sensitive to the drugs' effects on the stomach, which can result in bleeding ulcers.

Battle depression. It can make people feel tired, unfocused, and mentally slow. In fact, depression in the elderly is often mistaken for Alzheimer's disease.

"Antidepressant medications do more than relieve the symptoms of depression," says Dr. Birge. They seem to affect the region of the brain (the hippocampus) that plays a key role in memory. "They also may stimulate the generation of nerve cells," he adds. By aiding in the repair of nerve cells, antidepressants may help restore memory and other mental functions that have degraded over time.

For more information on memory loss: Visit the Web site of the American Geriatrics Society at www.americangeriatrics.org. Or go to the Alzheimer's Association at www.alz.org.

multiple sclerosis

The symptoms seem mild at first. A little fatigue or weakness. An increase in frequency of urination. A "funny" feeling in the arms and legs that doesn't go away.

"For some, multiple sclerosis remains a relatively mild disease," explains Thomas Leist, M.D., director of the Multiple Sclerosis Center at Thomas Jefferson University Hospital in Philadelphia. Even when the disease takes a more serious course, symptoms tend to flare briefly, then improve or go for long periods of time into remission.

Multiple sclerosis (MS) is thought to occur when the immune system's defensive cells attack the sheath, or myelin, that insulates nerve fibers. The damage results in inflammation and scarring (sclerosis), which blocks nerve signal transmission.

MS usually strikes before age 40, and more than three-fourths of those newly diagnosed are women. It may be linked to viral infections, and people with affected relatives may be more susceptible than those without the family history.

There isn't a cure for MS, but with a combination of medications and home care strategies, most people can manage the symptoms.

For Immediate Relief

home remedies

Allow time for rest. Bone-weary fatigue is the hallmark of MS. "People have to figure out what their stamina levels are and make the necessary adjustments," says Dr. Leist. Get help with your physical household chores. Make arrangements to adjust your work schedule. "I advise people to have 40 minutes or an hour of quiet time at lunch in order to recharge their batteries," he adds.

Keep temperatures on the cool side. MS reduces the body's ability to tolerate heat. You'll probably find yourself setting the thermostat at a lower setting than you used to. If you get too hot when you do your usual exercise, switch to

when to see a doctor

If you have muscle weakness, persistent numbness, pins and needles, or persistent fatigue, see a doctor. These are among the earliest symptoms of multiple sclerosis (MS), says Thomas Leist, M.D., director of the Multiple Sclerosis Center at Thomas Jefferson University Hospital in Philadelphia.

If new or old symptoms occur after a period of remission: It's important to make sure that you don't have an infection. If you're having a relapse, you may need intravenous injections of anti-inflammatory drugs. The drugs are usually given for 3 to 5 days, says Dr. Leist. If this happens often, your doctor may want to review your immune-regulating regimen.

swimming or aquatherapy, Dr. Leist advises. The water will help to lower your body temperature.

Eat whole grains and other fiber-rich foods. Fiber helps to prevent constipation, a common symptom in those with MS.

Enjoy regular massages. Massage may help fight the muscle spasms that are often a symptom in MS, says Dr. Leist.

alternative therapies

Take vitamin C supplements. Women with MS have a high risk of urinary tract infections because the bladder doesn't always empty completely. Dr. Leist recommends taking 1,000 milligrams of vitamin C daily, unless there is a history of kidney stones. "It acidifies the urine and helps prevent infections," he says.

Try cranberry caplets. Available in health food stores, they contain substances that help reduce frequent urination—a bothersome symptom in those with MS. Dr. Leist recommends following the directions on the label. "You can't drink enough cranberry juice to get the same effects," he adds.

mind-body techniques

Join a support group. Or make an appointment to see a counselor. Research suggests that people with MS suffer from depression more than the general population. Remaining active and keeping a positive outlook on life will give you the energy that you need to cope with the illness.

medical options

Ease inflammation with steroids. During flare-ups, your doctor may give you injections of corticosteroids, medications that reduce inflammation and help decrease the severity and duration of symptoms.

Make sure you sleep well. If your sleep quality is good and the fatigue persists, medication can help. A study of 72 people with MS found that 85 percent had less fatigue when they took a prescription medication called modafinil (Provigil).

Long-Term Solutions

home remedies

Exercise often. It boosts energy and also increases bone density. People with MS are often sedentary, which weakens bones and raises the risk of fractures, says Dr. Leist. Low-impact aerobic exercises, such as walking or swimming, are good choices, he adds.

medical options

Control relapses with immune-regulating drugs. "Interferon beta-1a (Avonex), interferon beta-1b (Betaseron), and glatiramer (Copaxone) reduce the number of attacks by about a third and impact the course of the disease," says Dr. Leist.

For more information on multiple sclerosis: Visit the Web site of the National Multiple Sclerosis Society at www.nmss.org. Or go to the Web site of the Multiple Sclerosis Foundation at www.msfacts.org.

nausea and vomiting

Literally hundreds of illnesses and conditions—from food poisoning and stomach "flu" to pregnancy—can result in nausea or vomiting in women. Most of the time, the miserable sensations are simply your body's way of saying "no thanks."

If you ate tainted food at a "greasy spoon"–type diner, for example, your stomach would do everything possible to expel the offending substances. Even morning sickness is thought by researchers to be one of the body's defense mechanisms against contaminants in the diet.

Nausea can also be more serious. Sometimes, women feel nauseated and will vomit in response to medications administered during labor, surgery, or chemotherapy, although significant strides have been made in prescription medications that counteract these sometimes violent reactions.

"There is a whole new class of drugs available for chemotherapy, which have made it a completely different experience. We don't see the horrendous nausea and vomiting that we once did," says Barbara Goff, M.D., associate professor of obstetrics and gynecology at the University of Washington School of Medicine in Seattle.

In the vast majority of cases, nausea and vomiting will get better on their own. "It's horrible, but you just have to ride it out," says Alan L. Melnick, M.D., director of the joint residency program in family and preventive medicine at Oregon Health Sciences University in Portland.

Depending on the cause of the queasies, here's what doctors advise.

For Immediate Relief

Clear the air. Nausea can be worsened by strong odors. This is especially true during pregnancy, when many women become hypersensitive to smells. When your stomach is tossing and turning, open a few windows and keep the fresh air flowing. You may even want block the bottom of the bedroom door with a rolled towel or blanket to prevent odors from coming in, suggests Miriam Erick, a registered dietitian at Brigham and Women's Hospital in Boston and author of *No More Morning Sickness*.

Eat lightly. When your stomach is upset, eating large portions will trigger muscular contractions that will make the nausea worse. It's a good idea to eat small servings—just a few mouthfuls at a time—until you're feeling better.

when to see a doctor

If nausea or vomiting persists for more than 48 hours, or if you're having other symptoms, such as abdominal pain or blood in the vomit, see your doctor right away. You could have a more serious problem that requires medical attention, says Scott A. Fields, M.D., vice chairman of family medicine at Oregon Health Sciences University in Portland.

Indulge your food desires. Women with morning sickness should ask themselves whether any food or type of food seems remotely appealing during bouts of queasiness. Erick divides potential foods into categories such as salty, crunchy, sour, spicy, and cold and lets women find choices they can stomach. Even snack foods are fine for 1 to 2 days, says Erick, and better for you and your fetus than no food at all.

Keep it bland. Nibble on soda crackers, bread, or other bland foods, anything without a strong odor. Keeping a little food in your stomach will help absorb acids and reduce nausea-causing spasms, says Erick.

Sip slowly. If you've been vomiting, you're probably losing important electrolytes (minerals in the blood), which regulate muscle contraction, says Erick. You need to replace the liquids and minerals that were lost—but slugging down water or juice will make the nausea worse. It's better to sip small amounts of liquids—juice or broths—until your stomach is better. "Lemonade seems to work for some women," she says. "It could be the small amounts of potassium or its calorie content."

Wear a wristband. Available from mail-order catalogs and outdoor supply stores, acupressure wristbands put pressure on the inside of the wrist, which may prevent—or stop—nausea. In a Norwegian study of 97 women suffering from morning sickness, those who wore the bands recovered more quickly than those who didn't use them.

Take a stomach soother. Products that contain phosphorated carbohydrate solution (such as

Emetrol) will reduce stomach contractions and make the nausea more bearable.

Give ginger a try. A traditional remedy for motion sickness, ginger may also relieve nausea caused by morning sickness. The easiest way to use ginger is in supplement form: The recommended dose is two 500-milligram tablets three times daily. Or you can drink ginger tea, made by steeping 1 cup of boiling water over a teaspoon of freshly grated ginger for 10 minutes.

Eat peppermint candy. Or drink peppermint tea. It contains a chemical compound called menthol, which eases digestion and calms the stomach.

To make peppermint tea, crush 1 teaspoon of fresh peppermint leaves, cover with a cup of boiling water, and let it steep 10 minutes. You can drink the tea as often as necessary to get relief.

Learn to relax. Morning sickness and chemotherapy-associated nausea and vomiting may be calmed when you are calmed. Meditation, visual imagery, hypnosis, massage, and progressive relaxation techniques (systematically tensing and relaxing muscle groups) are options that may make you feel better emotionally and physically.

For Long-Term Prevention

Ask your doctor about vitamin B$_6$. If you experience severe nausea during pregnancy, your doctor may recommend taking vitamin B$_6$ supplements. There's some evidence that it's helpful, and dosages up to 50 milligrams daily have been shown to be safe during pregnancy.

Talk to you doctor about medications. If you've suffered from motion sickness in the past, you may want to ask your doctor for a prescription drug to help alleviate the symptom, says Scott A. Fields, M.D., vice chairman of family medicine at Oregon Health Sciences University in Portland. There are several to choose from that you can take before embarking on cruises or long drives.

overactive bladder

The bladder's job is simple. It stores urine, a mixture of water and wastes excreted by the kidneys, then squeezes it out of the body when it's full.

The bladder's signaling mechanisms are equally simple. When it starts filling up, pressure on its muscular walls triggers nerve signals, which tell you that it's time to use the bathroom.

In women with overactive bladders, however, there's often a problem with the nerves or with the bladder muscle itself. Rather than wait until it's full, the bladder sends out "gotta go" signals when even a tiny amount of urine trickles in. This creates an overwhelming need to urinate, even if you've just used the bathroom.

Many things can cause a hair-trigger bladder, including urinary tract infections and injuries—which may occur during vaginal childbirth—that affect the muscles or nerves, says Abraham N. Morse, M.D., assistant professor of urogynecology at the University of Massachusetts Medical School in Worcester.

Doctors estimate that fewer than 50 percent of women with bladder control problems get help from their doctors. This is unfortunate because nearly everyone can achieve good bladder control with a few simple strategies.

For Immediate Relief

home remedies

Cut back on caffeine. A study of 259 women with overactive bladders found that those who consumed the most caffeine had the highest risk of experiencing bladder instability, a condition doctors call urge incontinence.

"Caffeine is a major bladder irritant," explains Dr. Morse. "When people switch to decaf, they usually get a lot better."

Quit smoking. The nicotine in cigarettes affects more than the lungs. "The nerve receptors in the bladder that stimulate contractions are called nicotinic receptors," says Dr. Morse. "You can imagine what smoking does to them."

Avoid spicy foods. Eating high-octane salsa or other spicy foods can stimulate bladder contractions and cause uncomfortable sensations of urgency, says Gary Lemack, M.D., assistant professor of urology at the University of Texas Southwestern Medical Center in Dallas. Citrus fruits and juices may have a similar effect, he adds.

Pass up cranberry juice. "A lot of women drink cranberry juice because they've heard it prevents urinary tract infections," says Dr. Morse. "The problem with cranberry juice is that it can irritate the bladder and make it more sensitive."

Drink "flat" water. The carbon dioxide bubbles in fizzy water and soft drinks make the urine more acidic, which can trigger the urge to urinate, says Dr. Morse.

THREE THINGS I TELL EVERY FEMALE PATIENT

ABRAHAM N. MORSE, M.D., assistant professor of urogynecology at the University of Massachusetts Medical School in Worcester, gives the following advice for coping with an overactive bladder.

1 SEE A "BLADDER TRAINER." Ask your doctor to refer you to a physiotherapist who specializes in pelvic floor exercises. You'll also receive instruction in bladder drill training, to help your bladder hold urine longer.

2 DON'T LOOK FOR AGGRESSIVE TREATMENTS. Women with overactive bladders rarely require surgery. They often have success with simpler approaches, such as Kegel exercises and bladder training.

3 PUT YOUR MIND AT EASE. Poor bladder control is embarrassing and uncomfortable, but it doesn't have to be permanent. Nearly all women who work with their doctors will gain full or partial control, usually within weeks. ∎

Squeeze the urge away. The next time you feel as though you have to urinate immediately, tighten the same muscles that you'd use to stop urine in midflow, says Dr. Morse. If you do this several times in succession, the feelings of urgency will often go away.

Don't drink at bedtime. It's not uncommon for people with overactive bladders to wake up on damp sheets in the morning. "I advise people to stop drinking water or other beverages after 8:00 P.M.," says Dr. Lemack.

alternative therapies

Try acupuncture. There's some evidence that stimulating an acupuncture point above the ankle can override intense urges to urinate. The treatment makes sense in theory because there's a nerve above the ankle that has branches leading to the bladder, Dr. Morse explains.

mind-body techniques

Quiet your mind. The next time you experience a sudden urge to urinate, "breathe deeply, calm yourself down, and have confidence that you're not going to make a mess," says Dr. Morse. If you can calm yourself for about 30 to 60 seconds, there's a good chance that the urge will go away, he explains.

For Long-Term Relief

home remedies

Put your bladder on the clock. "The best treatment for urge incontinence is what we call bladder drill training," says Dr. Morse. Urge in-

when to see a doctor

In general, if the need to urinate interferes with your daily activities or your sleep, see a doctor.

If you're having large accidents rather than small leaks, see your doctor right away. Losing large amounts of urine may be a sign of nerve damage or other neurological problems, says Gary Lemack, M.D., assistant professor of urology at the University of Texas Southwestern Medical Center in Dallas.

If you see blood in the urine: You might have a urinary tract infection that is irritating the bladder. Tumors in the urinary tract can also cause bleeding along with urgency.

If you feel as though your bladder never completely empties: This means that the nerves or muscles that control the bladder probably aren't working the way they should. You're also more likely to develop urinary tract infections.

continence occurs when you are unable to hold back urinating when the urge to void is present. The rules are simple: Rather than rush to the bathroom when your bladder tells you to, you go only at certain times.

"You would start out by going to the bathroom every 20 minutes, whether you need to go or not," says Dr. Morse. "In between, you have to try to hold it, even if it means leaking a little. Most people can make it for 20 minutes, and it gets you thinking more about the time than about your discomfort."

Once women can comfortably hold their urine for 20 minutes, they begin increasing the time.

"People feel that if they don't go to the bathroom immediately, they're going to leak later. Breaking this behavior cycle is very important and very effective," says Dr. Morse.

Most women can get to the point where they're urinating, by the clock, about every 3 hours. "When you get to that point, you're done," says Dr. Morse.

Do Kegel exercises. They're a powerful strategy for calming an overactive bladder because they strengthen the pelvic floor muscles—the same muscles that give you urinary control, says Dr. Lemack.

Kegels are done by squeezing the muscles that you use to stop and start the flow of urine. Clench and relax the muscles about 10 times, and repeat this exercise several times daily. "Women who do these exercises daily almost always gain a significant amount of control," says Dr. Lemack.

mind-body techniques

Reduce the tension in your life. "We're not sure why, but in younger women especially, those who have very stressful lives often suffer from urgency," says Dr. Lemack.

Take a hint from your bladder: Unwind. Give yourself an hour each day to do something that's just for you, like taking a long walk, watching some television, or going to a movie or museum. "Doing whatever it takes to reduce stress is probably the best solution for many women," Dr. Lemack adds.

medical options

Calm the bladder with medication. The prescription drug oxybutynin chloride (Ditropan) relaxes the bladder muscle and also reduces irritation, says Dr. Morse. One of its side effects is that it sometimes causes a dry mouth, however. Talk to your doctor to see if this medication is right for you.

Give the bladder a jolt. Research has shown that it may be possible to stop those irregular bladder contractions by hitting them with precise amounts of electricity for 20 to 30 minutes. This technique is known as functional electrical stimulation.

A probe is inserted into the vagina, where it releases an electrical current that stimulates nerves that lead to the bladder. "It can dramatically reduce the way the bladder responds to signals," says Dr. Morse.

Ask your doctor about InterStim therapy. You've heard of pacemakers for the heart, but now doctors are investigating similar devices for controlling urinary urges. A surgically implanted InterStim system sends electrical signals to the nerves that regulate bladder function.

"The electrical pulses act as a distraction to a trigger-happy bladder," explains Rodney Anderson, M.D., professor of urology at Stanford University.

The patient is given a remote control to turn stimulation up or down as needed. In studies, Dr. Anderson and others found that it completely eliminated incontinence in almost half of the patients studied.

For more information on urge incontinence and an overactive bladder: Point your browser to the Web site of the Simon Foundation for Continence at www.simonfoundation.org.

overactive thyroid

You can think of hormones produced by the thyroid gland as the fuel that keeps you going. When the thyroid gland produces the proper amount of hormones, your vital functions hum along at the proper speed. If the gland is overactive, on the other hand, it's like stepping on the accelerator. Your heart rate goes up, you may be nervous or excitable, and your body will gobble calories in order to fuel your high-speed metabolism.

The most common cause of an overactive thyroid gland, called hyperthyroidism, is Graves' disease, an immune system disorder that disrupts the gland's ability to regulate its hormone output. Hyperthyroidism can also be triggered by a viral infection called viral thyroiditis.

"Viral thyroiditis clears up on its own, although we may give medications to temporarily reduce the heart rate and reduce the pain of the inflammatory process," says Shahla Nader, M.D., professor in the department of internal medicine at the University of Texas–Houston Medical School.

However, most people with hyperthyroidism will need medical treatment to get their hormones under control.

For Immediate Relief

home remedies

Have your doctor review your medications. Some prescription medications, including a heart

drug called amiodarone (Cordarone), contain large amounts of iodine. This can stimulate the thyroid gland to produce excessive amounts of hormone, says Dr. Nader.

Get plenty of calcium. People with high levels of thyroid hormone in the blood may lose bone calcium at an accelerated rate. Your doctor may advise you to eat plenty of leafy greens, fortified juices or cereals, low-fat dairy products, and other calcium-rich foods.

The loss of calcium doesn't occur quickly, however. It's mainly an issue for people whose hyperthyroidism has gone untreated for a long time, Dr. Nader explains.

alternative therapies

Take an herbal combination. In Europe, a common treatment for early-stage thyroid problems is to drink an herbal tea that combines bugleweed with lemon balm. Used in combination with medical treatment, the tea can help control the amount of hormone produced by thyroid cells.

To make a tea, combine 2 teaspoons of lemon balm with 1 teaspoon of bugleweed in a cup of hot water. Let the herbs steep for 10 minutes, and drink the tea several times a day.

medical options

"Burn out" the gland. When hyperthyroidism is caused by Graves' disease, your doctor will probably recommend treatment with radioactive iodine. Taken orally, the iodine is absorbed by the gland, where it releases radiation that destroys hormone-producing cells.

"Usually a single dose will correct the overactivity," says Dr. Nader.

The one problem with radioactive iodine is that it typically destroys so much of the gland that levels of thyroid hormone drop too low. Most people who undergo the treatment will take thyroid-replacing hormones for the rest of their lives, says Dr. Nader.

Consider surgery. Some people aren't able (or willing) to take radioactive iodine. Surgery to remove the gland is an effective alternative, says Dr. Nader.

Stop the symptoms. Because high levels of thyroid hormones can put excessive strain on the heart and circulatory system, your doctor may give you medications—usually beta-blockers, such as Inderal or Lopressor—to slow the heart rate and take the strain off the arteries until other treatments take effect.

For Long-Term Relief

home remedies

If you smoke, give it up. People with Graves' disease who smoke appear to have a higher risk of developing blindness or other eye problems related to this condition, says Dr. Nader.

medical options

Take antithyroid drugs as directed. They gradually reduce symptoms by curtailing the thyroid gland's output of hormones. "We advise pregnant women to use medications and absolutely avoid exposure to radioactive iodine," says Dr. Nader.

The drugs propylthiouracil (which is suitable for pregnancy) and methimazole (Tapazole) are generally taken for a year and then discontinued. In some cases, this eliminates the problem for good. In about 50 percent of cases, however, people will have relapses that will require additional treatment, Dr. Nader says.

when to see a doctor

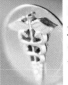

If your appetite has increased, but you're losing weight, see your doctor right away. This is one of the first signs of an overactive thyroid gland, says Shahla Nader, M.D., professor in the department of internal medicine at the University of Texas–Houston Medical School.

If your eyes are protruding, or if you feel as though there's sand in your eyes: These may be symptoms of Graves' disease.

If you're experiencing depression or mood swings and you've never had these problems before: It's not uncommon for people to be diagnosed with depression when they actually have an unrecognized thyroid problem, and it is worthwhile to check out the thyroid.

parkinson's disease

The symptoms of Parkinson's disease are so mild at first that many people don't bother calling their doctors. They may be a little shaky, or tired more often. Their handwriting may change, or they may be irritable or depressed for no apparent reason. If they have trouble getting out of a chair, they just assume that they're getting a little creaky with the passing years.

Even though Parkinson's disease often progresses at a snail's pace, there's no stopping it. Over time, nerve cells in a part of the brain called the substantia nigra become impaired or die. They're unable to produce a chemical called dopamine, which allows the brain to direct the body's complex movements. The result can be muscle stiffness or tremors that gradually get more and more severe.

No one's sure what causes the neurons to die off. Some people may have a genetic tendency to develop Parkinson's disease—but only if they're exposed to environmental "triggers." What these triggers might be, however, remains a mystery, says Richard B. Dewey Jr., M.D., associate professor of neurology and director of the Clinical Center for Movement Disorders at the University of Texas Southwestern Medical Center in Dallas.

There isn't a cure for Parkinson's disease, but there are a number of strategies for relieving symptoms and supplying the brain with the dopamine that it needs.

For Immediate Relief

home remedies

Exercise as much as you can. One study found that people with early to mid-stage Parkinson's disease who exercised twice a week had strength increases of 41 percent and improvements in coordination of 42 percent, according to lead researcher Iris Reuter, M.D., of the department of clinical neurosciences at King's College Hospital in London.

when to see a doctor

If you have persistent, involuntary trembling or quivering that seems to be getting worse, see a neurologist right away. This is known as a tremor, the classic symptom of early-stage Parkinson's disease, says Richard B. Dewey Jr., M.D., associate professor of neurology and director of the Clinical Center for Movement Disorders at the University of Texas Southwestern Medical Center in Dallas.

If you're having symptoms on one side of the body: Both Parkinson's disease and stroke tend to occur "unilaterally." If you're having symptoms on both sides of the body, you may have a different type of neurological problem.

If you're taking medications and notice an increase in symptoms: People with Parkinson's may need to have their dosages of medication adjusted as often as every 3 months.

Stay active, both socially and physically. "There's a tendency for people with Parkinson's to get very sedentary," says Dr. Dewey. "They need to stay active because it will help them maintain their normal lifestyles as long as possible."

Eat a high-fiber diet. It helps prevent constipation, a common symptom in those with Parkinson's disease.

"Physical activity is the most important thing for preventing constipation," Dr. Dewey adds. "If you sit on a couch all day, you'll never have normal bowel movements."

Get regular massages. Massage reduces muscle pain and stiffness, and it also helps people relax. "Anything that people with Parkinson's can do to relax is helpful because stress can aggravate the symptoms," Dr. Dewey explains.

medical options

Start treatment with a dopamine agonist. If you've recently been diagnosed with Parkinson's disease, your doctor will probably give you a prescription for dopamine agonists, medications that simulate the effects of dopamine in the brain.

People who take these drugs will often have a complete remission of symptoms for 1 to 3 years. As the drugs become less effective, your doctor will probably supplement your treatment with a medication called levodopa (or l-dopa).

"Most people will eventually wind up taking a combination of the two drugs," Dr. Dewey says.

For Long-Term Relief

home remedies

Eat protein late. Dietary protein blocks some of the effects of levodopa therapy. Your doctor may recommend that you follow a protein "redistribution" diet, in which most of the protein in your diet is consumed at night, when a temporary loss of mobility won't be as bothersome.

For more information on Parkinson's disease: Visit the Web site of the National Parkinson Foundation at www.parkinson.org.

phlebitis

Greece is renowned for its sunny climate, delicious yet healthy cuisine, and an ancient language that's unusually precise. Take the word "phlebitis": It's derived from the Greek word for vein (*phleb*), and the suffix for inflammation (*itis*). It's hard to get clearer than that.

Phlebitis usually occurs when a blood clot inside a vein causes painful inflammation, says John Blebea, M.D., associate professor of vascular surgery at the Pennsylvania State University College of Medicine and medical director of the Vascular Diagnostic Laboratory in Hershey. When the inflammation occurs in veins deep beneath the skin, it's called deep venous thrombosis; this condition is extremely serious and until recently required hospitalization. More often, the problem occurs in veins that are closer to the skin. Known as superficial phlebitis, it may cause pain, redness, or localized swelling. The area may be warm to the touch and feel painful when you're walking.

Women with varicose veins have a higher risk of developing superficial phlebitis because the blood in their legs flows more slowly and irregularly, making it more likely to form clots, says Dr. Blebea. Women are more likely than men to get phlebitis because they tend to be more likely to have varicose veins.

Anything that interferes with circulation can potentially cause phlebitis: hormone replacement therapy or the use of birth control pills can be risk factors; so can smoking, especially in combination with birth control pills, or a sedentary lifestyle. "Pregnancy also puts a woman at risk for phlebitis or deep venous thrombosis," Dr. Blebea adds. The levels of estrogen and progesterone then are higher than normal, which increases the risk of clotting. In addition, as the uterus gets larger and heavier, it puts pressure on veins in the abdomen, which decreases bloodflow to the legs.

Superficial phlebitis is more of an annoyance than a serious health problem, but the pain in the legs can be very uncomfortable, and in some cases take weeks to clear up. It also increases the risk that clots will occur in "deeper" veins in the future. To reduce inflammation and get blood moving again, here's what doctors advise.

For Immediate Relief

home remedies

Cool the area. When the veins first start to act up, applying an ice pack or a cool compress will temporarily reduce inflammation and relieve the pain, says Dr. Blebea. He recommends using compresses made with an aluminum acetate solution (Domeboro), available at pharmacies. "Such compresses to the affected area are often useful for the first several days," he says.

Take ibuprofen. "It will reduce the inflammation, which will improve the pain," says Dr. Blebea. For the first week that your legs are hurting, take 400 milligrams of ibuprofen three times daily, or every 4 to 6 hours, he advises.

Put your feet up. In order to reduce the swelling and lessen your discomfort, elevate your legs when you're not walking. This can be done

when to see a doctor

If you have an area on a leg that is red, swollen, or painful, see your doctor right away. Even if you don't have varicose veins, these symptoms could mean that you have phlebitis or deep venous thrombosis, says John Blebea, M.D., associate professor of vascular surgery at the Pennsylvania State University College of Medicine and medical director of the Vascular Diagnostic Laboratory in Hershey.

"You cannot distinguish between superficial phlebitis and a clot in the deep-vein system, which is potentially life threatening without the appropriate treatment," says Dr. Blebea.

If you do have a blood clot in a deep vein, your doctor will most likely give you a prescription for "blood-thinning" medications, which will keep the clot from getting bigger while your body works to dissolve it. Surgery or clot dissolution is usually required only when leg swelling is severe.

by simply putting a pillow under them while you relax on the couch or in bed, or using a step stool when sitting on a chair. A recliner-type chair is ideal for phlebitis patients, says Dr. Blebea.

Walk, run, dance, or swim. In fact, any type of exercise that flexes the calf muscles can help prevent the progression of phlebitis. When muscles in the legs contract, they put pressure on the veins that can literally push blood uphill, says Dr. Blebea. He warns, however, to hold off on most activity for about a week, or until the pain has diminished.

For Long-Term Relief

home remedies

Wear compression stockings. The best ones are available by prescription. They apply precise amounts of pressure to the legs, which can reduce swelling and pain. "If you're on your feet a lot, compression stockings can sometimes improve bloodflow and help to prevent recurrent phlebitis," Dr. Blebea adds. "If you already have it, you should be wearing them every day once the worst of the pain is over and you are able to put them on comfortably."

Wear flats instead of heels. The problem with high heels is that they restrict the movements of muscles in the legs. When you wear flats or shoes with low heels, every step you take pushes blood upward to the heart.

For more information about phlebitis: Point your browser to the Web site of the American Venous Forum at www.venous-info.com.

phobias and panic attacks

Fear can save your life. When you see a suspicious stranger on the street or when a large, angry dog is coming your way, fear makes your heart beat faster and prepares your mind and muscles for action.

But irrational fear can wreak havoc on your life. Millions of women (and men) suffer from panic attacks—overwhelming sensations of anxiety that come without warning and for no good reason. Others are terrified by things that shouldn't be all that scary, like riding in elevators or browsing in a shopping mall.

Doctors aren't sure what causes panic attacks. They're probably linked to disruptions in a part of the brain called the hippocampus. "These are people who may be more sensitive than they should be to perceptions of potential danger," says Jack G. Modell, M.D., professor of psychiatry at the University of Alabama in Birmingham.

If one or both of your parents suffered from phobias, you're more likely to have them, too. Women may experience phobias more than men and tend to generally feel more vulnerable.

Don't allow your fears to take control of your life. With a combination of therapy, medications, and a variety of coping strategies, almost everyone can get them under control.

For Immediate Relief

home remedies

Hold your breath for 10 seconds. "It allows carbon dioxide to build up in the body, which reduces hyperventilation and other symptoms of anxiety for some people," says Kelly Conforti, Ph.D., a clinical psychologist and manager of psychotherapy services at the Mental Health Center at the University of New Mexico Health Sciences Center in Albuquerque.

Get up and leave. People tend to experience panic attacks at certain times or in certain situations, such as when they're in a crowded place. "Just leaving the situation and going somewhere else can reduce levels of panic," says Dr. Modell.

In the long run, it's better to get the problem under control than to "run" when you start feeling anxious, Dr. Modell adds. "But to get relief from a particular attack, getting away is a reasonable thing to do."

mind-body techniques

Play a mind game. Nearly everyone gets anxious when they feel that people around them are judgmental or dominant. "Try imagining that the person is a turkey, or even the back end of a horse," Dr. Modell advises. "You'll be less nervous when you take the situation less seriously and see the person in a different light."

medical options

Sedate your fears. If you need to occasionally get your fears under control—because you're about to take a plane trip, for example—ask your doctor if a sedative would help, Dr. Modell suggests. Prescription sedatives won't eliminate fears,

THREE THINGS I TELL EVERY FEMALE PATIENT

KELLY CONFORTI, PH.D., a clinical psychologist at the University of New Mexico Health Sciences Center in Albuquerque, gives the following advice for stopping panic attacks.

1 **BREATHE SLOWLY AND DEEPLY.** "A lot of panic symptoms are triggered by hyperventilation," Dr. Conforti says. When you force yourself to breathe no more than eight to 12 times a minute, you'll reduce the amount of oxygen in your body, which will help stop you from hyperventilating.

2 **BREATHE INTO A PAPER BAG.** It increases blood levels of carbon dioxide, thereby reducing feelings of anxiety and panic.

3 **DRINK LESS COFFEE.** For some people, as little as 200 milligrams of caffeine—about the amount in two cups of coffee—can stimulate the feelings of panic attacks. ■

but they will temporarily reduce feelings of anxiety and help you cope with the moment. Sedatives that are commonly used for phobias and panic attacks include lorazepam (Ativan), diazepam (Valium), clonazepam (Klonopin), and alprazolam (Xanax). These medications may cause drowsiness and driving impairment, so use with care, cautions Dr. Modell.

Block panicky feelings. Many people avoid sedatives because they dislike feeling less alert than usual. An alternative is to take a prescription drug called a beta-blocker. "Beta-blockers don't do much from the neck up, but they block the body's response to fear," says Dr. Modell. They may cause dizziness, he adds.

For Long-Term Relief

home remedies

Get to know what scares you. People are most frightened by things that seem unfamiliar and alien. Dr. Modell advises women to learn everything they can about the things that frighten them most.

If you're afraid of flying, read up on how airplanes work and what pilots do to control them. If you're afraid of spiders or snakes, learn about their natural habits. "When you understand that snakes aren't going to run up and chase you, you'll realize that the fears may be excessive and unreasonable," Dr. Modell says.

medical options

Confront your fears. One of the best ways to overcome phobias is with a technique called "exposure and response prevention." You'll work with a therapist or psychologist, who will expose you, in a slow and controlled way, to the things that scare you most.

Suppose you're afraid of spiders. Your therapist might begin by talking about spiders. Then she'll show you pictures of spiders. Finally, she might ask you to be in the same room with a spider.

"You gradually increase the intensity of the ex-

when to see a doctor

If your heart is racing, you're perspiring, and you're having trouble breathing, seek urgent care immediately. The symptoms of panic attacks and heart attacks are very similar, says Jack G. Modell, M.D., professor of psychiatry at the University of Alabama in Birmingham.

If you've just started having panic attacks, and you've never had them before: A number of medical problems, including hypoglycemia (low blood sugar), can trigger symptoms that feel like panic. The side effects from medications, including decongestants, can also simulate the sensations of panic attacks.

If you're having panic attacks more than a few times a month or if you've avoiding normal activities because you're afraid of attacks: You'll want to see a mental health professional, who will help you find ways to prevent anxiety from interfering with your life.

posure while teaching coping skills," Dr. Conforti explains. About 80 percent of those who practice this technique will experience partial or even total relief from their fears.

Consider SSRI antidepressants. Even if you don't suffer from depression, this type of medication (selective serotonin reuptake inhibitor) can help reduce the frequency and intensity of panic attacks and phobias. The drugs are usually taken for about 6 months, at which point your doctor may wean you from the medication. In some cases, the panic attacks will stop for good, although many people will continue to take small doses of the medication to prevent recurrences.

For more information on phobias and panic attacks: Visit the Web site of the National Institute of Mental Health at www.nimh.nih.gov.

pneumonia

A generation ago, people were terrified of pneumonia, and for good reason. It was the leading cause of death in the United States until the mid-1930s, and even today, it's among the top 10 causes of mortality among women over 25.

Pneumonia refers to a number of infections and inflammatory conditions affecting the lungs. Most cases of pneumonia are caused by bacteria, but they also can be caused by pollutants, viruses, fungi, or tiny organisms called mycoplasmas. Pneumonia often occurs after a bout of the flu, when the lungs are already inflamed and weakened.

Pneumonia can cause shaking chills, a high fever, chest pain, difficulty breathing, and discolored mucus. It's essential to see a doctor because pneumonia can potentially cause permanent lung damage and may be fatal for some people, says Anne L. Davis, M.D., a pulmonologist and associate professor of medicine at New York University School of Medicine and an attending physician at Bellevue Hospital, both in New York City.

The only way to definitively diagnose pneumonia is to have a chest x-ray, along with laboratory tests to determine what type of pneumonia you have. You'll probably need medications to knock out the infection, says Dr. Davis. In the meantime, here are a few ways to reduce the discomfort right away.

For Immediate Relief

home remedies

Eat chicken soup. It's not just an old wives' tale. Chicken soup really does help ease respiratory infections, including pneumonia. It helps thin airway secretions, so you can breathe more easily.

Inhale steam. It moisturizes dry tissues in the airways and helps loosen mucus in the chest. The easiest way to steam your airways is to take a long, hot shower or bath. Or you can fill a pot with water and bring it to a boil. Carefully, remove the pot from the stove and place it on a protected table or counter. Drape a towel over your head to create a type of sauna, and breathe in the steam. Be sure to keep your face a safe distance from the scalding-hot water so you don't get burned.

To make the steam even more effective, add a few drops of eucalyptus oil to the pot. Eucalyptus has been used for centuries as a natural expectorant. Look for it at a health food store or pharmacy.

alternative therapies

Breathe easier with thyme. Herbalists recommend this flavorful kitchen herb for treating coughs caused by pneumonia and other respiratory infections. It thins mucus in the airways and makes coughs more "productive."

To make a tea with thyme, steep 2 teaspoons of dried herb in a cup of hot water for 10 minutes. You can drink the tea several times a day.

medical options

Call your doctor. When pneumonia is caused by bacteria, you're going to need antibiotics. They work very quickly and will usually start easing symptoms within a few days. You'll have to take them longer than that—usually for 10 days—to ensure that all the bacteria are destroyed.

For Long-Term Relief

home remedies

Eat a lot of fruits and vegetables. Some of the best are spinach and kale, which are rich in vitamins A and C, and tomatoes, broccoli, and strawberries, which provide even more vitamin C. These and other nutrients in these foods strengthen the immune system, which will help you heal more quickly.

While you're shopping for vegetables, be sure to stock up on carrots. Researchers at the USDA Human Nutrition Research Center on Aging at

THREE THINGS I TELL EVERY FEMALE PATIENT

STEVEN MOSTOW, M.D., professor of medicine and infectious diseases and associate dean at the University of Colorado Health Sciences Center in Denver, gives the following advice to patients who are suffering from pneumonia.

1 **BE PATIENT.** Pneumonia doesn't go away quickly, says Dr. Mostow. Many people won't feel fully recovered for weeks or even a month.

2 **TAKE IT EASY.** When you have pneumonia, your lungs can't absorb as much oxygen as they should. It's a good idea to avoid strenuous activity until you're completely better.

3 **WATCH OUT FOR RELAPSES.** It's not uncommon for pneumonia to get better for a while, then suddenly get worse. If you find that you're getting short of breath after you've been recovering, or if you have a recurrent fever, see your doctor right away. ■

Tufts University found that eating as little as $1\frac{1}{2}$ to 2 carrots daily significantly increased immune cell activity.

Avoid cigarette smoke and alcohol. Both of them tend to suppress the ability of the immune system to cope with the infection, says Steven Mostow, M.D., professor of medicine and infectious diseases and associate dean at the University of Colorado Health Sciences Center in Denver.

raynaud's phenomenon

t hardly takes courage to pull a tray of ice cubes from the freezer or pluck a newspaper from a snow-covered lawn—unless you have Raynaud's phenomenon, a mysterious condition in which changes in temperature cause the fingers or toes to turn cold and tingly, sometimes for hours at a time.

It's natural for blood vessels to temporarily constrict when you're exposed to cool temperatures. In those with Raynaud's, however, the vessels overreact and stay shut longer than they should. The prolonged lack of circulation causes the skin to turn white from a lack of blood, then blue as the tissues run out of oxygen, and then pink when circulation eventually resumes.

There are two forms of Raynaud's: the "primary" form, which means that there isn't an underlying disease that's causing the symptoms, and the "secondary" form, in which the symptoms are caused by other problems, such as scleroderma, a connective tissue disorder.

Most people with primary Raynaud's don't mind it all that much, says Filemon Tan, M.D., Ph.D., assistant professor of internal medicine and rheumatology at the University of Texas–Houston Medical School.

"It can be bothersome, but it's rarely serious," says Dr. Tan. "It doesn't take people long to learn how to prevent the attacks."

For Immediate Relief

home remedies

Thrust your hands under warm running water. It will stop an attack almost instantly. "By the time you get your hands under the tap, the attack may have just about run its course anyway," Dr. Tan adds.

Use a cup holder. Holding a cold can of soda or even a glass of ice water can trigger attacks in some people with Raynaud's. You may want to spend a few dollars for a plastic or foam cup holder, which will keep your fingers from getting chilled.

Buy a pair of lined mittens. They trap body heat better than gloves. Pull them on whenever you're going outside in cold weather—or, if necessary, when you're taking something out of the refrigerator or freezer, says Dr. Tan.

Bundle up. It's not enough just to protect your hands and feet. For people with Raynaud's, the blood vessels may shut down when any part of the body is exposed to cold, says Dr. Tan.

Dressing in layers is the best way to stay warm during the cold months. Wear a T-shirt under a shirt under a sweater under a jacket.

alternative therapies

Warm your feet with hot pepper. It doesn't work for everyone, but you may want to try an old folk remedy for Raynaud's: Mix a little red pepper with talc and cornstarch and sprinkle it in your socks. The "hot" chemical in peppers, called capsaicin, may help to stimulate bloodflow and help keep your feet warm. If your

when to see a doctor

 If emotional stress triggers Raynaud's attacks even when your hands or feet are warm, or there's swelling, joint redness, muscle weakness, tight or puffy skin over the hands, or unusual skin rashes: You may have secondary Raynaud's, a potentially more serious form of the disease, says Filemon Tan, M.D., Ph.D., assistant professor of internal medicine and rheumatology at the University of Texas–Houston Medical School. These symptoms may indicate an underlying tissue disease, Dr. Tan says.

If the attacks happen more than once a day or if the symptoms persist for more than a few minutes: The persistent lack of bloodflow could lead to serious tissue damage, including gangrene.

If the fingertips have turned black, ulcerations have developed on the tips, or you've lost all feeling: You may have suffered tissue damage, and you need to see a doctor immediately.

mouth or eyes come in contact with the pepper, burning and irritation may result. People sensitive to capsaicin may develop a rash, Dr. Tan cautions.

medical options

Get prescription relief. If you have frequent Raynaud's attacks or if the attacks are unusually painful, your doctor may prescribe a medication that will help keep the blood vessels open. These might include oral medications, such as calcium-channel blockers, or topical treatments, such as nitroglycerin cream.

"People who live in warm climates, such as here in Houston, may only have to take the medication in winter," Dr. Tan adds.

For Long-Term Relief

home remedies

If you smoke, try to quit. The nicotine in cigarettes causes blood vessels in the hands and feet to constrict, which may increase the frequency of attacks, says Dr. Tan.

mind-body techniques

Reduce the stress in your life. Exposure to cold may be more likely to trigger an attack if you're already tense and anxious. In rare cases, stress alone is enough to trigger an attack, says Dr. Tan.

There are dozens of effective ways for reducing stress, such as yoga, meditation, and feel-good activities such as going to movies or working in the yard.

repetitive strain syndrome

f you've ever slept with your arm in an uncomfortable position and awakened to feel tingling as blood returns to the hand, you've experienced one of the classic symptoms of repetitive strain syndrome.

Repetitive strain syndrome is an umbrella term for a group of conditions that includes carpal tunnel syndrome and tennis elbow. Carpal tunnel syndrome is the most serious form of repetitive strain, and it's very common in women.

The carpal tunnel is a narrow passage in the wrist, with the wrist bones on one end and the carpal ligament on the other. Within the tunnel are the flexor tendons and the median nerve. Problems begin when the outer layer of the flexor tendons, the synovium, swells and thickens.

"As it thickens, it takes up space in the carpal tunnel and starts to block the blood supply to the median nerve," explains Mary Lynn Newport, M.D., associate professor of orthopedic surgery at the University of Connecticut Health Center in Farmington. Without adequate bloodflow, nerve damage begins.

The first symptoms of carpal tunnel syndrome include tingling, numbness, burning, or pain in the hands. The symptoms tend to be worse in the morning. In some cases, the hands get so weak that women can't hold a cup of coffee.

Many things can cause carpal tunnel syndrome. Women who repeat the same motions over and over again—while typing, for example, or working on cash registers or assembly lines—have a high risk of developing carpal tunnel syndrome. In fact, women are seven times more likely than men to get it, partly because of hormonal fluctuations that lead to fluid retention. "When tissues in the hands retain fluid, the synovium swells, which pinches the median nerve," Dr. Newport explains.

when to see a doctor

If you have persistent numbness or tingling in the hands, or if pain doesn't go away: Contact your doctor right away. There's a good chance you have carpal tunnel syndrome, and quick treatment will help ensure that it doesn't get worse, says Mary Lynn Newport, M.D., associate professor of orthopedic surgery at the University of Connecticut Health Center in Farmington.

If the pain gets progressively worse or if it interferes with your normal activities: Your doctor may recommend injecting steroids into the injured area to reduce inflammation. Steroid injections sometimes cure the problem, but more often they're used to provide short-term relief (up to 3 months, in some cases).

If steroids or other medications don't bring relief: You may need surgery to cut and release the band of ligaments at the bottom of the carpal tunnel. This provides more space for the nerve and tendons to move freely, without compression of the nerve.

Carpal tunnel syndrome can often be reversed as long as it's treated before permanent nerve damage occurs. Here are some of your options.

For Immediate Relief

home remedies

Ice it right away. As soon as you start having wrist pain, put a cold pack—or ice cubes wrapped in a towel—on the back of the wrist. Applying cold for 10 to 15 minutes at a time, several times a day, will constrict blood vessels and reduce inflammation in the wrist, says M. Patricia Howson, M.D., assistant chief in the department of orthopedics at Kaiser Permanente in Redwood City, California.

Take over-the-counter pain relievers. Aspirin, ibuprofen, and other analgesics reduce the body's production of prostaglandins, chemicals that increase pain and inflammation.

Use wrist splints. Available in drugstores, splints keep the wrists flat and straight, which reduces strain and helps the injury heal more quickly. "Wear the splint as often as possible," says Dr. Howson. "It's especially important to wear it at night because many people sleep with their hands curled up."

Long-Term Solutions

home remedies

Stretch your hands. Stretching increases blood-flow and flushes out accumulated fluids. "Use one hand to stretch and pull the fingers back on your other hand," Dr. Newport suggests.

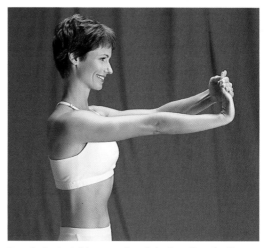

Regularly stretching your hands by bending the fingers backward is one of the best ways to prevent carpal tunnel syndrome and to help it heal more quickly.

Avoid prolonged wrist motions. "If you're sitting in front of a computer all day, get up every hour and make a few phone calls or do some filing," says Dr. Newport. "The key is to use different muscles in your hands and fingers."

Make your workstation wrist-friendly. If you spend a lot of time at a desk or workstation, take a few minutes to arrange things in a strain-reducing manner. For example:

- Adjust the computer monitor so that it's at eye level. If it's too low or too high, you'll hold your body in unnatural positions that can increase strain on the wrists, says Dr. Newport.

- Relax your shoulders, keep your feet comfortably flat on the floor, and sit in a chair that helps to hold your back straight.

- Hold your wrists straight when you type; your elbows should be bent at a 90-degree angle.

Cut back on dietary salt. The average American consumes more than 3,000 milligrams of salt daily, a lot more than the upper limit of 2,400 milligrams that doctors recommend. High intakes of dietary salt can lead to fluid retention, which increases pressure on the median nerve responsible for carpal tunnel pain, says Dr. Howson.

Some of the saltiest foods include cheeses, chips, fast food, and packaged and convenience foods. It's worth reading food labels and stocking up on low-sodium foods whenever possible, says Dr. Howson.

Keep your wrists in neutral. When you're doing things that seem to be causing pain, take a look at your hands. There's a good chance that they're tensed, with the wrists bent, says Dr. Howson. "Try to keep the wrists straight whenever possible," she advises. "You want to avoid keeping them in a bent, flexed, or twisted position for long periods of time."

Use your entire hand for gripping. When you hold items with just your thumb and fingers, you're working muscles that share the same nerve supply as the carpal tunnel, which further fatigues the area. "Use your whole hand, including the palm and fingers, when gripping an object," says Dr. Howson.

Get your body moving. "We don't exactly know why, but studies have shown that regular aerobic exercise may prevent carpal tunnel syndrome, in addition to slowing its progress," says Dr. Newport.

alternative therapies

Take vitamin B$_6$. "We don't have scientific studies to prove it, but vitamin B$_6$ does seem to help some people," says Dr. Newport. If you're having wrist pain, try taking 50 milligrams of vitamin B$_6$ twice daily for 6 weeks to see if it helps, she advises.

For more information about repetitive strain syndrome: Visit the Web site of the American Academy of Orthopedic Surgeons at www.aaos.org.

respiratory allergy

I f women with respiratory allergies spent their lives in a bubble—if their kids never brought home stray pets and dust disappeared with a dirty look—then sneezes and watery eyes would be as rare as winning the lottery.

But we live in the real world. Indoors and out, allergy-causing substances are everywhere. Dogs and cats are covered with dander. There are dust mites, molds, and pollen-filled winds, any one of which can put your respiratory system on red alert.

"Most people believe that outdoor allergens cause the biggest problems, but indoor allergens actually have the greatest impact because people spend most of their time inside," says Bill Berger, M.D., clinical professor in the division of allergy and immunology at the University of California, Irvine; vice president of the American College of

Allergy, Asthma, and Immunology; and author of *Allergies and Asthma for Dummies*. In fact, indoor air can sometimes cause greater symptoms than the air outside, he adds.

Some women suffer from respiratory allergies only during hay fever season, but for many others, the misery persists all year. Doctors call this perennial allergic rhinitis, and it's easy to diagnose because women with allergies often have "allergic shiners"—dark circles under the eyes that are caused by increased bloodflow near the sinuses.

You can't cure respiratory allergies, but there are many ways to ease the symptoms—or even stop them entirely.

For Immediate Relief

home remedies

Take advantage of antihistamines. They block the effects of histamine, the body chemical that causes sneezing, wheezing, and other respiratory symptoms. Over-the-counter products that contain antihistamines—such as diphenhydramine (like Benadryl) and chlorpheniramine (like Chlor-Trimeton or Dristan Cold Multi-Symptom Formula)—can be very effective, although they may cause drowsiness or a dry mouth in many of the people who use them.

To get the benefits of antihistamines with few or no side effects, your doctor may advise you to use a prescription nonsedating product, such as loratadine (Claritin) or fexofenadine (Allegra).

Use decongestants as necessary. Pharmacy shelves are packed with over-the-counter decongestant sprays, which relieve nasal congestion by shrinking blood vessels in the nose and reducing swelling. These medications are very effective for short-term relief—but don't use more than the recommended dosage, and certainly not on a regular basis, and never for more than 3 to 5 days in a row. People who overuse nasal decongestants often experience a "rebound effect," in which the stuffiness comes back with a vengeance as soon the medications are discontinued.

Get dust mites out of your life. These tiny creatures live in house dust, and they thrive in sheets, pillowcases, mattresses, drapes, and carpets. In fact, many people with allergies also test positive for sensitivity to dust mites. To get rid of mites:

- Dust thoroughly at least once a week. Wipe every surface with a damp cloth, including the tops of door and window frames. Be especially vigilant about cleaning the bedroom because you spend more time there than in any other room.

- Cover heating and air conditioning vents with filters, available at home supply stores. Look for HEPA filters, which will trap mites and other allergy-causing particles.

- Vacuum the house once a week, preferably with a vacuum cleaner equipped with a HEPA filter. Hardwood, tile, and linoleum floors are easier to keep dust-free than is carpeting.

- Wear a dust mask whenever you're cleaning or raising dust in the house.

■ Wash your bedding weekly in hot water. Dust mites can't survive high temperatures. As long as the hot water in your house is 130°F or hotter, it will kill mites as well as their eggs.

Keep pollen out. To keep allergy-causing pollens out of the house, you may want to keep the windows closed in the spring and summer, and use the air conditioner instead.

Stay inside during peak hours. During the allergy season, airborne pollen counts are highest in the early morning and in the evening. You may want to schedule your days so that you're inside during those times.

medical options

Talk to your doctor about nasal sprays. If you can't seem to control your allergies with home care, you may want to consider using a steroid nasal spray that contains beclomethasone (such as Vancenase). Within the first 24 hours, steroid nasal sprays reduce inflammation and irritation in the lining of the nose, which can reduce nasal congestion and drippiness and make it easier to breathe.

Another nasal spray commonly used is cromolyn sodium (Nasalcrom). Nasalcrom is available without a prescription and is used to prevent or treat the symptoms of seasonal and chronic allergic rhinitis. Your doctor may decide to prescribe a nasal antihistamine spray called azelastine (Astelin), which is used to treat the symptoms of allergic rhinitis.

Consider immunotherapy. If your allergies are severe and you can't seem to get relief, your

"False" Allergies

You can be pretty sure you have respiratory allergies if your nose starts running every spring or if your symptoms tend to get worse during the semiannual housecleaning. But what if your symptoms flare up even when you haven't been around pets, pollen, or dust?

You could have a condition called nonallergic vasomotor rhinitis, which basically means that your nose is overly sensitive, even in the absence of allergies.

"Just as some women blush more easily than others, some get stuffy or congested when they're exposed to things such as spicy foods or cold air," says Bill Berger, M.D., clinical professor in the division of allergy and immunology at the University of California, Irvine; vice president of the American College of Allergy, Asthma, and Immunology; and author of *Allergies and Asthma for Dummies*.

Many things can trigger nonallergic vasomotor rhinitis. Possible culprits include changes in temperature or weather, tobacco smoke, paint fumes, and even the smell of newspapers.

Oral antihistamines and other oral allergy medications may not help if you have nonallergic vasomotor rhinitis, says Dr. Berger. Your doctor will probably advise you to use azelastine (Astelin), a nasal antihistamine spray that has been approved by the FDA for the treatment of this condition. ■

doctor may recommend a procedure called immunotherapy, or allergic desensitization. You'll work with an allergist, who will give you a series of injections that contain tiny amounts of the allergens that bother you. Over time, your body will become less and less sensitive. Immunotherapy therapy won't necessarily eliminate allergies, but it can make your symptoms much more tolerable.

when to see a doctor

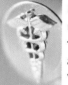

If you can't control sneezing, a runny nose, or other allergy symptoms with home care, make an appointment to see an allergist. You may need skin tests to determine what, exactly, you're allergic to, says Bill Berger, M.D., clinical professor in the division of allergy and immunology at the University of California, Irvine; vice president of the American College of Allergy, Asthma, and Immunology; and author of *Allergies and Asthma for Dummies*. Once you've identified the problem, it will be easier to find ways to avoid it, he explains.

If your symptoms include persistent headaches, fever, or fatigue: What appear to be allergy symptoms may be caused by an underlying ear or sinus infection.

If you've had allergies for years, and they seem to be getting worse: Long-term allergies can increase the risk for nasal polyps, growths in the nasal passages that can interfere with breathing. Your doctor will examine the inside of your nose to make sure that the breathing passages are clear.

For Long-Term Relief

home remedies

Keep a little distance from dogs and cats. Millions of Americans are allergic to proteins found in the saliva, urine, and skin cells of dogs and cats. All pets produce these proteins. There's no such thing as a "hypoallergenic" pet—although cats with dark coats do appear to cause more symptoms than those with white or light-colored coats.

If your dog or cat sleeps in the bedroom with you, chances are you're inhaling tremendous amounts of allergens every night, says Frank Virant, M.D., an allergist and clinical professor of pediatrics at the University of Washington in Seattle. At the very least, you should put your pet's bed in another part of the house.

You'll do even better if your dog or cat spends more time outside, adds Linda B. Ford, M.D., an allergist in Omaha, Nebraska, and past president of the American Lung Association.

If possible, wash your pets every 1 to 2 weeks. A plain-water wash may reduce the number of allergic-causing particles from the coats of dogs and cats, says Clifford W. Bassett, M.D., assistant clinical professor of medicine at the State University of New York Health Science Center in Brooklyn and an attending physician and faculty member of New York University School of Medicine.

Keep your furnishings simple. Overstuffed chairs and couches are wonderful to sit on, but over time they trap—and hang on to—large amounts of dust mites, animal dander, and other allergy-causing particles. The same is true of heavy drapes, feather pillows, and textile wall hangings. In fact, animal dander sticks to your clothing, your hair, and the walls of your house.

You'll do better if you furnish your home with products made from wood, leather, plastic, or vinyl, says Laurie Blevins Fowler, M.D., allergy clinic director and assistant professor of surgery and child health at the University of Missouri HealthCare in Columbia. Be aware that some women with chemical sensitivities may have reactions to plastic or vinyl products as well.

For more information about respiratory allergies: Visit the Web site of the American Academy of Allergy, Asthma, and Immunology at www.aaaai.org.

restless legs syndrome

The word "restless" doesn't begin to describe the sensations that people with restless legs syndrome may experience nearly every night.

Try "creeping." "Crawling." "Burning and aching." Once the feelings strike, the only way to get relief is to move your legs—which means that instead of sleeping, you may spend part of your nights stretching, pacing, or marching in place.

Doctors aren't sure what causes restless legs syndrome. They suspect that it's linked to an imbalance of chemicals in the brain or spinal cord, or possibly to problems with peripheral nerves in the legs or feet, says Nancy Foldvary, D.O., a neurologist and director of the Sleep Disorders Center at the Cleveland Clinic Foundation in Cleveland.

Restless legs syndrome is more common in women, and it tends to worsen over time. It's unlikely to cause serious physical problems, but people often complain of insomnia or daytime sleepiness because they don't get all the sleep that they need, Dr. Foldvary says.

To give your legs the "rest" they need, here's what doctors advise.

For Immediate Relief

home remedies

Massage your legs. It's probably the quickest way to relieve the sensations, especially if you use vigorous pressure to knead and rub the muscles.

"Stimulation of the legs seems to be effective in some people," says Dr. Foldvary.

Stretch your muscles. Any kind of leg movement will help reduce the uncomfortable sensations, says Dr. Foldvary. One helpful exercise is to briefly stand with your back against a wall and your knees bent, as though sitting in a chair. This stretches and tires the muscles, which will often temporarily relieve the feelings.

"It's very helpful for people just to stretch their ankles by extending their feet while they're lying in bed," Dr. Foldvary adds. "It's also helpful for some people to get out of bed and move. The movement somehow inhibits the uncomfortable sensations."

Avoid caffeine and alcohol. It's not clear why, but people who quit drinking alcoholic or caffeinated beverages sometimes have a significant reduction in restless legs symptoms.

Keep your mind busy. The next time your legs get restless, try giving your full attention to mental activities, such as doing crosswords or playing a video game. It may reduce or eliminate the discomfort.

For Long-Term Relief

Get more iron in your diet. Studies have shown that people with low blood levels of iron may be more likely to develop restless legs syndrome— and the lower their iron levels, the worse the symptoms get.

"There are people whose symptoms go away

when to see a doctor

If you're extremely tired during the day even though you felt as though you slept well the night before, or if you have insomnia, call your doctor. People with restless legs syndrome often experience jerky leg movements while they sleep, which can prevent them from entering the deeper sleep stages, says Nancy Foldvary, D.O., a neurologist and director of the Sleep Disorders Center at the Cleveland Clinic Foundation in Cleveland.

If your leg discomfort is accompanied by persistent fatigue, or if you're also having heavy menstrual bleeding: You could be suffering from iron deficiency anemia, which may cause or contribute to the discomfort.

after they start taking iron supplements," says Dr. Foldvary.

People with low levels of iron may be advised to take 45 milligrams of iron daily until their blood levels of this important mineral return to normal. After that, you'll want to make sure to get the Daily Value of 18 milligrams of iron—by taking a multivitamin and also by eating lean meats, fortified cereals, or other iron-rich foods.

Take a B-complex supplement. People who don't get enough folate, vitamin B_{12}, or other B vitamins may experience nerve problems (neuropathies), which have been linked to restless legs syndrome, says Dr. Foldvary. Follow the directions on the label.

Ask your doctor about medications. As recently as 10 years ago, sedatives were the main drugs used to treat restless legs syndrome. The medications helped, but people who took them often felt tired and "hungover" in the morning. Today there are many more choices available, says Dr. Foldvary.

Your doctor may prescribe a medication called levodopa. Used to treat Parkinson's disease, it also can relieve restless legs syndrome by increasing brain levels of a chemical called dopamine. Other helpful prescription medicines include pergolide (Permax), ropinirole (Requip), pramipexole (Mirapex), and gabapentin (Neurontin).

For more information on restless legs syndrome: Visit the Web site of the Restless Legs Syndrome Foundation at www.rls.org.

rheumatoid arthritis

A majority of women will develop some form of arthritis by the time they reach their 60th birthdays. Most will experience "wear-and-tear arthritis," or osteoarthritis, a condition that causes pain and stiffness as cartilage that cushions one or more joints breaks down over time. Less common, and potentially much more serious, is rheumatoid arthritis, which occurs when the body's immune system "mistakenly" attacks tissues in the joints and other parts of the body.

Rheumatoid arthritis has been called a whole-body illness. In addition to causing joint pain, it may result in fatigue, fever, weight loss, and even anemia.

It's not clear what causes rheumatoid arthritis, but there's definitely a genetic factor: In other words, it's an inherited disease, and women are $2\frac{1}{2}$ times more likely than men to get it. Unlike wear-and-tear arthritis, which affects primarily middle-aged and older adults, rheumatoid arthritis often strikes in the twenties and thirties.

Like osteoarthritis, rheumatoid arthritis affects multiple joints in the body. The symptoms may be limited to pain and stiffness, although in many cases the joints will also be swollen and warm to the touch, says Michael Lockshin, M.D., director of the Barbara Volcker Rheumatology Center at the Hospital for Special Surgery in New York City. Rheumatoid arthritis can worsen very quickly. In some cases, in fact, it can permanently damage joints in as little as 1 year. Quick treatment is important, both to halt the progression of the disease and to ease the painful symptoms.

For Immediate Relief

home remedies

Use over-the-counter painkillers. A class of medications called nonsteroidal anti-inflammatory drugs, which includes aspirin and ibuprofen, is considered the first-line treatment for arthritis-related pain and stiffness, says Dr. Lockshin.

Warm the joints. Applying heat to the sore joints can be very soothing, especially in the morning, when joints are stiffest. The easiest way to heat the joints is to lounge in a hot bath or shower. Or, using warm water (not above 90°F), you can moisten a towel or fill up a hot-water bottle and hold it to the affected area. When the towel or hot-water bottle cools, wet or fill it up again and repeat the treatment.

Ease pain with wax. If you're having trouble with joints in the hands or feet, you may want to try a "paraffin bath," in which the joints are coated with a warm, waxy coating. The wax delivers long-lasting heat to relieve stiffness and pain. Mail-order catalogs and some pharmacies sell Crock-Pot–like devices that heat paraffin to the appropriate temperature.

Exercise as much as you can. Regular exercise improves circulation to the joints, increases strength, and raises levels of brain chemicals that reduce pain. It's among the best treatments for rheumatoid arthritis, says Dr. Lockshin.

"You don't want to do aggressive exercise right away," he adds. "In the beginning, a woman could do gentle, range-of-motion exercises, such as stretching. If she has neck pain, she could slowly roll her head around in a circle 10 times twice a day. If she has wrist pain, she could simply open and close her hands slowly 10 times twice a day. As she becomes more limber, she could move to more aerobic exercises."

Consider modest weight lifting. When combined with range-of-motion and aerobic exercises, weight lifting can reduce pain and possibly help prevent long-term damage. However, be sure to talk to your doctor before lifting weights. He or she may advise you to work with a physical therapist, who will design a workout to strengthen the areas where you need the most help.

when to see a doctor

If you're experiencing pain or swelling in three or more joints and the symptoms persist for more than a week, see a rheumatologist. There's a good chance you have rheumatoid arthritis, and quick treatment is essential to slow the progression of the disease, says Michael Lockshin, M.D., director of the Barbara Volcker Rheumatology Center at the Hospital for Special Surgery in New York City.

If joint pain is accompanied by fever, fatigue, or other whole-body symptoms: You may need prescription medications to help reduce the body's overactive immune response.

Take ashwagandha. An herb, it contains chemical compounds that reduce inflammation. The recommended dose is 3 to 6 grams of dried ashwagandha root daily in a decoction (boiled down), or 6 to 12 milliliters of liquid extract per day.

Or try guggul. A resin extracted from an Indian desert-dwelling tree, guggul supplements have been shown to have powerful anti-arthritic and anti-inflammatory effects. The recommended dose is 500 milligrams of standardized guggul extract (standardized to guggul lipids), taken internally twice daily.

Drink 3 to 4 cups of green tea every day. It's rich in polyphenols, chemical compounds that appear to prevent inflammatory cells from getting into joints to do damage. Green tea also is rich in the antioxidant vitamins C and E, nutrients that "neutralize" joint-damaging molecules in the body called free radicals.

The polyphenols in green tea may help prevent the condition from getting started. In a study at Case Western Reserve University in Cleveland, laboratory mice were given the amount of polyphenols found in 3 to 4 cups of green tea. Fewer than half of the animals developed rheumatoid arthritis, compared with 92 percent of those given only plain water.

See a rheumatologist at the first sign of symptoms. A recent study from UCLA concluded that seeing a specialist is the gold standard strategy for treating rheumatoid arthritis. Among patients whose care did not include a rheumatologist, only 50 percent received the level of care recommended by the American College of Rheumatology, such as annual doctor visits, blood tests, and drug monitoring.

Use the heavy hitters. Many people with rheumatoid arthritis can control their symptoms for years or even decades with over-the-counter analgesics. As the disease progresses, however, prescription medications are often essential—either to "calm" the immune system or to relieve painful (and joint-damaging) inflammation, says Dr. Lockshin. Some of the drugs that are commonly used include prednisone, methotrexate (Rheumatrex), hydroxychloroquine (Plaquenil), cyclosporine (Sandimmune or Neoral), and gold salts (Solganal).

Women with rheumatoid arthritis are often hesitant to commit themselves to long-term treatment with prescription drugs, but it's worth doing. In a Canadian study of 119 people with rheumatoid arthritis, half were given prescription medication; the others took a sugar pill. After 9 months, all the participants were free to use any treatment that they required. The researchers found that those in the early-treatment group had significantly less pain and improved joint mobility at follow-up evaluations 3½ years later.

For Long-Term Relief

home remedies

Eat more fish. Or talk to your doctor about taking fish oil supplements. Studies have shown

---

THREE THINGS I TELL EVERY FEMALE PATIENT

MICHAEL LOCKSHIN, M.D., director of the Barbara Volcker Rheumatology Center at the Hospital for Special Surgery in New York, offers this advice for women with rheumatoid arthritis.

BE PERSISTENT. Because rheumatoid arthritis can cause so many different symptoms, it may take months before it's identified with certainty. "If you're in pain and your regular doctor isn't helping, see a rheumatologist, who will examine you for rheumatoid arthritis," says Dr. Lockshin.

REPORT ALL CHANGES IN SYMPTOMS. It's normal for women with rheumatoid arthritis

to have periods of relatively little pain, followed by flare-ups. It's important to report all changes to your doctor—such as having persistent fever when in the past you've only had joint pain. Changes in symptoms may mean that you need different medications or treatments to get the problems under control.

BE PREPARED FOR UPS AND DOWNS. "There will be good times and bad times," says Dr. Lockshin. "We can usually minimize the bad times by using the proper medications." ■

that the omega-3 fatty acids in fish oil can help relieve joint swelling and morning stiffness. Your doctor may advise you to take eight to 10 capsules of fish oil daily—about the amount that you'd get in a 6-ounce serving of salmon or other fatty fish.

Fish oils don't work overnight, however. Research has shown that they have to be used daily for about 12 weeks to get results.

Stretch out with yoga. It's among the best ways to improve your range of motion by restoring flexibility and improving circulation to the joints. Improved circulation is important because it brings more oxygen and nutrients to the damaged joints.

Yoga has other benefits as well. It relaxes muscles and stimulates the release of endorphins, painkilling chemicals produced by the body. Mentally, yoga has a calming, relaxing effect.

Most health clubs offer yoga classes, from beginning to advanced. If you're just starting out, check with your doctor before signing up for yoga. You'll be advised to start out slowly in order to build strength and flexibility. Eventually, you'll want to work up to 40 to 60 minutes of yoga daily. That may sound like a lot, but rheumatoid arthritis is a serious condition, and the time you spend doing yoga will be time well spent.

For more information about rheumatoid arthritis:
Visit the Web site of the American College of Rheumatology at www.rheumatology.org. Or go to the Web site of the Arthritis Foundation at www.arthritis.org.

sciatica

Nearly all women get back pain on occasion, and usually it clears up on its own. A related condition—and one that's potentially more serious—is sciatica, an irritation of the lumbar nerves in the lower back.

"The most common symptoms of sciatica are numbness, tingling, and weakness or pain in the leg or foot," says Stephen Hochschuler, M.D., clinical instructor at the University of Texas Health Science Center in Dallas, founder and chairman of the Texas Back Institute in Plano, and author of *Treat Your Back without Surgery*.

Sciatica is associated with pressure or inflammation of nerves—which in turn is often associated with a bulging or herniated disk.

Surgery is sometimes required to relieve pressure on the nerves, but often you can ease the painful inflammation with a combination of medications and simple home remedies.

For Immediate Relief

home remedies

Ice the injury. As soon as sciatica pain begins, apply ice wrapped in a towel to the lower back for 15 minutes several times a day. Continue applying ice for 48 hours. It numbs the area and constricts blood vessels, reducing swelling and inflammation, says Dr. Hochschuler.

Follow cold with heat. "After 48 hours, apply heat to the area," Dr. Hochschuler advises. It increases circulation and removes pain-causing toxins from the tissues. Put a heating pad or hot-water bottle wrapped in a towel on your lower back for 15 minutes at a time, and repeat the treatment throughout the day, he advises. Be careful not to burn the skin.

Drink eight to 10 glasses of water daily. It's another way to help remove the inflammatory (and painful) toxins from the body, says Dr. Hochschuler.

Exercise in water. Swimming or simply wading in a heated pool is probably the best exercise for sciatica. "The warmth of the water prevents the muscles from going into spasm and putting more pressure on the nerves," says Dr. Hochschuler. Stop if pain increases, however.

Take one to two regular-strength aspirins or ibuprofen four times daily. The drugs relieve inflammation as well as pain, says Dr. Hochschuler.

medical options

Take oral steroids, if prescribed. Available by prescription, steroids are considered the gold standard for reducing inflammation. They have side effects, however, so they're used only when home treatments aren't effective.

Ask your doctor about "injection therapy." When sciatica doesn't get better on its own, your doctor may recommend injections that combine an anesthetic with a powerful anti-inflammatory drug. Injected around the injured nerve, the medications reduce pain and swelling and may eliminate the need for surgery.

Long-Term Solutions

home remedies

Get physical therapy. It's among the best ways to prevent future episodes of sciatica because it

---

WHAT WORKS FOR ME

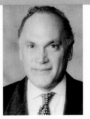

STEPHEN HOCHSCHULER, M.D., *is a clinical instructor at the University of Texas Health Science Center in Dallas, founder and chairman of the Texas Back Institute in Plano, and author of* Treat Your Back without Surgery—*and he's suffered from sciatica for 16 years. Here's how he keeps it under control.*

I take ibuprofen whenever I feel the leg pain. I avoid any lifting during that time, and I try to avoid any stresses or strains on my back.

When I do have to lift something, I always bend at the knees, no matter what the object is. I also wear a back support because I have to stand and operate for up to 7 hours at a time. I also keep my weight down, drink lots of water, and exercise. I vary my exercise routine by riding a bike, hiking, and skiing. ∎

when to see a doctor

If the numbness, tingling, or leg pain lasts more than 2 weeks, see your doctor. Long-term sciatica may not get better without medical treatment, says Stephen Hochschuler, M.D., clinical instructor at the University of Texas Health Science Center in Dallas, founder and chairman of the Texas Back Institute in Plano, and author of *Treat Your Back without Surgery*.

If the pain is accompanied by a loss of bladder or bowel control: This means the nerve injury is potentially serious, and you may require surgery to prevent it from getting worse. It is an emergency and needs treatment immediately.

strengthens the back and makes it less prone to injuries.

Rest before you lift. "If you've been on a long car ride, don't get out of the car right away and unload your luggage," says Dr. Hochschuler. "You don't want to add stress by lifting heavy objects. Get out of the car, stretch, and relax a bit. Then unload your luggage."

Lift with your legs. "Many women bend at the waist to lift heavy objects, which stresses the lower back," says Dr. Hochschuler. "Get close to the object and bend your knees—don't stoop over." Lift using your legs and knees, not your back.

shingles

Chickenpox is a common disease of childhood. Once the itchy red spots disappear, most of us just assume that the infection is gone for good, and rarely give it a second thought.

Unfortunately, the virus that causes chickenpox, a member of the herpes family, often returns for an encore long after the infection is gone. The virus leaves the skin and disappears deep into the nerves. Years or decades later, the virus may reactivate and rise to the surface, causing a painful rash with blisters known as shingles.

During its first stage, shingles causes a deep, burning pain somewhere in the skin. You may also have a fever or headache. As the infection

progresses, you develop red skin lesions, which quickly blister. The rash and blisters most commonly appear on the trunk of your body, but they may also occur around one eye, on the face or scalp, inside the mouth, or down an arm or leg. The blisters develop over several days and last 7 to 10 days before crusting. They may be very painful. You may also experience intense pain even if there isn't any rash.

"One of my patients told me that the pain was so bad that she wanted to jump off the roof," says John W. Edelglass, M.D., associate clinical professor of dermatology at Yale University School of Medicine.

The one good thing about shingles is that this

second bout of the chickenpox virus will probably be your last. However, women whose immune systems are weaker than they should be—because of underlying medical problems, for example—can get shingles again. And the big problem with shingles is that the pain often persists long after the sores have healed. This nerve pain, called postherpetic neuralgia, can drag on for months or even years.

Once you're infected with the virus, there's no way to get rid of it since it lives in the nerves forever. You can, however, reduce the pain of outbreaks with simple home care. There are also a number of medications that can dramatically reduce the pain and shorten the duration of the illness, says Dr. Edelglass.

For Immediate Relief

home remedies

Relieve pain with a compress. The quickest way to soothe rashes or sores caused by shingles is to apply a compress made with Burow's solution (like Domeboro). The solution reduces pain and also dries the sores, which helps them heal more quickly, says Dr. Edelglass. Prepare the compress by first mixing Domeboro powder or tablets with water according to the package directions. Dr. Edelglass recommends using a clean cloth, such as a piece of old linen, saturating it in the solution, and gently squeezing out the excess. Apply the compress to the affected area repeatedly over 10 minutes, resaturating the cloth if nec-

THREE THINGS I TELL EVERY FEMALE PATIENT

JOHN W. EDELGLASS, M.D., associate clinical professor of dermatology at Yale University School of Medicine, gives women this advice for reducing the discomfort of shingles.

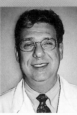

1

GET PLENTY OF REST. Shingles can take quite a toll on the body. You will need plenty of rest in order to recover. Take it easy and let others pamper you for a while.

KEEP YOUR DISTANCE—SOMETIMES. Shingles itself is not contagious, so you can't give or catch it. However, shingles is caused by the chickenpox virus, which means that a child or adult who has not had chickenpox in the past could

potentially be infected by someone with shingles. When you have the rash or blisters, avoid close contact with anyone who has never had chickenpox, Dr. Edelglass advises. Once the blisters have crusted over, the danger has passed.

2

SEE A DERMATOLOGIST. Internists and family practice physicians may not be as familiar with shingles as dermatologists are, which means they could miss the diagnosis and delay treatment, says Dr. Edelglass. You're better off seeing a dermatologist as soon as symptoms begin, when you feel a persistent one-sided burning or pain in the skin, and especially if blisters begin to appear. ■

3

essary. If the solution stings the skin, dilute it with more water. Repeat the compresses two to four times a day, as needed for comfort.

Cool the skin. "In addition to the Burow's solution, you may apply a lotion called Sarna," says Dr. Edelglass. "It contains menthol, which can cool and soothe the skin."

Enjoy an oatmeal soak. If you don't want to bother with compresses or lotions, you can ease rashes and sores by taking a lukewarm (not hot) bath. Sprinkle a cup or two of colloidal oatmeal (like Aveeno) into the water, Dr. Edelglass advises. Soak for 10 to 15 minutes, two to four times a day, until you feel better. "You can also use oatmeal bar soap," he adds. "Oatmeal is very soothing to the skin."

Take a painkiller. Aspirin, ibuprofen, naproxen, and other over-the-counter analgesics reduce skin inflammation as well as pain, says Dr. Edelglass.

medical options

Take antiviral medication. The severity and duration of shingles attacks can be significantly reduced if you take prescription antiviral drugs within 1 to 2 days after the blisters erupt. Drugs such as valacyclovir (Valtrex) and famciclovir (Famvir) help prevent the virus from reproducing, which can reduce or even eliminate postherpetic neuralgia, says Dr. Edelglass.

For Long-Term Relief

home remedies

Apply hot pepper cream. If you still feel pain after the blisters have healed completely, your doctor may recommend an over-the-counter topical analgesic cream containing capsaicin (like Zostrix and Capzasin). Capsaicin is a chemical compound made from hot pepper extract. "You will feel a temporary burning or tingling sensation, which may last for 3 to 4 days," Dr. Edelglass explains. "Capsaicin essentially swamps the nerve endings, thereby gradually reducing the deeper nerve pain caused by the virus."

Apply a thin coating of the cream to the affected area, gently rubbing it into the skin, three to four times a day as needed. Wash your hands when you're finished to avoid getting the cream into your eyes or other sensitive areas. Do not use on sensitive skin, such as the face or groin, or on open sores. If you experience too much irritation or if the burning sensation lasts longer than 3 to 4 days, stop using it and consult your doctor.

For more information about shingles and postherpetic neuralgia: Visit the Web site of the National Institute of Neurological Disorders and Stroke at www.ninds.nih.gov.

sore muscles

Muscles are tough, flexible bands of tissue. They can stretch and contract to a remarkable degree, but they aren't impervious to damage. When you've done something too vigorously and feel sore the next day—like digging up your flower bed in the spring—it's because the muscles have developed tiny tears.

"The muscle becomes inflamed, and the inflamed tissue releases histamines and prostaglandins, chemicals that irritate nerves and cause soreness, says Priscilla Clarkson, Ph.D., professor of exercise science and associate dean of the School of Public Health and Health Sciences at the University of Massachusetts in Amherst.

As you would expect, soreness usually occurs when you've worked your muscles harder than they're accustomed to—either because you're doing a new activity, such as playing tennis for the first time in 20 years, or because you did too much too fast, such as sprinting when you usually jog.

Muscle soreness isn't likely to be serious, and it usually fades within a few days. But it can have long-term consequences: Among women who begin a new exercise program, soreness is among the reasons for giving it up. So if you're hoping to achieve long-term fitness goals—or simply want to move without grimacing—it's worth taking quick action to relieve soreness and protect the muscles from additional damage.

For Immediate Relief

home remedies

Take aspirin or ibuprofen. Don't assume that these medications are lightweights just because you can buy them over the counter. They're among the best remedies for stopping muscle pain as well as swelling.

WHAT WORKS FOR ME

WILLIAM O. ROBERTS, M.D., *staff physician at MinnHealth Family Physicians in White Bear Lake, Minnesota, and spokesman for the American College of Sports Medicine, is serious about getting regular exercise—and sometimes he overdoes it. Here's his secret for relieving soreness fast.*

When I cross-country ski out West, I give my muscles a strenuous workout, and sometimes I

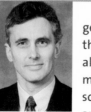

get a little sore. I soak in the hot tub at the spa or at the hotel I'm staying at. I also take 400 IU of vitamin E and 250 milligrams of vitamin C. The research is scant on this, but I suspect that taking antioxidant nutrients reduces damage to the muscles when you're doing unaccustomed exercise. ∎

Ice the area. "As soon as you feel the soreness, immediately place an ice pack—or even a bag of frozen vegetables—on the area for about 20 minutes," says William O. Roberts, M.D., staff physician at MinnHealth Family Physicians in White Bear Lake, Minnesota, and spokesman for the American College of Sports Medicine. You can protect your skin by putting a damp cloth between it and the ice pack or bag of frozen vegetables. "Ice reduces swelling and soreness, slows bleeding from muscle tears, and reduces bruising."

If you don't have an ice pack, it's fine to apply ice cubes wrapped in a damp washcloth or towel. Repeat the treatment once an hour until the pain is better, Dr. Roberts advises.

Give muscles some time off. If you keep doing whatever made your muscles sore in the first place, tears will get larger and you'll hurt even more later on. "Rest your sore muscles for 24 to 48 hours after they start to ache," says Dr. Roberts.

Speed healing with heat. Within a day or two after the soreness begins, it's a good idea to apply a heating pad or a hot-water bottle wrapped in a washcloth or towel to the area for about 20 minutes at a time. Heat increases circulation, which helps flush toxins from the area. It also speeds the body's natural repair process.

"I'm a big fan of sitting in a hot bath or a hot tub," says Dr. Roberts.

Look for distractions. Studies have shown that when people concentrate on pain, the muscles contract even more, increasing soreness. So don't dwell on the discomfort. Get your mind off the pain—by listening to music, watching TV, or simply curling up with a good book.

THREE THINGS I TELL EVERY FEMALE PATIENT

WILLIAM O. ROBERTS, M.D., staff physician at MinnHealth Family Physicians in White Bear Lake, Minnesota, and spokesman for the American College of Sports Medicine, treats a lot of women with muscle pain. He always gives his patients this special advice.

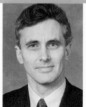

1 **EAT SMART.** "If you eat a healthful diet, you will have an adequate energy supply for the muscles to work properly," he advises. For optimal muscle health, he advises minimizing the intake of meat and saturated fat, and eating more fish, legumes, whole grains, and fruits and vegetables.

2 **ALWAYS STAY ACTIVE.** "You decrease your chances of damaging the muscles if you exercise regularly," says Dr. Roberts.

3 **PACE YOURSELF.** A lot of women get hurt when they've been less active than usual, then overdo it. During the winter, for example, it's common for women to be somewhat sedentary. Then, on the first warm day, they charge outside and tear up the yard or go for a long run. The muscles aren't used to the exertion, which can result in painful tears. Always start slowly to give your muscles time to adjust, Dr. Roberts advises. ■

Get a massage. "It breaks up scar tissue and helps remove waste products, such as lactic acid, from the site," says Dr. Roberts. This is important because lactic acid increases pain and slows the time it takes for injured muscles to heal.

To find a qualified massage therapist near you, contact the American Massage Therapy Association at the toll-free number (888) 843-2682, or at (847) 864-0123, or go to the association's Web site at www.amtamassage.org.

alternative therapies

Drink yarrow tea. Available in pharmacies and health food stores, yarrow contains an oil that eases muscle spasms and reduces inflammation. To make a tea, steep 1 teaspoon of dried yarrow in a cup of boiling water for 10 minutes. Strain and drink. You can drink the tea several times a day until you're feeling better.

For Long-Term Prevention

home remedies

Get regular exercise. The muscles are more likely to stay loose and limber when you exercise regularly, which can prevent painful tissue tears, says Dr. Roberts.

"Try to work out for at least 30 minutes 5 days a week," he advises. For overall muscle fitness, aerobic exercises—such as walking, biking, and swimming—are hard to beat. "Activities that involve jumping or pounding, such as jumping rope, can be uncomfortable and may lead to injury," he adds.

Give the muscles time to adjust. "Start a training program gradually," says Dr. Clarkson.

when to see a doctor

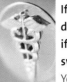

If you have muscle soreness that doesn't get better in a few days or if there's an unusual amount of swelling or pain, call your doctor. You could have torn a ligament or even fractured a bone, says Priscilla Clarkson, Ph.D., professor of exercise science and associate dean of the School of Public Health and Health Sciences at the University of Massachusetts in Amherst.

If your urine is brown, see your doctor immediately. A severely damaged muscle resulting from overexertion can cause excessive proteins to leak out into the blood and tax your kidneys, sometimes causing them to shut down.

If the muscle pain is accompanied by a fever, a rash, or whole-body aches and pains: It's not uncommon for muscle pain to be a sign of Lyme disease, a bacterial infection that requires treatment with antibiotics.

"Listen to your body. If you feel pain or discomfort, stop. Don't overexert yourself."

Warm up and cool down. Even if you're in good shape, plunging right into physical activity without giving the muscles time to warm up may increase the risk of soreness.

Start by doing your usual activity at a lower intensity than usual, says Michele Stanten, fitness editor at *Prevention* magazine. For example, if you normally jog at a 10-minute-mile pace, slow it down at first. This gets your body ready for exercise by stretching the muscles and increasing bloodflow. After about 5 minutes, you can pick up the pace to your regular intensity.

Whole-Body Stretch

This is one of the best all-around stretches for preventing soreness.

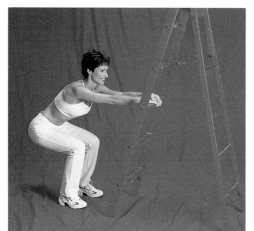

Hold on to a doorknob, a pole, or something else sturdy. Your feet should be shoulder-width apart, with the toes pointing forward. Slowly sit back into a squat, keeping your knees over your ankles. Lower yourself as far as you comfortably can—but don't bend your knees beyond 90 degrees (left).

Slowly drop your chin toward your chest and round your back (below). Hold the position, take six to eight slow breaths, then slowly return to the starting position.

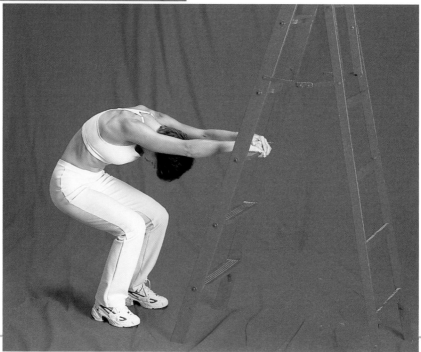

When you're ready to call it quits, don't just stop. If you do, lactic acid and other waste products of metabolism will remain in the muscles. Instead, gradually decrease the intensity of the exercise for about 5 minutes—for example, by dropping down to a slower jog, then to a brisk walk, and finally to a plain walk.

Save a few minutes for stretching. A lot of men and women alike stretch before they exercise, which may be the wrong thing to do.

Stretching *after* exercise may be better for improving flexibility while minimizing the risk of overstretching and damaging the muscle tissue. A postexercise stretch is a great way to reduce—and prevent—muscle soreness. It is most effective if you do it right after you've been exercising, when the muscle tissue is warm.

For more information about muscle soreness: Visit the Web site of the American College of Sports Medicine at www.acsm.org.

sore throat

All sorts of things can cause a sore throat, from air pollution or postnasal drip to talking too long and too loud around people who are smoking. Most of the time, however, sore throats are caused by the same thing that causes cold and flu: a virus that makes itself at home for a few days, causing inflammation and irritation. Women are no more prone to sore throats than men are, and sore throats usually clear up on their own. Here's how to reduce the discomfort in the meantime.

For Immediate Relief

home remedies

Gargle with salt water. It's an old folk remedy, but it's still one of the best ways to soothe a sore throat. Mix $1/4$ teaspoon of salt in $1/2$ cup of warm water, and gargle several times a day.

Suck on hard candy. It increases the flow of saliva and helps moisturize irritated tissues in the

throat, says Anne L. Davis, M.D., a pulmonologist and associate professor of medicine at New York University School of Medicine and an attending physician at Bellevue Hospital, both in New York City. Medicated lozenges are even better because they contain a mild anesthetic that temporarily numbs the throat, she says.

Add honey to your tea. It soothes tissues in the throat and helps prevent further irritation. The tea itself is beneficial because it helps moisturize dry, irritated tissues, says Dr. Davis.

Drink a lot of water. One reason sore throats hurt so much is that the inflamed tissues have lost their usual moisture, making them dry and irritated. The best way to remoisturize tissues is from the inside: Drink at least eight full glasses of water daily—more if you can.

Eat plenty of citrus fruits. They might sting a bit going down, but they're rich in vitamin C, which has been shown to shorten the severity and duration of colds. Vitamin C also strengthens the body's ability to resist pain-causing viruses.

Breathe steam. It fills the throat and airways with moisture and provides almost instant relief. The easiest way to inhale steam is to take a long, hot shower. Or you can plug in a vaporizer. To make the steam even more effective, add a few drops of eucalyptus oil to the diffuser. It breaks up congestion, which makes it easier to breathe when you have a cold or the flu. Look for eucalyptus oil at health food stores and pharmacies.

when to see a doctor

If your throat is so sore that swallowing is extremely painful or if your voice is wheezy or you're having trouble breathing, call your doctor immediately. Sore throats are sometimes caused by a condition called epiglottitis, a dangerous throat infection that can shut down the airway and make it impossible to breathe, says Anne L. Davis, M.D., a pulmonologist and associate professor of medicine at New York University School of Medicine and an attending physician at Bellevue Hospital, both in New York City.

If your throat is sore and you also have a high fever: You could have strep throat, a bacterial infection that requires treatment with antibiotics.

If you've recovered from a sore throat but then relapse with achy joints, fever, or a sharp pains that may mimic cardiac trouble: It's possible that you had strep throat, and it's now causing a secondary condition called rheumatic fever. Rheumatic fever can damage the heart, so it's essential that you see a doctor right away.

Take acetaminophen. It quickly reduces pain and swelling when you have a sore throat, says William J. Hall, M.D., president of the American College of Physicians–American Society of Internal Medicine in Philadelphia and chief of general medicine of the geriatrics unit, professor of medicine, pediatrics, and oncology at the University of Rochester School of Medicine department of medicine in New York. Aspirin and ibuprofen are also helpful, but they're more likely to cause stomach upset or other side effects, says Dr. Hall.

Use an anesthetic spray. There are many over-the-counter products that contain small amounts of local anesthetics. Sprays such as Chloraseptic are short-lasting, but they reduce pain almost instantly, says Dr. Hall.

alternative therapies

Gargle with echinacea. Numb an achy throat with echinacea, an immune-boosting herb that makes it easier to recover from infections. Mix ¼ to ½ teaspoon of echinacea tincture with 8 ounces of warm water. (You may swallow the solution after gargling.) Repeat several times a day as needed.

Coat your throat with slippery elm. It's been used for hundreds of years to ease sore throat pain. Taken in tea or lozenge form, slippery elm coats tissues with a smooth, slick barrier that reduces irritation. To make the tea, pour ½ cup of boiling water over 1 teaspoon of powdered slippery elm bark. Sip tea throughout the day to soothe the irritated throat. Purchase lozenges at the health food store, and follow the label instructions. Make certain the primary ingredient is slippery elm; some products are slippery elm in name only.

sprains

The joints in your body are held together with tough, fibrous cords of tissue called ligaments. Ligaments, which support the joints and keep them stable, have a certain amount of give. But when they're stretched too hard or suddenly, they get inflamed and irritated—sprained, in other words.

"Ligament sprains are always related to some form of injury," says Kim Fagan, M.D., a sports medicine physician who teaches in the internal medicine residency programs at Carraway Methodist Medical Center and Baptist Healthcare System in Birmingham, Alabama. "The most common ligament injuries involve the ankle, and they're generally the result of twisting types of injuries, such as when you jump and land on the side of the foot."

Sprains are rarely serious, but they're painful and slow to heal. You may find yourself limping and grimacing for a week or more. To reduce the discomfort and help sprains heal more quickly, here's what experts advise.

For Immediate Relief

home remedies

Take a rest. Whether you sprained an ankle while playing tennis or jammed your wrist while working in the yard, the most important thing is to stop what you're doing—immediately. If you keep putting pressure on the joint, you'll increase the pain and inflammation, and slow the time it takes to heal.

Apply ice. "The key to treating a sprain is to get ice on it immediately. Ice reduces the swelling, which will reduce pain," says Dr. Fagan.

If you don't have a cold pack, fill a plastic bag with ice cubes or take an unopened bag of frozen peas, wrap it in a thin towel, and hold it on the area for 20 minutes at a time. Repeat the treatment four times a day until the pain is gone, says Dr. Fagan.

Wrap it tightly. Use an Ace bandage or elastic wraps to bind the area over the sprain, says Dr. Fagan. This technique, called compres-

when to see a doctor

If you've sprained a joint and the pain is severe, or if the pain doesn't get better in a few days, make an appointment to see your doctor. You may have torn a ligament or even broken a bone, and surgery might be needed to repair the damage, says Kim Fagan, M.D., a sports medicine physician who teaches in the internal medicine residency programs at Carraway Methodist Medical Center and Baptist Healthcare System in Birmingham, Alabama.

If you notice little or no improvement in the swelling or the ability to move or use the joint after couple of days or if you're unable to bear weight on the affected joint, consult your doctor. These are red flags that mean the sprain might not get better without medical treatment, says Dr. Fagan.

sion, helps reduce swelling and pain. Don't make the bandage so tight that you cut off circulation, Dr. Fagan adds. It should be just tight enough that you can barely lift the edge to look underneath.

Elevate the joint. If you've sprained your wrist, try to keep your hand elevated above chest level to reduce swelling. For your ankle, put a pillow underneath the calf.

Continue following the rest, ice, compression, and elevation therapy for 24 to 48 hours or for as long as there is swelling, advises Dr. Fagan.

Take aspirin or ibuprofen. Apart from reducing pain, they also decrease the inflammation associated with the injury, which may help the sprain heal more quickly, says Dr. Fagan.

For Long-Term Prevention

home remedies

Strengthen the joints. When muscles in the ankle and other joints are strong, there's less stress on the ligaments, which reduces the risk of sprains. Because ankle sprains are so common, it's worth focusing on this area to build up your strength.

"Simple heel raises are a good form of ankle strengthening," says Dr. Fagan. Stand with your toes on the edge of a stair or a curb, your heels suspended over the edge. Rise on your toes, pause at the top, then lower your heels. Try to repeat the exercise 10 to 15 times, once or twice a day. "As you get stronger, you can do one leg at a time," says Dr. Fagan.

Watch where you're going. Sprains often occur when people accidentally step off a curb or into a hole in the yard. "Walk on familiar territory so you can avoid the pitfalls," says Dr. Fagan. "Also, try to walk where it's well-lit so you can see where you're going."

Stretch first. Before you exercise, it's a good idea to warm up slowly—by going up and down on your toes, for example, or bending your wrist backward and forward.

temporomandibular disorder

Of all the joints in the body, the jaw probably has the heaviest workload. Every time you eat, drink, talk, or yawn, this joint moves smoothly up and down.

At least, that's what's supposed to happen. "If there is uneven stress because the muscles and joint are out of alignment, the muscles can shorten, tighten, and go into spasm, causing temporomandibular disorder," says Richard H. Price, D.M.D., consumer advisor for the American Dental Association.

Apart from jaw pain, temporomandibular disorder (TMD) can result in clicking or popping sounds, pain that extends to the neck or shoulders, and sometimes headaches or hearing problems. It's not clear why, but studies suggest women are $1\frac{1}{2}$ to 2 times as likely as men to suffer from TMD.

Many things can cause the disorder. A severe injury to the jaw or joint and arthritis resulting from an injury are two clear causes. Habits such as resting your chin against your hand or another object may lead to TMD. That's why violin players may be prone to the disorder, notes Dr. Price. Some experts suggest that stress can cause or aggravate TMD since people who clench or grind their teeth can develop long-lasting jaw pain. It can also be caused by a misalignment between the upper and lower teeth. Sometimes the problem is as simple as a cap or filling that isn't fitted properly: Your bite will be uneven, which puts uneven (and painful) pressure on the jaw joint, Dr. Price explains. Researchers now say TMD may be the result of a combination of behavioral, psychological, and physical factors.

TMD can be a chronic problem that requires dental treatment. But usually it's a temporary condition related to stress, says Dr. Price. When the stressful times are past, and you quit clenching your jaw or grinding your teeth, the pain will often disappear as well.

To relieve the discomfort right away, and to reduce the chances that it will become a long-term problem, here's what you can do.

For Immediate Relief

home remedies

Take some pain relief. When TMD comes on suddenly, the best approach is to take ibuprofen or naproxen. Both of these medications reduce inflammation as well as pain, says Dr. Price.

Chill the area. When you first start having jaw pain, hold a cold pack or a plastic bag filled with ice cubes on the area to relieve pain and inflammation. "You can also use a bag of frozen vegetables," says Dr. Price. The advantage of this approach is that the bag will mold itself around the contour of your jaw, putting the cold right where you need it, he explains. Whatever method you choose, just make sure to keep the bag wrapped in a thin towel to protect your delicate skin. Hold it on the area for 20 minutes. Continue the ice treatments three or four times a day for 2 to 3 days, or until the pain is relieved.

Apply heat—for chronic TMD. "Ice works for people with acute pain, but moist heat works better for those with chronic pain," says Dr. Price.

when to see a doctor

If you're having jaw pain and it's getting worse despite home treatments or if the symptoms come back over time, make an appointment to see your dentist: Since most TMD problems are temporary, the goal of therapy is to let the body heal itself through stress management and self-care practices. Your dentist may recommend anti-inflammatory drugs to help you deal with pain. But sometimes the joint itself is damaged, and surgery may be the only way to relieve the pain, says Richard H. Price, D.M.D., consumer advisor for the American Dental Association.

"Stand in a comfortably hot shower and let the water run over your jaw. You can also put a hot-water bottle or a heating pad on the jaw until you feel relief." Applying heat to the area will increase circulation and relax painful muscle spasms and is sometimes a part of the therapy to manage a chronic condition, he says.

For Long-Term Prevention

home remedies

Limit jaw movements. Opening the mouth too wide strains the joint and surrounding muscles, which can trigger TMD. It will also make the pain worse if you already have the disorder.

"If you feel a yawn coming on, try not to open your mouth so wide," says Dr. Price. Cut up sandwiches and other types of food into smaller pieces. If you have the disorder, choose foods that are easy to chew, such as fish or whole wheat bread instead of a steak or a bagel.

Quit chewing gum. Every time you chew gum, your jaw moves up and down far more than usual, and the extra movements can aggravate TMD symptoms. If you don't already have the condition, the added motions may be a contributing factor resulting in TMD, says Dr. Price.

Use a bite guard when you sleep or anytime you're under stress. Available from dentists, bite guards are made from heavy-duty acrylic, and they're customized to fit your mouth exactly. They more equally distribute force when you grind or clench your teeth, which reduces stress on the jaw joint, Dr. Price explains.

"Some people only need to wear them at night during stressful times, when they're having pain in the jaw," Dr. Price says. "Others may need to wear them every night." The guards can also be worn during the day. "If you always feel anxious and frustrated when you're stopped in traffic, wearing a guard will help 'untrain' the joint that's moving incorrectly as you clench or grind your teeth," he adds.

mind-body techniques

Control the stress in your life. When you're tense, you may grind your teeth while you sleep, or clench your jaw more than usual. Most people aren't even aware they're doing it, but over time it can lead to joint pain, says Dr. Price.

There's no easy way to unwind when life's pressures are getting to you. Dr. Price often refers people with the disorder for biofeedback training. "Specialists will teach you techniques that concentrate on relaxing and becoming more aware of what's happening in your body so that you can change an unconscious habit into a conscious action," he explains. "If you usually clench your teeth while waiting in the seemingly endless line at the toll booth, biofeedback will teach you to put yourself at ease and stop the movement." Other techniques that may be helpful include deep breathing, yoga, meditation, and listening to relaxation tapes. Regular exercise is an excellent way to dispel stress. So is taking time by yourself to just sit and think pleasant thoughts.

thinning hair

In some ways, women are luckier than men. Nearly all women will lose some of their hair over time, but they rarely develop bare spots. Even when their hair gets thinner, they can often disguise the changes by styling their hair differently or using shampoos and conditioners that "bulk" the hair and make it look thicker. Another plus is that when a woman's hair thins, the front hairline isn't lost, as with the telltale receding hairline that many balding men experience.

Despite these benefits, however, thinning hair can be a devastating experience for many women. "Even though they lose their hair differently, thinning hair may be more of a trauma for women because it is less socially acceptable," says Diana Bihova, M.D., a dermatologist in New York City. A number of different factors can contribute to hair loss in women, but fortunately there are options that can help slow, stop, or reverse thinning hair, or at least minimize its appearance.

It's normal for a woman to lose anywhere from 50 to 100 hairs daily. The hairs are usually replaced by new ones, which grow at the rate of about $1/2$ inch a month. As women get older and their estrogen levels fall, the rate of hair loss may slightly exceed the pace of replacement. Known as androgenic alopecia, this type of hair loss is caused by a combination of genetic factors and high levels of androgens circulating in the blood, hormones that affect hair follicles, says Dr. Bihova.

Trauma from accidents, divorce, and other stressful events—as well as physical problems, such as anemia, liver, or hypothyroid disease—may cause hair to get thinner. Solving hair loss problems involves addressing the underlying medical problem, as well as caring for your hair to minimize the visual impact of your condition.

For Immediate Relief

home remedies

Change your hair color. The chemicals in hair colors slightly roughen the surface of each hair. This gives hair more body, makes it look fuller, and helps disguise thin spots, says Linda Tam, owner of Linda Tam Salon in New York City.

Women who have fine hair to begin with will want to choose lighter hair colors, Tam adds. Light browns or blondes will blend with the color of the scalp and make the hair appear thicker.

Add highlights. "I often advise women to highlight their hair because it creates a sense of depth and makes the hair appear fuller," says Anelka Szaruga, an instructor at American Beauty Academy in Philadelphia.

Or use lowlights. Adding streaks of a color that are a shade or two darker than your natural hair color creates the optical illusion that your hair is thicker than it really is, says Justine Beech, director of color at Gavert Atelier salon in Beverly Hills, California.

Wash your hair less often. Every time you shampoo your hair, the cleansing agents remove oils and cause the hair to lie flatter. "If you wash your hair a little less often, maybe two or three times a week, it will have a little more body and fullness," Tam says. This is most effective if you have normal or dry hair. If it tends to be oily, wash your hair daily, as usual, and add styling gel before blow-drying to give extra body.

when to see a doctor

If your hair is thinning and you're premenopausal, see a dermatologist. Younger women who experience hair loss may have medical problems, such as hypothyroid disease or dermatological problems, says Diana Bihova, M.D., a dermatologist in New York City.

If you're taking a new medication and you're losing hair: A number of prescription and over-the-counter drugs—including diuretics, thyroid medication, and even ibuprofen—may trigger hair loss in some people.

If the hair loss occurs suddenly and you've developed bare patches: You could have a condition called alopecia areata, which is thought to be linked to family history as well as stress. This condition is often temporary, and your hair may start to grow back within a few months.

If your hair loss is a serious concern to you: According to Dr. Bihova, the stress some women experience due to thinning hair problems can create a vicious cycle that only contributes to increased hair loss.

Use protein-based conditioners. Check the label for ingredients called hydrolyzed animal proteins. Known as thickeners, the proteins coat the hair shafts and give the hair more thickness and heft.

"Women whose hair is thinning should use a lightweight conditioner," says Szaruga. "The lighter products don't bring the hair down next to the scalp as much as heavier conditioners."

Finish with a cold rinse. After washing and conditioning your hair, adjust the temperature so that cool water soaks your hair for a few minutes. A cold rinse seals in some of the conditioner, which will give your hair additional body and shine.

Put hair mousse to use. Mousse is a lightweight styling gel that adds a thin, oily coating to the hair shafts and makes them appear fuller, Tam says.

Wear your hair shorter. "One of the best things women can do is wear a shorter cut and style it with a body wave," Tam says. "When the hair is 2 or 3 inches long, it's a little more curly and is less likely to lie against the scalp and reveal the thin spots."

Go for a natural look. "I recommend that women wear their hair a little more messy and tousled, rather than always having it smoothly combed," Szaruga says. "They should definitely wear their hair above the shoulders, either for a layered look or in a shorter blunt cut. That will make it look fuller than before."

Use a blow-dryer. It roughens up the hair shafts and also causes the hair to rise higher off the scalp. To avoid damaging the hair shafts, set the dryer on "low" and hold it 6 to 10 inches away from your hair, Szaruga says.

Finish with a vinegar rinse. White vinegar makes hair shiny and gives it a thicker appearance. Mix 1 tablespoon of white vinegar and a pint of water in a spray bottle. Spritz it on after you've shampooed and conditioned your hair. Leave it on for about 3 minutes, then rinse. If you're concerned that the rinse may leave you smelling like a salad, use chamomile tea instead of water, suggests Beech. Soaking a chamomile tea bag in warm water before adding the vinegar cuts the smell significantly, says Beech, and seems to give more shine to the hair.

Long-Term Solutions

Eat a balanced diet. Women who go on crash diets, or those with eating disorders or other conditions that affect the body's intake of nutrients, may experience hair loss, says Dr. Bihova. Protein and iron are especially important for the hair to grow normally.

The best sources of protein include lean meats, low-fat dairy foods, and legumes and whole grains. For iron, enjoy lean meats and fish, and fortified cereal products.

Use minoxidil. Available over the counter, minoxidil (such as Rogaine and generic brands) is an effective treatment for androgenic alopecia.

"About a third of the people who use it will grow new hair, and another third will maintain the hair they have," says Dr. Bihova.

Available as a liquid, minoxidil is rubbed into the scalp twice daily. It's not an instant cure, Dr. Bihova adds. In fact, she recommends seeing a dermatologist for a correct diagnosis of your hair-thinning problem because while minoxidil works for many people, it won't help at all if you don't have androgenic alopecia. Some women who use minoxidil may start to see results in about 3 months, but for others it may take as long as a year, says Dr. Bihova.

When using minoxidil, be careful to keep it off your face, Dr. Bihova warns. "It may cause facial hair growth if you get it on your skin."

Unload some of the stress in your life. In order to conserve energy during stressful times, your body may slow the rate of hair growth. If you're burning the candle at both ends or dealing with stressful life events, you may want to spend some time unwinding with meditation, regular exercise, and other relaxing activities.

tinnitus

Tinnitus means "to ring," but that doesn't begin to describe the buzzing, clicking, roaring, or other sounds that people with this condition hear inside their heads.

Experts aren't sure what causes tinnitus, a condition in which the brain perceives sounds when no real sounds exist. They do know that exposure to loud noises can cause tinnitus. So can circulatory problems, buildups of earwax, or side effects from medications.

"It's also part of the aging process," says Gordon B. Hughes, M.D., professor in the department of otolaryngology and communicative disorders at the Cleveland Clinic Foundation in Cleveland. "For the vast majority of people, it's mild, occasional, and not especially bothersome."

Tinnitus can sometimes be eliminated by treating underlying medical problems. More often, people have to find ways to cope with the persistent noise. Here are various strategies to try.

For Immediate Relief

home remedies

Cut back on coffee or tea. The caffeine in these and other beverages constricts blood vessels and temporarily raises blood pressure, which can make the sounds of tinnitus louder, says Dr. Hughes. Alcohol may have a similar effect.

Mask the sounds. A hearing aid–like device called a masker creates sounds that are matched in pitch to the sounds of tinnitus. "At least half the people who use a masker find that it's more acceptable to listen to an external sound than the spontaneous internal noise," says Dr. Hughes.

Use a hearing aid. About 90 percent of those with severe tinnitus also suffer from hearing loss. Wearing a hearing aid makes the tinnitus less noticeable by boosting the real sounds around you.

Clean out the wax. Excessive earwax can impair hearing and make the sounds of tinnitus louder. One solution is to use over-the-counter eardrops that contain carbamide peroxide. "Used as directed on the label, they're a reasonable approach," says Dr. Hughes.

when to see a doctor

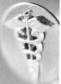

If you're taking medications and start experiencing tinnitus, talk to your doctor or pharmacist. A variety of over-the-counter and prescription drugs, including aspirin and some antibiotics, may cause ringing or other noises, says Gordon B. Hughes, M.D., professor in the department of otolaryngology and communicative disorders at the Cleveland Clinic Foundation in Cleveland.

If you've just started hearing ringing or other sounds: You may have an underlying medical problem that's causing tinnitus. Causes can include inner ear conditions and, in rare cases, tumors. Scientists have found a link between tinnitus, Lyme disease, and hyperacusis, a heightened sensitivity to normal sounds.

Ask your doctor about "double therapy." A study at the Shea Ear Clinic in Memphis found that more than 70 percent of the time, people who were treated with a combination of inner ear lidocaine injections and an intravenous dose of the same drug experienced at least partial relief from tinnitus.

"This treatment has been very successful for people whose tinnitus hasn't responded to anything else," says John J. Shea Jr., M.D., lead author of the study and chief otologic surgeon at the clinic.

Long-Term Solutions

Protect your ears. Because tinnitus may be triggered by loud noises, any additional assaults on your ears could worsen it. Try to avoid noisy activities, such as mowing the lawn or attending loud concerts. It's also helpful to wear earplugs. Music stores sell earplugs that are designed for musicians: They let in music and voices, but at a lower volume.

Reduce the sodium in your diet. Tinnitus is sometimes caused by a condition called Ménière's disease, which occurs when excessive amounts of fluid accumulate in the ear. People with this condition should restrict their daily sodium intake to 2,000 milligrams—by limiting the use of table salt and buying low-sodium soups, condiments, and other packed foods, says Dr. Hughes. "There's no question that physical and emotional stress aggravates tinnitus," he says. "If there's an obvious source of stress in your life, get counseling or find some other way to deal with it."

Consider antidepressants. Drugs that are used to treat depression may relieve tinnitus in some people. The medications don't work for everyone, however. They're effective only in those who are also suffering from depression, Dr. Hughes explains.

For more information on tinnitus: Go online and visit the Web site of the American Tinnitus Association at www.ata.org.

tooth discoloration

When you hear people describe teeth as "pearly whites," you have to wonder if their eyesight isn't quite what it should be.

It would be nice if teeth stayed white and unblemished, but that's not the way Nature made them. As the years go by, the teeth naturally take on a yellowish or grayish hue, says Lawrence Wolinsky, D.M.D., Ph.D., professor of oral biology and oral medicine at UCLA.

Part of the problem is the foods we eat. The outer layer of the teeth, the enamel, is more porous than it appears. When you eat highly pigmented foods or beverages, such as tomato sauce, red wine, and coffee, some of the color is absorbed by the enamel. "They'll slowly but surely cause the teeth to stain," says Dr. Wolinsky. Enamel can also be discolored by exposure to fluoride-rich water during the early years of tooth development.

Staining occurs in deeper portions of the tooth as well. These types of stains, which are commonly caused by childhood exposure to tetracycline antibiotics, are not easily removed and usually require the attention of a dentist.

Dentists have developed a variety of techniques to bring back the original white. There are also things you can do at home to make your smile brighter than ever. Choose what works best for you.

For Immediate Relief

Use whitening toothpastes. They may contain peroxides, which act as bleaching agents. "These pastes are good for minor surface stains," Dr. Wolinsky says.

Brush away the stains. Toothpastes that contain silica act as abrasives and help remove dingy stains, Dr. Wolinsky says. Baking soda mixed with a little water has a similar effect. "You don't want to use these products too often because they can wear away portions of the teeth," Dr. Wolinsky adds.

Use a bleaching gel. You can buy home bleaching kits at pharmacies. The kits include a bleaching agent, usually carbamide peroxide, and a mouthpiece. You fill the mouthpiece with gel

and wear it for an hour or two a day—or overnight for quicker results. For the first couple of weeks after treatment, you should avoid foods and beverages that can stain your teeth.

Home bleaching will brighten the teeth somewhat, but it may require a long time, usually several weeks, before you'll notice the results, Dr. Wolinsky says. Also, the mouthpieces rarely fit well. Some people experience gum irritation or other side effects from the chemicals.

Get a "power bleaching." Some dentists perform in-office bleaching, in which the teeth are coated with a highly concentrated bleaching gel. The gel "turns on" when it's exposed to special lights. "It can lighten your teeth by more than two shades in less than an hour," says Dr. Wolinsky.

when to see a doctor

If your teeth get sensitive when you use a bleaching gel, call your dentist. Some bleaches contain chemicals that remove water from the teeth, which irritates the nerves, says Lawrence Wolinsky, D.M.D., Ph.D., professor of oral biology and oral medicine at UCLA.

If there's a burning sensation in the gums that doesn't go away: The mouthpiece probably doesn't fit properly and is allowing the chemicals to irritate the gums.

If there's a generalized redness that extends to the cheeks or tongue: You may be having an allergic reaction to a chemical in the bleach.

Use a home treatment provided by your dentist. Unlike over-the-counter bleaching kits, those provided by dentists use stronger chemicals, and the mouthpiece is customized for a precise fit. "You usually apply them for an hour a day for 7 days," says Dr. Wolinsky.

Cover the stains. If your teeth are damaged or badly stained, your dentist may recommend covering them with veneers, ultrathin porcelain or plastic shells that are permanently attached to the teeth. The one drawback to veneers is cost: You can expect to pay as much as $1,000 per tooth.

Long-Term Solutions

home remedies

Always brush after meals. "It takes a long time for staining to occur," says Dr. Wolinsky. "If you're constantly removing film from the teeth by brushing, it will reduce the possibility of staining."

Rinse your mouth. When you don't have time to brush, a quick rinse will help prevent staining chemicals in coffee, wine, and other foods and beverages from penetrating the enamel.

Finish meals with a carrot. Along with apples, celery stalks, and other raw fruits and vegetables, carrots contain fiber, which gently "brushes" the teeth with every crunch, says Dr. Wolinsky.

Avoid staining foods. Instead of drinking red wine, switch to white. Drink green or herbal teas instead of black tea or coffee. "Avoiding or having smaller amounts of staining foods can make a difference," says Dr. Wolinsky.

For more information on tooth discoloration and other dental issues: See the Web site of the American Dental Association at www.ada.org.

ulcers

For a long time, ulcers were thought to be caused by stress. Hard-driving executives were almost proud to have them because ulcers supposedly meant that they were working long hours and putting the company's success above their own internal affairs.

Then, about 20 years ago, researchers discovered that the vast majority of ulcers are caused by infection with the bacterium *Helicobacter pylori*. Using its spiral shape as a microscopic bore, the bacterium burrows through the protective mucus that coats the stomach and part of the small intestine, allowing powerful stomach acids to damage the delicate layers underneath.

The result is an ulcer—a sore that's usually no larger than a pencil eraser but can cause a great deal of pain.

Most ulcers are caused by infections, but they can also be due to the long-term use of aspirin, ibuprofen, and similar drugs. Known as nonsteroidal anti-inflammatory drugs, or NSAIDs, the medications inhibit the body's production of chemicals needed to protect the stomach lining.

Most people with ulcers require treatment with antibiotics or other medications, says David Peura, M.D., professor of medicine and associate chief of gastroenterology and hepatology at the University of Virginia in Charlottesville. Whether or not you take drugs, however, there are a number of strategies for easing the pain of ulcers and helping them heal more quickly.

For Immediate Relief

home remedies

Avoid acidic or spicy foods. While an ulcer is healing, the acids in oranges, grapefruit, and other foods can cause a temporary burning sensation, says Dr. Peura. Fiery chili can make things worse. So can alcohol and caffeine. Once your ulcer is healed, however, you should be able to eat anything you want, Dr. Peura says.

when to see a doctor

If you experience stomach pain or a burning sensation, usually in the middle of the night or between meals: These are the classic signs of an ulcer, says David Peura, M.D., professor of medicine and associate chief of gastroenterology and hepatology at the University of Virginia in Charlottesville.

If your stools are black or tarry: This may be a sign that an ulcer is causing internal bleeding.

If you're tired all the time for no good reason: It's not uncommon for ulcers to bleed slowly, which can result in fatigue and other symptoms of iron deficiency anemia.

Suppress the acid. Over-the-counter medications called H_2 blockers—such as cimetidine (Tagamet) and ranitidine (Zantac)—cause the stomach to produce less acid, which can reduce the pain of ulcers and help them heal more quickly.

Try to relax. Even though emotional stress doesn't cause ulcers, it does increase the stomach's output of acids, which can make the pain of ulcers worse, says George Sachs, M.D., professor of physiology and medicine at UCLA.

You can't eliminate life's stresses, but you can find ways to cope with them a little better—by exercising regularly, practicing yoga or meditation, or simply giving yourself a little more time to relax. (For step-by-step action plans for starting an exercise plan and relieving stress, see chapters 5 and 7.)

medical options

Eliminate the infection. If tests show that your ulcer is caused by *H. pylori* bacteria, your doctor may recommend treatment with antibiotics. Once the organisms are gone, the ulcer will heal within a few weeks—and there's a good chance that it will never come back.

In addition to antibiotics, your doctor may prescribe H_2 blockers or another type of medication called proton pump inhibitors (PPIs) as part of the therapy. PPIs, such as esomeprazole (Nexium) and pantoprazole (Protonix), suppress acid production by halting the mechanism that pumps the acid into the stomach. Some treatment plans also include drugs that shield the stomach's mucous lining from acid damage.

Long-Term Solutions

home remedies

Switch pain relievers. People who take a lot of aspirin or other NSAIDs can develop potentially serious ulcers. This can happen to anyone, but it's most common in those 60 years and older.

Your doctor will probably advise you to switch to acetaminophen. It's just as effective as ibuprofen and aspirin, but it's much less likely to cause stomach irritation or ulcers, says Dr. Peura.

Snuff out the cigarette habit. Smoking increases the risk of ulcers, slows the rate at which they heal, and also makes them more likely to come back. There's even evidence that suggests that people who smoke are more likely to get infected with the ulcer-causing bacterium.

Giving up cigarettes isn't easy, of course. (For more information on giving up the habit for good, see chapter 8.)

urinary incontinence

Women who have gone through pregnancy and childbirth sometimes joke about the frequency of their bathroom stops. What they don't laugh about—or in some cases even discuss with their doctors—are the embarrassing "leaks" that may occur when they sneeze, laugh, or bend over to pick up a sock.

"Women might start noticing small stains or dampness on their underwear," says Gary Lemack, M.D., assistant professor of urology at the University of Texas Southwestern Medical Center in Dallas. "The leaks happen suddenly, usually with strenuous activity, such as lifting heavy objects."

More than 13 million Americans—most of them women—suffer from urinary incontinence, which is the inability to completely control the flow of urine. Incontinence often occurs after childbirth or menopause because women may lose strength in the muscles (the pelvic floor muscles) that support the bladder. The muscles that surround the urethra, the tube that carries urine from the body, can also weaken over time.

If this is happening to you, don't put up with it. Incontinence is *always* caused by underlying physical problems, says Dr. Lemack.

Incontinence may clear up on its own, but often it doesn't. The good news is that about 80 percent of women can reduce or eliminate incontinence with a combination of medical treatments and home care strategies.

For Immediate Relief

home remedies

Put your bladder on a schedule. "Go to the bathroom every 2 hours, even if you don't feel like you have to go," says Dr. Lemack. Women who practice "timed voiding" are less likely to leak urine accidentally.

Drink less coffee. Or at least switch to decaf. The caffeine in coffee and other beverages increases the body's output of urine. Caffeine also stimulates bladder contractions, which can lead to unexpected leaks, says Lily A. Arya, M.D., assistant professor of urogynecology at the University of Pennsylvania in Philadelphia. She advises limiting caffeine intake to 200 milligrams daily, which is the equivalent of two 6-ounce cups of coffee.

Use a tampon. If you find that you frequently leak urine when you cough, sneeze, or exercise, you might want to use a tampon even when you're not having your period. Tampons provide extra support for the bladder, which can prevent urine from escaping, says Mary Jane Minkin, M.D., clinical professor of obstetrics and gynecology at Yale University School of Medicine.

Follow the package insert guidelines for how long you can safely wear a tampon without increasing your risk of toxic shock syndrome—usually 4 to 8 hours.

Use pads as necessary. You don't want to depend on absorbent pads, such as sanitary napkins, because they don't solve the underlying problem. But if you find that you're nervous about having "accidents," absorbent pads can give you the confidence you need to get out and about, Dr. Lemack says. They're also helpful as an interim measure when you're working with your doctor to get your bladder under control.

Control allergies. Women who suffer from hay fever or other allergies may have flare-ups of incontinence due to coughing or sneezing. It's worth trying over-the-counter antihistamines during allergy season, says Dr. Lemack.

THREE THINGS I TELL EVERY FEMALE PATIENT

GARY LEMACK, M.D., assistant professor of urology at the University of Texas Southwestern Medical Center in Dallas, gives the following advice for coping with incontinence.

1

KEEP A "VOIDING" DIARY. For several weeks, record your bladder "habits." Write down how often (and how much) you drink, how many times you urinate, and how many "accidents" you have. The diary will help your doctor determine the best course of treatment.

DO KEGEL EXERCISES DAILY. "I advise people to do Kegels in conjunction with the voiding

diary in order to measure progress," Dr. Lemack says.

2

CONSIDER YOUR GOALS. For some women, the treatments used to control incontinence are more inconvenient than the symptoms themselves. If your goal is complete dryness, you may need to consider surgery or other medical treatments. On the other hand, if the leaks only happen once or twice a week, you might want to stick with simpler treatments, such as Kegel exercises or the occasional use of pads. ■

3

Cap the leaks. If you experience incontinence only occasionally, your doctor may recommend urethral caps, tiny disposable plugs that fit inside the urethra and hold back the flow of urine. When you need to use the bathroom, you remove the plug, then replace it when you're done.

"They can be helpful when there are certain activities that women want to participate in—for example, playing tennis once or twice a week—which they know make them leak," explains Abraham N. Morse, M.D., assistant professor of urogynecology at the University of Massachusetts Medical School in Worcester.

Discuss medications with your doctor. If you're taking diuretics (water pills) for high blood pressure or other conditions, you may have more trouble controlling your bladder. "Changing to a different drug or changing the timing of drug administration may be helpful," says Dr. Lemack.

Tighten the urethra. If you've lost strength in the urethra, your doctor may recommend periurethral injections, which add bulk to the tissue and increase urinary control. The injections are effective, but they may have to be repeated over time, says Dr. Lemack.

Consider a pessary. Made of rubber, a pessary is a device that slips inside the vagina and helps support the bladder. "Some are also designed to press the urethra, which can give additional control," says Dr. Morse. "Pessaries are helpful in some cases, but most women will gain better control with other methods." You'll need to speak to your gynecologist about whether a pessary is right for you.

Long-Term Solutions

Squeeze in some muscle training. One of the most effective strategies both for treating and preventing incontinence is to strengthen the pelvic floor muscles, says Dr. Morse. These are the same muscles you use when stopping urine flow in midstream.

All you have to do is clench and relax the muscles about 10 times, and repeat the series three times daily. The great thing about these exercises, called Kegel exercises, is that you can do them anytime: when you're lying in bed, watching TV, or standing in line at the grocery store.

Tighten at the right time. Kegel exercises are used mainly to prevent incontinence, but you can also use them to stop leaks before they start. "That means contracting your pelvic floor muscles in anticipation of a cough, laugh, or sneeze to prevent urine from leaking out, says Linda Brubaker, M.D., a urogynecologist at Rush System for Health in Chicago.

Practice with vaginal weights. The tricky part about Kegels is figuring out which muscles you need to contract. Your doctor may recommend vaginal weights, which slip inside the vagina, as a training tool. If you aren't clenching the right muscles, the weights will slip out, Dr. Minkin explains.

Meet with a urinary "coach." "For younger women, who are unlikely to have nerve damage

when to see a doctor

If the leaks are accompanied by sudden, uncontrollable urges to urinate, see your family doctor. You could have a urinary tract infection that's irritating the bladder, says Abraham N. Morse, M.D., assistant professor of urogynecology at the University of Massachusetts Medical School in Worcester.

If you're leaking urine and you also have pelvic pressure or lower back pain: You could have a condition called cystocele, which occurs when weakened pelvic floor muscles allows the bladder to sag into the vagina.

or severe incontinence, I encourage going to physical therapy for pelvic floor muscle training," says Dr. Morse. "In many cases they'll gain enough control to be satisfied with the results."

Maintain a healthful weight. Women who have too much padding around the middle may have excessive pressure on the bladder. Losing weight—by exercising regularly, reducing the amount of fat in the diet, and eating more fruits and vegetables—may reduce the pressure and improve urinary control, says Dr. Lemack.

medical options

Use a magnetic chair. The treatment involves sitting in a magnetized chair in a doctor's office for about 20 minutes once or twice a week. "It's a high-tech way of doing pelvic floor exercises," Dr.

Morse explains. "The magnetic field causes nerves in the pelvic floor to fire, which makes the muscles contract."

Or consider electrical stimulation. There's some evidence that applying mild doses of electrical stimulation can strengthen muscles and improve the bladder's "holding" ability. A probe is temporarily placed in the vagina or rectum, and precise amounts of electricity are applied to stimulate the nearby muscles, including those surrounding the urethra, Dr. Morse explains. You'll learn how to use the device at the doctor's office, then you'll be able take it home to use on a daily basis.

Take muscle-tightening medications. Over-the-counter medications that include alpha-agonists (such as Sudafed) tighten muscles in the "neck" of the bladder and also in the urethra, which can make it easier to control urine flow. The drugs aren't always effective, however, and they may cause side effects, so it's important to use them under the supervision of your doctor, Dr. Lemack adds.

Supplement your body's estrogen. The reductions in estrogen that occur at menopause can result in weakness in the urethra or bladder. "I will often start patients on an estrogen suppository or cream if they have evidence of vaginal weakness," says Dr. Lemack.

For more information on urinary incontinence: Visit the Web site of the Simon Foundation for Continence at www.simonfoundation.org.

urinary tract infections

About the only good thing you can say about urinary tract infections is that they're easy to treat and rarely serious.

The bad news is that they're extremely common. One in five women will get a urinary tract infection (UTI) at some time in her life, and some women get them again and again.

UTIs that occur in the bladder are called cystitis. Those that affect the urethra (the tube through which urine leaves the body) are called urethritis, and infections in the kidneys (the most serious kind) are called pyelonephritis.

UTIs usually occur when bacteria that live around the anus gain entry to the urethra and begin to multiply. Sexual intercourse is a common cause of UTIs, but women who aren't sexually active get them, too. The risk of infections rises after menopause, when declines in the body's estrogen levels make tissues in the vagina and urethra more vulnerable to bacterial assaults.

If you suspect that you have a UTI, you'll want to call or see your doctor right away. You can "diagnose" some UTIs based on symptoms alone; typical symptoms for cystitis, for example, include a burning sensation while urinating and a powerful urge to urinate even after you've used the bathroom. But your doctor may need to perform tests to ensure that the infection hasn't spread to other parts of the body, explains Sanjay Saint, M.D., assistant professor of medicine at the University of Michigan Medical School in Ann Arbor.

Once you start taking antibiotics, the discomfort will usually disappear within a day or two, Dr. Saint adds. After that, you can plan a strategy to prevent infections from coming back.

For Immediate Relief

home remedies

Ease discomfort with heat. Placing a hot-water bottle or heating pad on your lower abdomen will relieve uncomfortable cramps or pressure while you're waiting for antibiotics to take effect, says Larrian Gillespie, M.D., president of Healthy Life Publications in Beverly Hills, California, and author of *You Don't Have to Live with Cystitis.*

Avoid coffee or alcohol for a few days. They can irritate the urinary tract when you have an infection. Coffee and other beverages with caffeine also stimulate urination, which can increase discomfort, says Dr. Gillespie.

alternative therapies

Avoid acidic foods. Orange juice, strawberries, vinegar, and other foods with a high acid content may create a more favorable environment for bacteria in the bladder, says Dr. Gillespie. "Eating these foods when you have an infection can increase the irritation," she adds.

Put aside the soy sauce. Along with bananas, nuts, cheese, and wine, it contains biogenic amines, amino acids that affect sensory nerve fibers in the bladder. Eating these foods when you have an infection may increase urinary "urgency," says Dr. Gillespie.

medical options

Ask your doctor about supplemental hormones. If you're past menopause and have been getting frequent infections, you may be a good candidate for hormone replacement therapy. Taking low doses of estradiol, a form of estrogen, strengthens tissues in the urethra and vagina and helps prevent infections, says Dr. Gillespie.

Long-Term Solutions

home remedies

Wash away bacteria. Removing bacteria from the area around the urethra is among the best strategies for preventing UTIs, says Mary Jane Minkin, M.D., clinical professor of obstetrics and gynecology at Yale University School of Medicine. Wash the genital area before having sex—and remember to urinate before and after intercourse. After using the bathroom, wipe from front to back. This helps ensure that anal bacteria don't get moved toward the urethral opening.

Consider alternative forms of birth control. Women who use diaphragms have a higher risk of UTIs. If you use a diaphragm and have recurrent infections, discuss alternative forms of birth control with your doctor.

Drink eight glasses of water daily. Water won't stop an infection in progress, but it dilutes the urine and reduces the concentration of infection-causing bacteria, says Dr. Gillespie. Drinking

THREE THINGS I TELL EVERY FEMALE PATIENT

LARRIAN GILLESPIE, M.D., president of Healthy Life Publications in Beverly Hills, California, and author of *You Don't Have to Live with Cystitis*, gives the following advice for dealing with urinary tract infections (UTIs).

1

DON'T WAIT TO TAKE ANTIBIOTICS. They're extremely effective at stopping UTIs. Most women can be treated with a single "triple dose," which is more convenient than the older, weeklong regimens.

DRINK BAKING SODA MIXED WITH WATER. "It makes the urine more alkaline for about 24

hours, which takes away the acid environment that bacteria need to multiply," says Dr. Gillespie. When you first notice symptoms, mix ¼ teaspoon of baking soda in a glass of water and drink it once daily until your symptoms are improved, she advises.

2

EASE DISCOMFORT WITH THE "ORANGE" PILL. An over-the-counter medication called phenazopyridine (such as Pyridium or Urobiotic) is a dye that turns the urine orange. It decreases bladder irritability and can be taken along with antibiotics to ease discomfort. ■

3

water also promotes urination, which helps remove bacteria from the bladder.

Stay clean naturally. The use of douches, deodorant sprays, and other "feminine" products can irritate the urethra and promote infections. Washing with soap and water is more effective and less irritating.

alternative therapies

Drink a glass of cranberry juice daily. Cranberry juice contains chemical compounds called proanthocyanidins, which help prevent bacteria from sticking to cells in the urinary tract. Blueberries contain the same helpful substances, says Dr. Minkin.

medical options

Arrange a plan with your doctor. UTIs respond quickly to antibiotics, but you can get them only with a prescription—which means that you have to put up with symptoms until you can see your doctor. Women who get frequent UTIs sometimes arrange for their doctors to prescribe antibiotics over the telephone when symptoms first appear. This is a reasonable approach if the

when to see a doctor

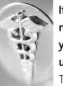

If you have flank pain, difficulty urinating, a burning sensation when you urinate, or frequent urges to urinate, see a doctor right away. These are classic symptoms of urinary tract infections, says Sanjay Saint, M.D., assistant professor of medicine at the University of Michigan Medical School in Ann Arbor.

If you have a flank pain, fever, chills, or nausea that accompanies the typical symptoms of a UTI: You could have a potentially serious kidney infection called pyelonephritis and must see a doctor right away.

If you feel pressure in the lower abdomen, and the urine has a strong smell: The infection could be in the bladder, a condition called cystitis.

infections are uncomplicated and your doctor is familiar with your health history, says Dr. Saint.

Dr. Saint led a study that looked at nearly 4,000 women with uncomplicated UTIs. The researchers found that those who had phone consultations with their doctors did just as well as those who came into the office for examinations.

vaginal dryness

At menopause, a woman's ovaries stop making estrogen, the hormone that stimulates the vaginal glands to produce lubricating moisture. The tissues lining the vagina become thinner, and the vagina may become dry enough to make sex uncomfortable.

"In addition to discomfort during intercourse, a woman who's menopausal may have a higher risk of vaginal infections because the natural vaginal environment changes," adds Debra Papa, M.D., assistant professor of obstetrics/gynecology at the University of Massachusetts Medical

School in Worcester. Also, the thinning of vaginal tissues makes women more susceptible to irritation or trauma, which may provide a gateway for an infection.

Women sometimes reach for petroleum jelly when they're feeling dry, but it's not a good choice: It acts as an irritant in the vagina.

Here are some better ways to enhance moisture and maintain your natural lubrication.

For Immediate Relief

home remedies

Use a water-based lubricant. Available over the counter, lubricants such as Astroglide and Replens help prevent dryness by replenishing moisture in the vagina. This reduces irritation and itching and decreases friction during intercourse, says Dr. Papa. They're also safe to use with condoms.

when to see a doctor

If you're getting recurrent infections, visit your gynecologist. Changes in the vagina's natural acidity can make women more prone to yeast and other infections, says Debra Papa, M.D., assistant professor of obstetrics/gynecology at the University of Massachusetts Medical School in Worcester.

If you're experiencing dryness even though you're premenopausal: Vaginal dryness is not a common complaint in younger women. If you're premenopausal and sex is uncomfortable for you, discuss this with your doctor.

Product ingredients vary, so it's best to follow instructions on the package on how to apply.

Switch tampons. Many premenopausal women find that vaginal dryness makes the use of tampons difficult or painful. You may want to try a brand that uses a cardboard or plastic applicator. Or use one that has a slimmer shape or a rounder tip, suggests Mary Jane Minkin, M.D., clinical professor of obstetrics and gynecology at Yale University School of Medicine.

To reduce irritation, it's fine to dab the tampon with a small amount of a water-based lubricant, Dr. Minkin adds.

Long-Term Solutions

home remedies

Stay sexually active. Having sex regularly maintains the elasticity of the vaginal tissues, which get dry at menopause.

Put out the cigarettes. Smoking constricts blood vessels and reduces vaginal circulation, which can cause a decrease in lubrication, says Dr. Papa.

medical options

Use an estrogen cream. Available by prescription, estrogen creams are applied directly to the vagina. They relieve dryness by strengthening vaginal tissue and promoting the ability of the glands to secrete adequate amounts of moisture, says Dr. Papa.

The creams initially need to be applied daily for several weeks, Dr. Papa advises. Then they're usually used two or three times a week. Follow your doctor's instructions or those that come in the package for dosage.

Use an estrogen ring. Estrogen creams are messy and inconvenient to apply, which is why some women opt for an estrogen ring. A diaphragm-like device, the ring is kept in the vagina for up to 3 months. It releases steady amounts of estrogen, keeping the vaginal environment healthy.

Consider oral estrogen. The medication in vaginal creams and rings mainly stays in the vagina—only small amounts enter the bloodstream. If you're postmenopausal, your doctor may recommend that you take oral estrogen.

Along with relieving vaginal dryness, supplemental estrogen helps prevent hot flashes and osteoporosis, a disease in which bones gradually become fragile and more likely to break. It may also help you to guard against heart disease. Women who still have a uterus need to take a progestin, along with estrogen, to offset the effects estrogen has on the lining of the uterus, Dr. Papa adds.

For more information about vaginal dryness and other conditions associated with menopause: Visit the Web site of the North American Menopause Society at www.menopause.org.

vaginal infections

The tropical rain forests are home to more species of life than any other location on earth. There's something about the warm, moist environments that allow many of nature's creatures to thrive.

Closer to home, quite a few organisms also thrive in a hothouse environment—which is why most women will get a vaginal infection at some time in their lives.

"The vaginal environment usually prevents infections by maintaining a balance between normal organisms and those that can cause infection," explains Debra Papa, M.D., assistant professor of obstetrics/gynecology at the University of Massachusetts Medical School in Worcester.

A fungus called *Candida albicans*, for example, is often present in the vagina. When the condi-

tions are right, it can multiply out of control and cause a yeast infection. It is estimated that at least 75 percent of women will get at least one yeast infection in their lifetime.

Infections can also be caused by bacteria, viruses, parasites, and species of fungus that are not the *albicans* type. Some infections are transmitted sexually. Others occur when offending germs on the outside of the body manage to get inside. An infection can also be a result of a disturbance in the vaginal environment due to antibiotics, douches, hormones, or stress. Regardless of how you get them, vaginal infections often cause a discharge along with intense irritation, itching, and odor.

Most vaginal infections can be treated with antifungal creams, antibiotics, or other medications.

In addition, there are things you can do to reduce the discomfort and prevent the infections from coming back.

For Immediate Relief

home remedies

Enjoy an oatmeal bath. Add colloidal oatmeal (such as Aveeno) to a warm bath and soak for a while. "Yeast infections especially can be pretty severe and intense," says Dr. Papa. "An oatmeal bath won't stop the infection, but it will relieve the itching and burning."

Let air circulate. Stay out of tight clothing while the infection is healing, Dr. Papa advises. At home, don't wear underwear under your skirt. "You want to keep the area dry, which will reduce the irritation," she says.

Sleep in just your nightie. Sleeping without underwear under your nightgown allows the area to "breathe," which reduces irritation and also makes it more difficult for yeast or other moisture-loving organisms to thrive.

Use a hair dryer. "When you have an infection, rubbing yourself dry with a towel can be uncomfortable," Dr. Papa says. She advises drying yourself with a hair dryer—set on low, of course.

medical options

Start with a checkup. If you've never had a vaginal infection before, don't assume that your symptoms are caused by yeast. Studies have shown that women often misdiagnose what they believe to be a yeast infection, which means that you could have a more serious infection that requires medical care.

Choose your medication. If you've had yeast infections in the past and you're sure that's what you have, it's fine to use an over-the-counter medication to treat it. Except in rare cases when yeast infections are caused by "resistant" organisms in the vagina, over-the-counter products work well, says Meg Autry, M.D., assistant professor of obstetrics/gynecology at the Medical College of Wisconsin in Milwaukee.

There are a number of products to choose from: creams, suppositories, and prefilled syringes. The active ingredient usually will be clotrimazole (such as Gyne-Lotrimin and Mycelex) or miconazole (Monistat). All of these products are effective for most *Candida albicans* infections. Just be sure to read the label. Different products may require that you use them for different lengths of time.

For most women, the 3-day treatments work just as well as those that are used for 7 days, Dr. Autry adds. Although, she adds, "a woman might have a species of yeast that can't be killed in 3 days." If your infection doesn't clear up after 3 days, you can try a 7-day product. If that doesn't work, you'll definitely want to see your doctor.

Reduce discomfort with a local steroid cream. The burning and itching sensations of yeast infections sometimes last for a week or more, even after using medication. To ease discomfort in the meantime, you may want to apply an over-the-counter cream containing hydrocortisone (such as Cortaid or Cortizone). Towelettes moistened with hydrocortisone are also available (Massengill Clean Relief). Your doctor may also prescribe a combination medicine, such as Lotrisone or Mycolog II, to treat the infection and relieve symptoms at the same time. These contain both a steroid and an antifungal.

Get a prescription. If your infection is caused by a resistant strain of yeast or other organisms, you'll probably need to take a prescription medication. For trichomoniasis, a sexually transmitted infection caused by the parasite *Trichomonas vaginalis*, your doctor may advise you to take oral metronidazole (Flagyl). Bacterial infections can also be treated with metronidazole (MetroGel-Vaginal) or with an antibiotic called clindamycin (Cleocin). Resistant strains of yeast usually succumb to a drug called terconazole (Terazol), says Dr. Autry.

For Long-Term Relief

home remedies

Wash with plain water. Nearly everyone enjoys scented soaps and bath oil, but you should avoid using these products even when you don't have an infection. The chemicals in them can irritate the vulvar tissues (the external parts of the genitals) and cause scratching. This may make it easier for infections to establish themselves, says Dr. Papa. Douches, too, can be irritating, so if you feel you must douche, use plain vinegar and water, advises Dr. Papa.

Change into something dry. After swimming or working out, change into dry clothing immediately afterward. It will make the vulvar and vaginal areas less hospitable to yeast.

Wear cotton panties. Unlike nylon and other synthetic fabrics, cotton allows air to get

THREE THINGS I TELL EVERY FEMALE PATIENT

MEG AUTRY, M.D., assistant professor of obstetrics/gynecology at the Medical College of Wisconsin in Milwaukee, gives the following advice to women who suffer from vaginal infections.

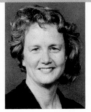

1 NEVER DOUCHE. "It's always bad," says Dr. Autry. "It changes the vaginal environment, and it also increases the risk of upper genital infections. There's some evidence that it may increase the risk of ovarian cancer as well."

2 BE GENEROUS WITH ANTIFUNGAL CREAMS. It's not uncommon for women with yeast infections to have inflammation outside the vagina. When applying a medicated cream, you may need to put it outside as well as inside the vagina.

3 GET CHECKED FOR DIABETES IF YOU HAVE FREQUENT INFECTIONS. This is especially true if you have any of the risk factors for diabetes, such as being overweight or having a family history of the disease. ∎

in and moisture to get out, which can reduce your risk of infections. If you wear panty hose, use the ones with cotton crotches. It's also a good idea to always wear comfortable, not tight-fitting, clothing.

Wipe microbes away. Vaginal infections can occur when bacteria that live around the anus migrate into the vaginal area. One way to prevent this is to wipe from front to back after urinating or having a bowel movement, says Dr. Papa.

Keep your blood sugar under control. Women with diabetes have an increased risk of vaginal yeast infections because they may have higher-than-normal levels of glucose (blood sugar), which can change the vagina's protective balance.

If you have diabetes, keeping your blood sugar levels stable—by eating a healthful diet, controlling your weight, and using medication, if necessary—is helpful in preventing infections from getting started, says Dr. Papa.

alternative therapies

Prevent infections with yogurt. Eating yogurt won't stop a yeast infection that's already in progress, but there's some evidence that it may reduce the risk of getting them in the future.

"The acidophilus in yogurt changes the vaginal pH," says Dr. Autry. In addition, when you eat yogurt that contains live bacterial cultures, the "good" organisms migrate into the vaginal canal and inhibit the growth of yeast. It may be especially helpful to eat yogurt when you're taking antibiotics. It replenishes the healthful organisms that are killed by the medication.

One 6-month study found that women who ate 8 ounces of live-culture yogurt daily were much less likely to develop yeast infections than those who didn't eat yogurt. "If you have recurrent infections, including yogurt in your diet is a good approach," says Dr. Autry.

Munch on mushrooms. In a small study, maitake, a delectable Japanese mushroom with scientifically proven immune-enhancing abilities, significantly eased the uncomfortable symptoms

when to see a doctor

If you get recurrent infections or have symptoms that don't improve after treatment with over-the-counter products: You may have a strain of yeast that requires treatment with prescription medications, says Debra Papa, M.D., assistant professor of obstetrics/gynecology at the University of Massachusetts Medical School in Worcester. You may also have a type of vaginal infection other than that caused by yeast.

If you develop a greenish or yellow discharge or lower abdominal pain: You could have a vaginal infection, one of which is called trichomoniasis, a sexually transmitted disease.

If you get a vaginal infection after having a new sex partner or if you've had multiple partners prior to the infection: Any symptom should be evaluated by your doctor.

of chronic yeast infections in all but one of the 13 women who participated in the study.

"The real culprit in chronic yeast infections is a depressed immune system, which I find to be a common problem for women who undergo constant stress," says herbalist Douglas Schar, Dip.Phyt., who conducted the study in his London clinic. "In my experience, raising a woman's immune function makes her less susceptible to chronic yeast infections."

Maitake is well-known for its ability to increase immune cell count and activity. In addition, it contains compounds that specifically inhibit or destroy *Candida albicans*, the organism that causes vaginal yeast infections. But watch out for some unwanted side effects: mannitol, the natural sugar found in maitake, causes gas and intestinal discomfort in some people.

medical options

Take care around your period. "The risk of almost all vaginal infections increases around the time of a woman's period because blood is an excellent culture medium," says Dr. Autry. "Sometimes women who get chronic infections may benefit from fluconazole (Diflucan) toward the end of their periods as a preventive measure."

For more information about vaginal infections: Visit the Web site of the National Women's Health Information Center at www.4women.org.

varicose veins

Women are much more prone to varicose veins than men, possibly because the female hormones estrogen and progesterone gradually weaken the vein walls, eventually reducing their ability to move blood uphill. No one knows the exact cause of this condition, but several factors may play a role. Women with a family history of varicose veins are much more likely to get them. Other factors that may cause or aggravate varicose veins include pregnancy, a lack of exercise, standing or sitting for long periods of time, crossing your legs, and obesity.

"By the time they're in their fifties, nearly one out of two women will have to contend with varicose veins," says Luis Navarro, M.D., attending physician at Beth Israel Medical Center and Lenox Hill Hospital, senior clinical instructor of surgery at the Mount Sinai School of Medicine, and director of the Vein Treatment Center in New York City.

The veins in the legs are in a constant struggle with gravity. It's easy for venous blood, the blood that's going back to the heart, to circulate from other parts of the body because the route it follows is usually downhill. But the venous blood that travels from the leg veins has to make an arduous uphill journey in order to reach the heart.

Sometimes the trip takes longer. If portions of the leg veins are weaker than they should be, or if tiny valves in the veins malfunction, blood tends to pool in the leg veins, causing them to bulge like little balloons. These areas of "stagnant" blood are called varicose veins.

Most varicose veins are the small, "spider" variety. They are blue or red in color and can resemble a tree branch or spider's web. These veins cover areas that range from very small to very large. Located close to the surface of the skin, they are usually found on the legs or face but may occur anywhere on the body and often coincide with larger varicose veins. Although spider veins may be unattractive, they rarely cause discomfort and you can pretty much ignore them.

Larger varicose veins, however, make the legs feel tired and sore. These blue, dark purple, or green veins may be raised above the skin's surface and are found most often on the backs of the calves or on the insides of the legs, anywhere from the groin to the ankle. They may be quite ropy, or bulging. In some cases the veins cause swelling in the legs or feet or around the ankles. Excess fluid leaks from the blood vessels into the tissues around the veins. The tissues become fragile, and the skin appears thin and may be inflamed. Open ulcers or sores may form and heal slowly.

Once varicose veins have formed, the only way to get rid of them is with surgery or other medical treatments. Most women don't need to do this because the discomfort of varicose veins, assuming there is any, can easily be managed with home remedies. In addition, there are a number of simple strategies that will help delay the veins' formation.

For Immediate Relief

home remedies

Change positions often. Varicose veins tend to cause the most discomfort when women have been standing or sitting for a long time, which allows the blood to pool. "Get up from your chair, or just get moving if you're standing, and walk around for a few minutes every 1 to 2 hours," Dr. Navarro suggests. "When you move, the calf muscles flex against the veins, which gets the venous circulation moving again."

Elevate your legs. When you raise your legs above the heart, blood that's pooled in the veins flows back into circulation, says Dr. Navarro. "You can put a couple of bricks or books under the legs at the foot of the bed, which will give some elevation. You can also sleep with a pillow or two under your feet. This will take the pressure off the veins and prevent the blood from pooling in the lower extremities." Putting your legs up while you're reading or watching TV is a good idea, too.

Wear compression stockings. Available from doctors and in pharmacies, stores that carry medical supplies, and department stores, compression stockings put precise amounts of pressure against the leg veins, which can reduce painful swelling. Compression stockings also help prevent varicose veins from getting worse.

"They essentially add an extra layer of muscle to your leg, which helps the calf and foot muscles move blood upward to the heart," says Dr. Navarro. Two of the best brands of compression stockings are Oroblu and Therafirm, he adds.

When buying compression stockings, here are a few things to keep in mind.

- Different stockings provide different amounts of compression, which is measured in millimeters of mercury (mmHg). For spider veins, you'll want stockings with moderate compression (15 to 20 mmHg). If the veins are bulging, use stockings with more compression (20 to 30 mmHg).

- Compression stockings come in different lengths: calf only, which extend to the knee; mid-thigh, which reach to the upper third of the thigh; full-thigh, which extend to the groin; and full-length panty hose. Choose a length that covers all of the veins that you want to compress.

alternative therapies

Take horse chestnut. Available in health food stores, this herb strengthens veins that have lost their elasticity, which can help ease discomfort. A number of studies have shown that women who take 250 to 312.5 milligrams of the standardized extract of horse chestnut twice daily will have considerable relief from symptoms.

medical options

Consider injections. If your legs keep hurting no matter what you do or if you're simply tired of looking at the unsightly veins, your doctor may recommend a procedure called sclerotherapy, in which a solution is injected into the varicose veins. The solution irritates the inner lining of the blood vessels, making the veins swell, close, and eventually disappear. This treatment can be used to eliminate both varicose and spider veins, as long as the main leg vein is not involved.

Apart from the prick of the needle, sclerotherapy is almost painless, although you may have some cramping for a day or two afterward. Since new veins may form, sclerotherapy is usually repeated every 2 to 4 years.

Talk to your doctor about other options. Doctors have recently developed a technique called the endolaser procedure, which uses lasers to seal and shrink the varicose veins, says Dr. Navarro. "It's done as an in-office procedure, using a local anesthetic," he explains, "and is used, when the main vein of the leg is affected, as a way to avoid surgery."

Varicose veins involving the main vein of the leg can also be shut down with the use of radio waves. In some cases, doctors advise removing the veins surgically. This is a more extensive pro-

when to see a doctor

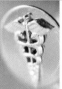

If leg pain wakes you up at night or if the area around varicose veins is swelling, itching, or scaling, make an appointment to see your doctor. It's possible that the tissues around the veins aren't getting enough blood and oxygen, or you may have circulatory or arterial problems. You may need medical treatment to remove or seal the veins, says Luis Navarro, M.D., attending physician at Beth Israel Medical Center and Lenox Hill Hospital, senior clinical instructor of surgery at the Mount Sinai School of Medicine, and director of the Vein Treatment Center in New York City.

cedure than simply sealing the veins, and it's usually recommended for large varicose veins that can't be controlled with the other treatments.

For Long-Term Prevention

home remedies

Exercise often. "It's my number-one tip for preventing varicose veins," says Dr. Navarro. "Try to exercise for 30 minutes at least three times a week. I recommend walking, running, swimming, bicycling, yoga, dancing, and tai chi. They are all great for circulation and building up the calf muscles."

Do toe raises. It's a good exercise for strengthening muscles in the feet and calves and also for removing pooled blood from the veins. Put your hand on a wall for support, and rise on your toes, as far as you can go. Hold the stretch for a moment, then lower yourself back down. "Do this for 5 to 10 minutes every day," suggests Dr. Navarro.

Get plenty of fiber in your diet. Women who eat a lot of whole grains, legumes, and other fiber-rich foods are much less likely to get constipated. This is important because constipation causes straining, which puts extra pressure on the leg veins.

While some studies have not found a consistent relationship between fiber, constipation, and the presence or severity of varicose veins, other research suggests that the diet of industrialized countries may be a risk factor.

"Studies have shown that in countries where people eat diets that are rich in fiber, the incidence of varicose veins is low," says Dr. Navarro. "When the same people come to Western countries and adopt a low-fiber diet, they have the same risk of developing varicose veins as the rest of the population." The optimal amount of fiber is 25 to 35 grams daily. All plant foods contain fiber. Some of the best include beans, peas, fruits, potatoes (with the skins on), berries, and whole grain breakfast cereals, such as Fiber One.

Eat less salt. The average American consumes more than 3,000 milligrams of sodium daily, a lot more than the Daily Value of 2,400 milligrams. "Consuming a lot of high-sodium foods causes inflammation and swelling, which makes the discomfort of varicose veins worse," says Dr. Navarro.

He advises women to buy low-sodium soups and other packaged foods and to avoid high-salt foods, such as luncheon meats and fast foods.

medical options

Ask your doctor to check your medications. Women who take supplemental hormones—either in the form of birth control or as hormone replacement therapy—sometimes develop varicose veins. Taking a lower dose will often provide the same benefits, but without the side effects, says Dr. Navarro.

For more information about varicose veins: Visit the Web site of the American Society for Dermatologic Surgery at www.asds-net.org. Other helpful Web sites are provided by the American College of Phlebology at www.phlebology.org and the American Academy of Dermatology at www.aad.org. You can also call the AAD at (888) 462-DERM.

Guidelines for Safe Use of Supplements

Vitamin and Mineral Supplements

Although serious side effects from vitamin and mineral supplements are not common, they can happen. The guidelines presented here are designed to help you use the supplements mentioned in this book safely and wisely.

Be sure to talk to your doctor before using any supplement if you have a chronic illness requiring medical supervision or medication. In fact, if you have any type of health problem, your doctor or pharmacist needs to know about any supplements you're taking before treating you with a prescription or over-the-counter medicine. If you are a woman who is pregnant, nursing, or attempting to conceive, do not use supplements unless under the supervision of your physician.

The vitamin and mineral doses listed below are the Daily Values or the suggested daily intakes (noted in *italics*). Also given below are the safe upper limits for adults, above which harmful side effects can occur. These amounts are the total from both food and supplements. Do not take more than the safe upper limit of any vitamin or mineral without first consulting your physician. (*Note:* mg = milligrams; mcg = micrograms; IU = international units.)

Nutrient	Daily Value (DV) or *Suggested Daily Intake*	Safe Upper Limit	Cautions and Other Information
CALCIUM	1,000 mg (the DV); *1,200 mg if over age 50*	2,500 mg	Taking more than 2,500 mg a day can cause serious side effects such as kidney damage. For best absorption, avoid taking more than 500 mg at one time. If you are over age 50, look for a formula that contains vitamin D as well as calcium since you may need more vitamin D than is supplied by a multivitamin alone. Some natural sources of calcium, such as bonemeal and dolomite, may be contaminated with lead and other dangerous or undesirable metals.
MAGNESIUM	400 mg	350 mg from supplements only	Check with your doctor before beginning supplementation in any amount if you have heart or kidney problems. Doses exceeding 350 mg a day can cause diarrhea in some people.
PANTOTHENIC ACID	10 mg	1,000 mg	A healthy, balanced diet provides enough of this nutrient to meet your body's needs.

Nutrient	Daily Value (DV) or *Suggested Daily Intake*	Safe Upper Limit	Cautions and Other Information
SELENIUM	70 mcg	400 mcg	Taking more than 400 mcg a day can cause dizziness, nausea, hair or nail loss, or a garlic odor on the breath or skin.
VITAMIN B₆ (pyridoxine)	2 mg	100 mg	Taking more than 100 mg a day can cause reversible nerve damage. When selecting a B-complex supplement, check the label for the amount of each ingredient to help you determine its safe use.
VITAMIN C	*100 to 500 mg* (DV is 60 mg)	2,000 mg	Taking more than 2,000 mg a day can cause diarrhea in some people. To help maintain levels of vitamin C throughout the day, take half of the recommended dose in the morning and half at night.
VITAMIN D	*400 IU (the DV), up to 600 IU if over age 70*	2,000 IU (50 mcg)	Taking more than 2,000 IU a day can cause headache, fatigue, nausea, diarrhea, or loss of appetite.
VITAMIN E	*100 to 400 IU* (DV is 30 IU)	1,500 IU (natural form, d-alpha-tocopherol) or 1,100 IU (synthetic form, from dl-alpha-tocopherol) supplements only	Because it acts like a blood thinner, consult your doctor before taking vitamin E if you are already taking aspirin or a blood-thinning medication, such as warfarin (Coumadin).
ZINC	15 mg	40 mg	Taking more than 40 mg a day can cause nausea, dizziness, or vomiting. When levels of zinc are elevated, the absorption of copper can become impaired.

Emerging Supplements

Reports of adverse effects from emerging supplements are rare, especially when compared with prescription drugs, and supplement manufacturers are required by law to provide information on labels about reasonably safe recommended dosages for healthy individuals. Be aware that the potency and dosing strategy can vary significantly among products.

You should note, however, that little scientific research exists to assess the safety or long-term effects of many emerging supplements, and some supplements can complicate existing conditions or cause allergic reactions in some people. For these reasons, you should always check with your doctor before taking any supplements.

We recommend that you take supplements with food for best absorption and to avoid stomach irritation, unless otherwise directed. Never take them as a substitute for a healthy diet since they do not provide all the nutritional benefits of whole foods.

And, if you are pregnant, nursing, or attempting to conceive, do not supplement without the supervision of a doctor.

Supplement	Safe-Use Guidelines and Possible Side Effects
COENZYME Q_{10}	Discuss supplementation with your doctor if you are taking the blood thinner warfarin (Coumadin). On rare occasions coenzyme Q_{10} may reduce the effectiveness of warfarin. Side effects are rare but include heartburn, nausea, or stomach upset, which can be prevented by consuming the supplement with a meal.
EPA (fish oil)	Do not take if any of the following apply: bleeding disorder, uncontrolled high blood pressure, use of anticoagulants (blood thinners) or regular aspirin, allergy to any kind of fish. People with diabetes should not take fish oil because of its high fat content. Increases bleeding time, possibly resulting in nosebleeds and easy bruising, and may cause upset stomach. Take fish oil, not fish liver oil, because fish liver oil is high in vitamins A and D—toxic in high amounts.
FIBER	Do not take if you are allergic to the source of fiber in the supplement, such as wheat or psyllium. Take under the supervision of your doctor if you have diverticulitis, ulcerative colitis, Crohn's disease, bowel obstruction, or any serious gastrointestinal disorder or if you are taking any medications. May cause gas or bloating.
FLAXSEED	If you are on medication, check with your doctor before supplementing with flaxseed because it may negatively affect absorption. Do not take if you have a bowel obstruction.
GLUCOSAMINE	May cause stomach upset, heartburn, or diarrhea.
GLUTAMINE	If you have problems with your kidneys or liver, check with your physician before supplementing.
QUERCETIN (bioflavonoid)	In some people, doses above 100 mg may dilate blood vessels and cause blood thinning. Should be avoided by individuals at risk for low blood pressure or problems with blood clotting.

Index

Underscored page references indicate boxed text. **Boldfaced** page references indicate photographs.

a

Abdominal fat
  activities for reducing and preventing, 303, 304, **305–9**, <u>305–9</u>, 310
  alcohol and, 310
  back pain and, 302
  clothing and, 303
  emotions and, 109
  fiber and, 310
  genetics and, 302
  lifestyle strategies in preventing, 302
  personal experience in reducing, <u>304</u>
  posture and, 303
  smoking and, 310
  stress and, 109, <u>303</u>
  tips for reducing, <u>310</u>
  water intake and, 302
Abdominal exercise, **82**, <u>82</u>
Abreva (cold sore cream), 345
Accutane, for pimples, 337
Ace bandage, for sprains, 477–78
ACE inhibitors, for high blood pressure, 176
Acetaminophen, in treating
  colds, 343
  fever, 377
  kidney stones, 420
  sore throat, 476
Acidophilus, 274
Acne, 335–37, <u>336</u>
Actigall, 391
Acupressure wristband, for nausea, 438
Acupuncture, in treating
  fibroids, 265
  overactive bladder, 441
  smoking cessation, 122
Acyclovir, <u>154</u>, 345
Adenosine triphosphate (ATP), 321
Age-related macular degeneration, 429
Aging, 2
  copper and, 54
  high blood pressure and, 14
  vitamin B_{12} and, 53

AHAs, 135–36, <u>136</u>
AIDS, <u>153</u>
Air travel, ear protection and, 369
Alcohol
  calories in, 94
  effects of, on
    abdominal fat, 310
    fertility, 254
    gout, 395
    heart disease, 41, 165
    hepatitis, 408
    high blood pressure, 174
    kidney stones, 421
    laryngitis, 423
    menopause, 292
    pneumonia, 453
    restless legs syndrome, 461–62
  food allergy and, 387–88
  moderate consumption of, 41
  multivitamins and, 53
  smoking cessation and, 123
Allegra, 399, 411, 458
Allergens, 398–99
Allergic desensitization. *See* Immunotherapy
Allergy
  allergens and, 398–99
  dust mite, 399, 458
  "false," <u>459</u>
  food, 385–90, <u>386</u>, <u>389</u>
  hay fever, 398–401, <u>400</u>
  hives, <u>62</u>, 410–12, <u>410</u>, <u>411</u>
  microfiber mask for outdoor, 400
  oral allergy syndrome, 401
  pet, 460
  pollen, 398–400, 459
  respiratory, 457–61, <u>459</u>, <u>461</u>
  test, 323
  treating, with
    antihistamines, 399
    herbs, <u>58</u>, 400
Almay skin products, 134
Aloe, for skin problems, <u>68</u>
Alpha-agonists, 492
Alpha hydroxy acids (AHAs), 135–36, <u>136</u>

f

W